ROADMAP TO POSTGRADUATE TRAINING IN PHARMACY

ROADMAP TO POSTGRADUATE TRAINING IN PHARMACY

P. Brandon Bookstaver, PharmD, BCPS (AQ-ID), AAHIVE
Associate Professor and Vice Chair
Department of Clinical Pharmacy and Outcomes Sciences
South Carolina College of Pharmacy – USC Campus
Columbia, South Carolina

Celeste R. Caulder, PharmD
Assistant Professor
Department of Clinical Pharmacy and Outcomes Sciences
South Carolina College of Pharmacy – USC Campus
Columbia, South Carolina

Kelly M. Smith, PharmD, BCPS, FASHP, FCCP
Associate Dean, Academic and Student Affairs
Associate Professor, Pharmacy Practice and Science
University of Kentucky College of Pharmacy
Lexington, Kentucky

April Miller Quidley, PharmD, BCPS
Clinical Pharmacist
Director, PGY-2 Critical Care Pharmacy Residency
Vidant Medical Center
Greenville, North Carolina

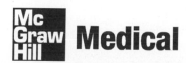 **Medical**

New York / Chicago / San Francisco / Lisbon / London / Madrid / Mexico City
Milan / New Delhi / San Juan / Seoul / Singapore / Sydney / Toronto

The *McGraw·Hill* Companies

Roadmap to Postgraduate Training in Pharmacy

1 2 3 4 5 6 7 8 9 DOC/DOC 18 17 16 15 14 13

ISBN 978-0-07-178875-5
MHID 0-07-178875-1

This book was set in Palatino by Aptara, Inc.
The editors were Michael Weitz and Christina M. Thomas.
The production supervisor was Catherine Saggese.
The index was prepared by Aptara, Inc.
Project management was provided by Abhishan Sharma, by Aptara, Inc.
The cover designer was Libby Pisacreta.
RR Donnelley was printer and binder.

This book is printed on acid-free paper.

Library of Congress Cataloging-in-Publication Data

Roadmap to postgraduate training in pharmacy / [edited by] P. Brandon Bookstaver . . . [et al.].
     p. ; cm.
   Includes bibliographical references and index.
   ISBN 978-0-07-178875-5 (soft cover : alk. paper) – ISBN 0-07-178875-1 (soft cover : alk. paper)
   I. Bookstaver, P. Brandon.
   [DNLM: 1. Education, Pharmacy, Continuing–United States. 2. Internship, Nonmedical
United States. 3. Vocational Guidance–United States.   QV 20]

615.1023–dc23   2012026827

McGraw-Hill books are available at special quantity discounts to use as premiums and sales promotions, or for use in corporate training programs. To contact a representative please e-mail us at bulksales@mcgraw-hill.com.

CONTENTS

SECTION I: Your GPS to Pharmacy Postgraduate Training / 1
Kelly M. Smith

SECTION II: How to Program Your GPS / 53
April Miller Quidley and P. Brandon Bookstaver

SECTION III: Turn Left, Turn Right: Choosing the Postgraduate Pathway for You / 207

Celeste R. Caulder and P. Brandon Bookstaver

REVIEWERS

Titilola Afolabi, PharmD Candidate
University of Tennessee Health Science Center College of Pharmacy
Memphis, Tennessee

Rachael R. Aletti, BS, PharmD
PGY-1 Pharmacy Practice Resident, Montefiore Medical Center
Bronx, New York

Yelena Atlasevich, PharmD
PGY-1 Acute Care Pharmacy Resident , University of California
San Diego Health System
San Diego, California

Harrison Bachmeier, PharmD
PGY-1 Pharmacy Practice Resident, Lee Memorial Health Systems
Fort Myers, Florida

Nicole K. Brogden, PharmD, PhD Candidate
Department of Pharmaceutical Sciences
University of Kentucky College of Pharmacy
Lexington, Kentucky

Shannon Buxell, PharmD
PGY-1 Pharmacy Practice Resident, Oregon Health & Science University
Portland, Oregon

Nitha K. Chou, PharmD Candidate
Massachusetts College of Pharmacy and Health Sciences
Worcester, Massachusetts

Toby Clark, RPh, MSc, FASHP
(Ret) Director of Hospital Pharmacy and Professor
University of Illinois at Chicago
Lead Surveyor, Accreditation Services, American Society of Health-System Pharmacists
(Adj.) Associate Professor, South Carolina College of Pharmacy
Medical University of South Carolina
Charleston, South Carolina

Margaret A. Croom, PharmD Candidate
South Carolina College of Pharmacy, Medical University of South Carolina
Charleston, South Carolina

Leanna Darland, PharmD Candidate
University of Louisiana at Monroe College of Pharmacy
Monroe, Louisana

McLisa V. Davis, BS, PharmD Candidate
University of Tennessee Health Science Center College of Pharmacy
Memphis, Tennessee

Kendra M. Demaris, PharmD
PGY-1 Drug Information Resident, Washington State University
Department of Pharmacotherapy, College of Pharmacy
Spokane, Washington

Vi P. Doan, PharmD Candidate
University of Houston College of Pharmacy
Houston, Texas

Kathryn Elofson, PharmD Candidate
University of Arizona, College of Pharmacy
Tucson, Arizona

Elizabeth K. Erlain, PharmD
PGY-1 Pharmacy Practice Resident, Froedtert Hospital
Milwaukee, Wisconsin

Amin Esmaily-Fard, PharmD Candidate
University of Houston College of Pharmacy
Houston, Texas

Leslie A. Esparza, PharmD Candidate
Washington State University College of Pharmacy
Spokane, Washington

Amy Francis, PharmD
PGY-1 Pediatric Pharmacy Resident, Huntsville Hospital
Huntsville, Alabama

Christina M. Gaard, PharmD, MPH
PGY-1 Pharmacy Practice Resident
Clement J. Zablocki Veterans Affairs Medical Center
Milwaukee, Wisconsin

Sandra Garner, PharmD, BCPS, FCCP
Associate Professor, Department of Clinical Pharmacy and Outcome Sciences
South Carolina College of Pharmacy, Medical University of South Carolina
Charleston, South Carolina

Kara B. Goddard, PharmD
PGY-2 Emergency Medicine Pharmacy Resident, Grady Health System
Atlanta, Georgia

Drayton A. Hammond, MBA, PharmD Candidate
South Carolina College of Pharmacy, Medical University of South Carolina
Charleston, South Carolina

Christopher Hilty, PharmD
PGY-1/2 Health System Pharmacy Administration Resident,
   Methodist University Hospital
Memphis, Tennessee

C. Morgan Honeycutt, BS, PharmD Candidate
University of Tennesssee Health Science Center College of Pharmacy
Knoxville, Tennessee

Farah Kablaoui, PharmD Candidate
South Carolina College of Pharmacy, University of South Carolina
Columbia, South Carolina

Ohannes V. Kandilian, PharmD Candidate
University of California, San Diego Skaggs School of Pharmacy and
   Pharmaceutical Sciences
San Diego, California

Minou Khazan, PharmD, PhD
PGY-2 Critical Care Pharmacy Resident, Palmetto Health Richland
Columbia, South Carolina

Christine K. Kim, PharmD
PGY-1 Drug Information Resident, Scott & White Memorial Hospital
Temple, Texas

Huda-Marie Kuttab, PharmD Candidate
Chicago College of Pharmacy, Midwestern University
Chicago, Illinois

Ryan Markham, PharmD Candidate
University of Georgia College of Pharmacy
Athens, Georgia

Amanda M. Memken, PharmD
PGY-1 Pharmacy Practice Resident, Palmetto Health Richland
Columbia, South Carolina

Kelly Monteen, PharmD Candidate
University of Tennesssee Health Science Center College of Pharmacy
Knoxville, Tennessee

Erin K. Morrison, PharmD
PGY-1 Pharmacy Practice Resident, Blount Memorial Hospital
Maryville, Tennessee

John Muchka, BS, PharmD
PGY- 1 Pharmacy Practice Resident, Froedtert Hospital
Milwaukee, Wisconsin

Caitlin R. Musgrave, PharmD
PGY-1 Pharmacy Practice Resident, Medical University of South Carolina
Charleston, South Carolina

M. Jill Odom, PharmD
PGY-1 Community Pharmacy Resident, Kennedy Pharmacy Innovation Center &
    Barney's Pharmacy
Kennedy Pharmacy Innovation Center & Barney's Pharmacy
Augusta, Georgia

Adebayo Ogunniyi, MPA Candidate, PharmD Candidate
University of Kentucky College of Pharmacy
Lexington, Kentucky

Ann Palm, PharmD
PGY-1 Pharmacy Practice Resident, Froedtert Hospital
Milwaukee, Wisconsin

Samantha Pelham, PharmD Candidate
Harrison School of Pharmacy, Auburn University
Auburn, Alabama

Breanne K. Peyton, PharmD Candidate
University of Louisiana at Monroe College of Pharmacy
Monroe, Louisana

Ngoc-Diep T. Pham, PharmD Candidate
Pacific University, School of Pharmacy
Hillsboro, Oregon

John Radosevich, PharmD
PGY-1 Pharmacy Practice Resident, The University of Arizona Medical Center
Tucson, Arizona

Kristina E. E. Rokas, PharmD Candidate
South Carolina College of Pharmacy, University of South Carolina
Columbia, South Carolina

Adrian Sandoval, PharmD Candidate
Texas A&M Health Science Center, Rangel College of Pharmacy
Kingsville, Texas

Brittany M. Schmidt, PharmD Candidate
The Ohio State University College of Pharmacy
Columbus, Ohio

Anokhi Shah, PharmD
PGY-1 Managed Care Pharmacy Resident, University of Pittsburgh
  Medical Center Health Plan
Pittsburgh, Pennsylvania

Caitlin Shamroe, PharmD Candidate
South Carolina College of Pharmacy, University of South Carolina,
Columbia, South Carolina

Tiffany R. Shin, PharmD
PGY-2 Ambulatory Care Pharmacy Resident, The Ohio State University
  College of Pharmacy
Columbus, Ohio

Karen Shin, PharmD Candidate
University of Minnesota, College of Pharmacy
Minneapolis, Minnesota

Lindsay A. Sorge, PharmD
PGY-1/2 Pharmaceutical Care Leadership Resident,
  University of Minnesota College of Pharmacy
Minneapolis, Minnesota

Brad M. Stevens, PharmD Candidate
University of Pittsburgh School of Pharmacy
Pittsburgh, Pennsylvania

Pearl Stier, PharmD
PGY-1 Pharmacy Practice Resident, Department of Pharmacy Practice,
  Midwestern University Chicago College of Pharmacy
Chicago, Illinois

Jessica Stover, BS, PharmD Candidate
University of Houston College of Pharmacy
Houston, Texas

Paul M. Stranges, PharmD
PGY-1 Pharmacy Practice Resident, Department of Pharmacy Services
University of Michigan Hospitals and Health Centers
Ann Arbor, Michigan

Christina L. Tan, PharmD Candidate
University of Houston College of Pharmacy
Houston, Texas

Stephanie Tears, PharmD Candidate
University of Florida College of Pharmacy
Gainesville, Florida

Maria Miller Thurston, PharmD, BCPS
PGY-2 Ambulatory Care Pharmacy Resident, University of Georgia
    College of Pharmacy
Charlie Norwood Veterans Affairs Medical Center
Athens, Georgia

J. Elliot Turner, PharmD
PGY-1 Pharmacy Practice Resident, Palmetto Health Richland
Columbia, South Carolina

Brittany N. White, PharmD Candidate
University of Tennessee Health Sciences Center College of Pharmacy
Knoxville, Tennessee

Cyle E. White, PharmD Candidate
University of Tennessee Health Sciences Center College of Pharmacy
Knoxville, Tennessee

Matthew L. Wolf, PharmD Candidate
University of Michigan College of Pharmacy
Ann Arbor, Michigan

Danielle M. Yates, PharmD
PGY-1 Pharmacy Practice Resident, Blount Memorial Hospital
Maryville, Tennessee

CONTRIBUTORS

Alison L. Apple, DPh, MS
System Director of Pharmacy, Methodist Le Bonheur Healthcare
Director of Pharmacy, Methodist University Hospital
Associate Professor
Department of Clinical Pharmacy
University of Tennessee College of Pharmacy
Memphis, Tennessee

John A. Armitstead, MS, RPh, FASHP
System Director of Pharmacy Services
Lee Memorial Health System
Fort Myers and Cape Coral, Florida

James R. Beardsley, PharmD, BCPS
Assistant Director of Pharmacy, Wake Forest Baptist Health
Adjunct Assistant Professor
Wake Forest School of Medicine
Winston-Salem, North Carolina

Marialice S. Bennett, BSPharm, RPh, FAPhA
Professor of Clinical Pharmacy
Director, Ambulatory and Community Care Residency Programs
The Ohio State University College of Pharmacy
Columbus, Ohio

P. Brandon Bookstaver, PharmD, BCPS (AQ-ID), AAHIVE
Associate Professor and Vice Chair
Department of Clinical Pharmacy and Outcomes Sciences
South Carolina College of Pharmacy – USC Campus
Columbia, South Carolina

Celeste R. Caulder, PharmD
Assistant Professor
Department of Clinical Pharmacy and Outcomes Sciences
South Carolina College of Pharmacy – USC Campus
Columbia, South Carolina

John S. Clark, PharmD, MS, BCPS, FASHP
Director of Pharmacy Services, PGY-1 Residency Program Director
University of Michigan Hospital and Health Centers
Clinical Assistant Professor
University of Michigan College of Pharmacy
Ann Arbor, Michigan

Elizabeth A. Coyle, PharmD, FCCM, BCPS
Director, PGY-2 Infectious Diseases Residency
UHCOP/Cardinal Health
Infectious Diseases Clinical Specialist, MD Anderson Cancer Center
Assistant Dean of Assessment and Clinical Associate Professor
University of Houston College of Pharmacy
Houston, Texas

Charles E. Daniels, BSPharm, PhD, FASHP
Pharmacist-In-Chief
UC San Diego Medical Center
Associate Dean of Clinical Affairs
UC San Diego Skaggs School of Pharmacy
La Jolla, California

Jessica R. Daw, PharmD, MBA
Clinical Pharmacy Manager and Director, PGY-1 Managed Care Residency
University of Pittsburgh Medical Center Health Plan
Pittsburgh, Pennsylvania

Heather M. Draper, PharmD, BCPS
Associate Professor
Department of Clinical Pharmacy
University of Tennessee College of Pharmacy
Knoxville, Tennessee

Lea S. Eiland, PharmD, BCPS
Associate Clinical Professor and Associate Department Head
Harrison School of Pharmacy, Auburn University
Huntsville, Alabama

Stefanie P. Ferreri, PharmD, BCACP, CDE, FAPhA
Clinical Associate Professor
Division of Pharmacy Practice and Experiental Education
UNC Eshelman School of Pharmacy, University of North Carolina at Chapel Hill
Chapel Hill, North Carolina

Jeffrey J. Fong, PharmD, BCPS
Clinical Pharmacy Specialist
UMass Memorial Medical Center
Assistant Professor
Massachusetts College of Pharmacy and Health Sciences
Worcester, Massachusetts

Brad S. Fujisaki, BSPharm, PharmD
Interim Assistant Dean for Faculty Development and Assistant Professor
School of Pharmacy, Pacific University
Hillsboro, Oregon

Jacob P. Gettig, PharmD, MPH, BCPS
Assistant Dean for Postgraduate Education and
    Associate Professor of Pharmacy Practice
Midwestern University, Chicago College of Pharmacy
Downers Grove, Illinois

Morton P. Goldman, PharmD, BCPS, FCCP
Consultant, American Pharmacotherapy, Inc.
Pittsburgh, PA

Nancy H. Goodbar, PharmD, BCPS
Assistant Professor of Pharmacy Practice
Presbyterian College School of Pharmacy
Clinton, South Carolina

Mary M. Hess, PharmD, FASHP, FCCM, FCCP
Associate Dean, Student Affairs
Jefferson School of Pharmacy
Philadelphia, Pennsylvania

Michael D. Hogue, PharmD, FAPhA
Associate Professor and Chair
Department of Pharmacy Practice
McWhorter School of Pharmacy, Samford University
Birmingham, Alabama

Tibb F. Jacobs, PharmD, BCPS
Clinical Pharmacist, Department of Family Medicine
LSU Health Shreveport
Associate Professor of Pharmacy Practice
University of Louisiana at Monroe - Shreveport Campus
Shreveport, Louisiana

Melissa D. Johnson, PharmD, MHS, AAHIVE
Assistant Professor of Medicine
Division of Infectious Diseases & International Health
Duke University Medical Center
Durham, North Carolina

Pamela R. Maxwell, PharmD, BCPS
Clinical Manager, Solid Organ Transplant, University Transplant Center, University
Health System & University of Texas Health Center
Director, PGY-2 Solid Organ Transplant Pharmacy Residency
Department of Pharmacy Services, University Health System
San Antonio, Texas

Lena M. Maynor, PharmD, BCPS
Director, PGY-2 Internal Medicine Pharmacy Residency
Clinical Assistant Professor and Director of Advanced Pharmacy Practice Experiences
West Virginia University School of Pharmacy
Morgantown, West Virginia

Ola Oyetayo, PharmD, MSc, BCPS
Clinical Pharmacist - Cardiology, Scott and White Healthcare
Assistant Professor
Department of Pharmacy Practice
Irma L. Rangel College of Pharmacy, Texas A&M Health Science Center
Temple, Texas

Asad E. Patanwala, PharmD, BCPS
Clinical Assistant Professor
Department of Pharmacy Practice & Science
University of Arizona College of Pharmacy
Tucson, Arizona

Ann M. Philbrick, PharmD, BCPS
Assistant Professor
Department of Pharmaceutical Care and Health Systems
University of Minnesota College of Pharmacy
Minneapolis, Minnesota

Beth Bryles Phillips, PharmD, FCCP, BCPS
Clinical Pharmacy Specialist, Ambulatory Care
Director, PGY-2 Ambulatory Care Pharmacy Residency
Charlie Norwood VA Medical Center
Clinical Associate Professor
University of Georgia College of Pharmacy
Athens, Georgia

Melissa Pleva, PharmD, BCPS, BCNSP
Clinical Pharmacist and Director, PGY-2 Critical Care Pharmacy Residency
University of Michigan Hospitals and Health Centers
Adjunct Clinical Assistant Professor
University of Michigan College of Pharmacy
Ann Arbor, Michigan

Maria C. Pruchnicki, PharmD, BCPS, CLS
Director, PGY-2 Ambulatory Care Pharmacy Residency
Associate Professor of Clinical Pharmacy
Division of Pharmacy Practice and Administration
The Ohio State University College of Pharmacy
Columbus, Ohio

April Miller Quidley, PharmD, BCPS
Clinical Pharmacist
Director, PGY-2 Critical Care Pharmacy Residency
Vidant Medical Center
Greenville, North Carolina

Daniel M. Riche, PharmD, BCPS, CDE
Cardiometabolic Clinic Coordinator
The University of Mississippi Medical Center
Assistant Professor
School of Pharmacy, School of Medicine
University of Mississippi
Jackson, Mississippi

Kelly M. Smith, PharmD, BCPS, FASHP, FCCP
Associate Dean, Academic and Student Affairs
Associate Professor, Pharmacy Practice and Science
University of Kentucky College of Pharmacy
Lexington, Kentucky

Todd D. Sorenson, PharmD, FAPhA
Director, Ambulatory Care Pharmacy Residency
Professor
Department of Pharmaceutical Care and Health Systems
University of Minnesota College of Pharmacy
Minneapolis, Minnesota

Colleen M. Terriff, PharmD, BCPS (AQ-ID), AAHIVE
Clinical Pharmacist
Deaconess Hospital
Clinical Associate Professor
Washington State University College of Pharmacy
Spokane, Washington

Melissa L. Theesfeld, PharmD
Assistant Professor and Director of Experiential Education
Department of Pharmacy Practice
Concordia University Wisconsin School of Pharmacy
Mequon, Wisconsin

Andrew P. Traynor, PharmD, BCPS
Assistant Professor and Director of Residencies and Practice Development
Department of Pharmacy Practice
Concordia University Wisconsin School of Pharmacy
Mequon, Wisconsin

Sharon Jung Tschirhart, PharmD, BCPS
Clinical Pharmacy Specialist, Geriatrics
Director, PGY-2 Geriatric Pharmacy Residency
South Texas Veterans Health Care System, San Antonio, Texas
Clinical Assistant Professor
The University of Texas College of Pharmacy
Austin, Texas

Anne M. Tucker, PharmD, BCNSP
Clinical Associate Professor
Department of Clinical Sciences and Administration
University of Houston College of Pharmacy
Houston, Texas

Suzanne Turner, PharmD
Education and Residency Coordinator
Lee Memorial Health System
Fort Myers and Cape Coral, Florida

PREFACE

You *could* try it, but I wouldn't recommend it. Yes, you *could* try to climb an icy mountain in the dark without a map, a light, or any specialized equipment, but I wouldn't recommend it. The likelihood of success is low; the likelihood of a painful ending is high. In the same way, I would not recommend that you try to navigate the process of achieving postgraduate pharmacy training without significant assistance. The process is too complicated and the stakes are too high to just blindly go forth. Fortunately, help has arrived! *Roadmap to Postgraduate Training in Pharmacy* is a comprehensive text that can help every pharmacy student successfully embark on their journey toward pursuing postgraduate training. This is a "must read" for all students considering the trip. The authors provide an insightful description of the postgraduate training experience and offer guidance on how to navigate the process from the decision point to pursue further training to the post-match transition from student to resident.

As a residency program director, I have the privilege of interacting with many wonderful students each year who desire to pursue postgraduate training. Some candidates are truly impressive. They know where they are going, why they are going there, and how to conduct themselves along the way. Others . . . not so much! Unfortunately, each year our selection committee interacts with unprepared students and reads through less than impressive application packets, and we lament, "Didn't this person get any help?" In recent years, the residency selection process has become very competitive. At my institution, we currently have a ratio of over 40 applicants for every PGY-1 residency position. How do you position yourself to be the "1" who is selected rather than the other "39"? Follow the advice in this book! It is written by knowledgeable authors who stem from a variety of institutions and practice sites throughout the country. Most have extensive experience on both sides of the table—they have invested time *mentoring* students to be strong residency candidates and they have been involved in *selecting* candidates for residency programs. They know what it takes to do well. Constructive reviews of all content from current fourth-year residency-bound students and pharmacy residents helped to mold this valuable resource.

I hope that two things become apparent to you as you read this book. First, I hope you realize how much all of the authors want you to be successful as you consider this next stage of your training. That was the impetus behind the book. Second, I hope you realize that we think this journey is worth pursuing. It is a very exciting time to be a pharmacist. The opportunity for pharmacists to make a difference in patients' lives has never been greater. However, to provide the level of care that our patients and other healthcare providers require, pharmacists must be as well trained as possible. Postgraduate training is the most efficient way of obtaining the necessary quality training your future patients deserve. Yes, you may have to reduce your earning potential for a year or two, but the rewards will last throughout the rest of your career.

So what are you waiting for? There is an exciting path set before you, and thanks to this text, you now have guide to help you along the way. So, read the book and start the journey. It's an adventure you won't want to miss.

—*James R. Beardsley, PharmD, BCPS*

COMMON ABBREVIATIONS

AACP	American Academy of Colleges of Pharmacy
ACCP	American College of Clinical Pharmacy
ACPE	Accreditation Council for Pharmacy Education
AMCP	Academy of Managed Care Pharmacy
APhA	American Pharmacists Association
APPE	Advanced Pharmacy Practice Experiences
ASHP	American Society of Health-System Pharmacists
ASHP COC or COC	ASHP Commission on Credentialing
ASHP MCM	ASHP Midyear Clinical Meeting
CMS	Centers for Medicare and Medicaid Services
CPRP	Community pharmacy residency programs
DUE	Drug-use evaluations
ED	Emergency department
FDA	Food and Drug Administration
GMAT	Graduate Management Admission Test
GPA	Grade point average
GRE	Graduate Record Exam
ICU	Intensive care unit
IPPE	Introductory Pharmacy Practice Experiences
IRB	Institutional Review Board
MBA	Masters of Business Administration
MHA	Masters of Health Care Administration
MPH	Masters of Public Health
MS	Masters of Science
MSCR	Masters of Science, Clinical Research or Clinical and Translational Research
MTM	Medication Therapy Management
NCPA	National Community Pharmacists Association
NMS	National Matching Service
P&T	Pharmacy and Therapeutics (referring to P&T committee)
PEOR	Pharmacoeconomics and outcomes research
PGY-1	Postgraduate Year One (reference to pharmacy residency)
PGY-2	Postgraduate Year Two (reference to pharmacy specialty residency)
PhD	Doctor of Philosophy
PhORCAS	Pharmacy Residency Online Centralized Application Service
PHS	U.S. Public Health Service
PN	Parenteral nutrition
PPS	Personnel placement service
PRN	Practice and Research Network
RPD	Residency program director
SCCM	Society of Critical Care Medicine
VA or VAMC	Veterans Affairs Medical Center

Your GPS to Pharmacy Postgraduate Training

• *Kelly M. Smith*

The Maturation of Postgraduate Pharmacy Training 1

Alison L. Apple

The most uniformly structured postgraduate pharmacy training programs are pharmacy residencies. They too are the most prevalent in the United States pharmacy career development model, and thus residency training serves as the focus of this chapter.

BIRTH ANNOUNCEMENT—IT'S A . . . RESIDENCY!

While you may discover pharmacy residency programs in a variety of settings (e.g., hospital, community, and managed care), the origins of residency training began in the hospital over 70 years ago. Postgraduate programs, originally referred to as internships, began in the early 1930s to train pharmacists in hospital pharmacy management. Harvey A. K. Whitney, one of the founders of the American Society of Hospital Pharmacists, established the first of these internship programs at the University of Michigan Hospital. The American Society of Hospital Pharmacists developed standards for internship training in 1948; however, it wasn't until 1962 that the initial accreditation process and residency standards were developed, and the term "internship" was replaced with "residency."[1]

> "I had no idea that pharmacy residency training has been around for over 60 years!"
>
> *Brittany W. – Pharmacy Student, Tennessee*

If you were a pharmacist enrolled in one of the first accredited residency programs, you would be learning to lead and manage hospital pharmacies. However, in the 1970s, as clinical pharmacy practice evolved, so did the development of clinical pharmacy residencies. The early clinical residencies were often associated with colleges of pharmacy as post-Doctor of Pharmacy training programs. For approximately 20 years, there were two types of residencies: clinical and general. It wasn't until 1993 that the American Society of Health-System Pharmacists (ASHP) developed a single standard for residency training called the Pharmacy Practice Residency with an emphasis on pharmaceutical care. Also between the 1970s and early 1990s, the first accreditation standards in specialty areas of practice were developed. These specialty programs grew at a rapid pace in the 1980s and 1990s; by the late 1990s, there were 15 recognized areas of specialized training.[2] During this time period, some students entered specialty training directly after the completion of pharmacy school.

IT'S ALL IN THE NAME

The next significant change in residency training occurred in 2005 with the development of the current Postgraduate Year One (PGY-1) and Postgraduate Year Two (PGY-2) residency standards. The terminology was adopted to clearly indicate the stepwise, progressive nature of pharmacy residency training, as well as to mirror the terminology used in other disciplines (e.g., medicine) so that external audiences would no longer be confused by the pharmacy practice and specialized terms. In practical terms, this new approach formalized the official requirement for completion of a PGY-1 residency prior to pursuing advanced training, hereafter known as a PGY-2 residency. While today's emphasis on PGY-1 residencies is to develop the skills necessary to provide patient-centered medication therapy management and serve as the foundation for advanced residency training (see Chapter 14), as a PGY-1 resident you will also be learning about improving the medication-use system, developing leadership, practice management and project management skills, providing education/training, and utilizing medical informatics.[3] In turn, the purpose of PGY-2 residency programs is for "the pharmacist to develop accountability; practice patterns; habits; and expert knowledge, skills, attitudes, and abilities in the respective advanced area of pharmacy practice."[4] (see Section III Introduction.)

FINDING THE RIGHT MATCH

ASHP implemented a residency match for the first time in 1979, but it wasn't until 1994 that the National Matching Service was engaged in the process. The "Match" is a mechanism to ensure a fair recruitment and selection process for both the residency programs and applicants. The requirement for all accredited programs, including community, managed care, and PGY-2 programs, to participate in the matching program was implemented in 2007. Prior to this time, only PGY-1 hospital and health-system residency programs were required participants (see Chapter 11).

BREAKING DOWN BARRIERS

Residency training in practice settings outside the hospital setting began much later than hospital-based programs. Community pharmacy residency program development began in the early 1980s. Between 1982 and 1986, there was significant activity within the American Pharmacists Association

(APhA) to standardize the vision for community residency programs and promote the development of residencies in community practice. In 1986, APhA began the Community Pharmacy Residency Initiative and published the programmatic essentials for community pharmacy residencies. These initial guidelines defined objectives in management, drug distribution, clinical services, drug information, home health care, and long-term care. In 1997, the guidelines were updated to emphasize patient care. The first APhA-ASHP community pharmacy residency accreditation standards were approved in 1999,[5] while the current PGY-1 standard for community residency training was implemented in 2007 (see Chapter 15).[6] Many of the community residencies today are sponsored by colleges of pharmacy in collaboration with community pharmacy practice sites.

The first managed care residency programs began emerging in the early 1990s. During this time period, ASHP developed two standards for managed care residencies: Residency Training in Pharmacy Practice (with emphasis on managed care) and Residency Training in Managed Care Pharmacy Systems. The Academy of Managed Care Pharmacy (AMCP), a long-time supporter of residency training, partnered with ASHP in 1998 for the accreditation of managed care pharmacy residencies. The first jointly written standard, *Accreditation Standard for Managed Care Pharmacy Practice Residencies*, was released soon after this agreement was reached. The current PGY-1 Managed Care Accreditation Standard, also developed collaboratively by AMCP and ASHP, was implemented in 2008. According to the current standard, "PGY1 residents in managed care pharmacy are trained to deliver pharmaceutical care utilizing three practice models: 1) individual patient care in which the pharmacist communicates findings and recommendations to those health care providers who provide care directly to the patient; 2) care provided to targeted groups of patients in which the pharmacist designs, conducts, monitors and evaluates the outcomes of organized and structured programs; and 3) population care management in which the pharmacist develops and implements medication-use policy" (see Chapter 16).[7]

KEEPING SCORE

As of 2012, there are four PGY-1 accreditation standards (pharmacy practice, community, managed care, and international), with the international standard joining the residency "family" in 2010. This latest standard was developed in response to a desire for other countries to have their programs accredited by ASHP, but recognizing the varying approaches each country takes to pharmacy degree program requirements and licensure (important elements of the residency standard). Since its approval, the international residency standard has been used to accredit a program in Saudi Arabia, and other programs are poised to follow (see Chapter 26). A common residency standard is in place for all PGY-2 programs, with specialty-defined outcomes, goals, and objectives for 18 areas of PGY-2 residencies. Additionally, there is a set of broadly applicable outcomes, goals, and objectives that can be applied to unique areas of practice that lack their own specific set (e.g., pharmacogenetics).

TABLE 1-1 • Distribution of PGY-2 Programs (February 2012)[8]

Type of PGY-2 Program	Number of Programs	Percentage of Total (%)
Critical care	96	19.3
Oncology	71	14.3
Ambulatory care	57	11.5
Infectious diseases	46	9.3
Pediatric	39	7.9
Internal medicine	25	5.0
Psychiatric	24	4.8
Health-system pharmacy administration	22	4.4
Solid organ transplant	20	4.0
Cardiology	18	3.6
Geriatric	13	2.6
Drug information	12	2.4
Informatics	10	2.0
Pharmacotherapy	6	1.2
Medication use safety	6	1.2
Palliative care and pain management	5	1.0
Nutrition support	3	0.6
Nuclear medicine	1	0.2
Other (e.g., emergency medicine and pharmacogenetics)	23	4.6
Total	497	

A look back at the ASHP Online Residency Directory in February 2012 revealed 866 PGY-1 residencies, with 753 (87%) in hospitals, health systems, and clinics; 76 (8.8%) in community; and 37 (4.3%) programs in managed care pharmacy practice settings.[8] Table 1-1 illustrates the distribution of accredited PGY-2 programs by area of specialty, including programs that have or will soon be seeking accreditation (e.g., candidate and pre-candidate). Beyond these two cohorts are 2-year residency programs, which combine the features of both PGY-1 and PGY-2 training into a 2-year period, often in concert with a master's degree. In February 2012, 2-year programs numbered: 29 in health-system pharmacy administration, with 25 offered in conjunction with a master's degree; 12 in pharmacotherapy; 1 in informatics; and 1 in medication systems and operations (considered a unique specialty area).

Although program growth has been significant, it has not kept up with the increasing number of applicants. Since 2003 there has been a steadily increasing gap between the number of applicants and the number of available resident positions. By 2011, this number had grown to 954, and was also evident for PGY-2 residency capacity. This same trend held for PGY-2 applicants as well. The reasons for growth in applicants are multifactorial, believed to be a result of increasing number of graduates from schools of pharmacy, policy

> "Knowing that the demand for residency positions far exceeds the number of programs available is a motivator to work hard to set myself apart from the hundreds of residency applicants."
>
> *Brittany W. – Pharmacy Student, Tennessee*

positions by national pharmacy organizations in support of residency training, and the state of the economy.[9]

Given the capacity divide amidst the growing professional need to complete a residency or other postgraduate training (see Chapter 2), now is the time for you to chart the course for your professional development. Examine your own goals, identify the training you need to reach them, strategize how you can best position yourself to be competitive for that training, and then begin the journey.

Chapter Takeaways

▶ Pharmacy residency training has been in existence in the United States for over 60 years.

▶ Current standards require completion of a PGY-1 residency prior to training in a specialized area of practice.

▶ Residency training exists in hospitals and health systems, as well as in community and managed care pharmacy practice sites.

▶ Demand for residencies far exceeds the available programs, particularly for PGY-1 programs in hospitals and health systems.

ROLE FOR THE MENTOR

Share the history of pharmacy residency training and your own residency journey with the pharmacy student.

Explain the purpose of PGY-1 residency training and the need for this training prior to specialized training.

Help the pharmacy student understand the current capacity issues with residency training so that he/she can understand the imperative for making themselves competitive in the search for residency training.

References

1. American Society of Hospital Pharmacists. Definitions of pharmacy residencies and fellowships. Am J Hosp Pharm. 1987;44:1142–1144.
2. Ray MD. Pharmacy residency training: Proposal for a fourth wave. Am J Health Syst Pharm. 1997;54:2116–2121.
3. ASHP Accreditation Standard for Postgraduate Year One (PGY-1) Pharmacy Residency Programs. American Society of Health-System Pharmacists Web site. http://www.ashp.org/DocLibrary/Accreditation/ASD-PGY-1-Standard.aspx. Accessed February 26, 2012.

4. ASHP Accreditation Standard for Postgraduate Year Two (PGY-2) Pharmacy Residency Programs. American Society of Health-System Pharmacists Web site. http://www.ashp.org/DocLibrary/Accreditation/ASD-PGY-2-Standard.aspx. Accessed February 16, 2012.

5. Stolpe SF, Adams AJ, Bradley-Baker LR, Burns AL, Owen JA. Historical development and emerging trends of community pharmacy residencies. Am J Pharm Educ. 2011;75(8): article 160.

6. Accreditation Standard for Postgraduate Year One (PGY-1) Community Pharmacy Residency Programs. American Society of Health-System Pharmacists Web site. http://www.ashp.org/DocLibrary/Accreditation/ASD-PGY-1-Community-Standard.aspx. Accessed February 26, 2012.

7. Accreditation Standard for Postgraduate Year One (PGY-1) Managed Care Pharmacy Residency Programs. American Society of Health-System Pharmacists Web site. http://www.ashp.org/DocLibrary/Accreditation/ASD-Managed-Care-Standard.aspx. Accessed February 26, 2012.

8. ASHP Online Residency Directory. American Society of Health-System Pharmacists Web site. http://accred.ashp.org/aps/pages/directory/residencyProgramSearch.aspx. Accessed February 25, 2012.

9. Teeters J. The current landscape of pharmacy residency training. American Society of Health-System Pharmacists Web site. http://www.ashp.org/DocLibrary/Accreditation/PRC2011/Current-Landscape.aspx. Accessed February 25, 2012.

What's in It for Me? Benefits of Postgraduate Training 2

John S. Clark and Melissa Pleva

The types and numbers of postgraduate training options available to you are seemingly endless. Yet, the reasons for you to delay entry into the job market may not be quite as numerous. You've probably had a hard enough time describing why it takes 4 years in pharmacy school, much less the education you had before that, to become a pharmacist. And now, you want, need, or are compelled to do more? Know that thousands of pharmacy students and even existing practitioners have worked through this debate before you, and the debate may rage long after you graduate. Yet, there are compelling reasons to invest more in your own career beyond your PharmD degree. We went to the source, the rich source of information that is our Postgraduate Year One (PGY-1) and Postgraduate Year Two (PGY-2) pharmacy residents, who provided some data for this chapter. Was it a formal study? No. However, mixing their thoughts with ours provides a well-rounded rationale for postgraduate training.

Before we proceed further, remember that, beyond residencies, there are other types of postgraduate education that can be considered, including graduate degrees. Specific programs offered, their structure and design, and numbers of programs are discussed in Chapter 25. Another option for graduates includes fellowships (see Chapter 24). Both graduate training and fellowship training can have a focus on research, while certain degree options will focus on measurement of clinical services or have a leadership orientation.

WHY COMPLETE POSTGRADUATE TRAINING?

In determining if a residency is right for you, consider what activities suit you best for your career. You may thrive on working with a healthcare team, be energized by seeing a patient's hemoglobin A1c drop from 11% to 6.5% after your months of work with them, or be drawn to working with pharmacy students and other trainees to help them flourish under your watchful eye. Residencies and other postgraduate training often provide you the flexibility in choosing a position that allows you to be involved in activities like these or others that interest you. However, the personal investment of a residency admittedly includes the issues of decreased salary (initially), decreased sleep, opening yourself up to feedback on your performance from all angles (but at least there are no more grades), and sacrificing some activities that you might normally do (movies, dinners out, exercise) while you are training. Those same sacrifices hold true for students in graduate school or those participating in fellowships; in fact, those periods of time often far surpass the duration of a residency year (or two). However, the career and professional development you experience in postgraduate training is exponential.

Knowing yourself, what you value and deem important, and what you wish to invest in and obtain from your career are critical to any steps you take as you embark on your professional journey. No longer will you have an academic advisor instructing you about the specific courses you will need to take to reach your goal of entering pharmacy school. Instead, you finally have some choices, but this newfound freedom may be a bit daunting or at least unfamiliar territory. Now is the time for you to seize the opportunity to figure out who you want to be in the future, and then have the courage to follow the steps to reach those goals. Not all newly graduating students feel able to choose residency or other postgraduate training due to the need to repay student loans or other personal obligations.

SO, WIFM . . . WHAT'S IN IT FOR ME?

Postgraduate training is designed to provide you with additional knowledge, skills, abilities, and attitudes needed for your career. Let's break those elements down a bit more to remove the educational mumbo jumbo.

Postgraduate training provides the opportunity to develop skills in clinical practice, research or project management, depth of knowledge, confidence in decision making, and the opportunity to specialize. Postgraduate pharmacy experiences are tied to more responsibility than you have as a student, but with more guidance from preceptors or faculty mentors than you would receive if you went directly into practice, research, or academia. On the surface, it may look like a residency is just an extension of your pharmacy school rotations. But, remember that residents are licensed pharmacists who are in the trenches, immersing themselves in all that they can to exponentially improve. The opportunity for you to focus on your career development in such a manner will likely never come along again, so think about additional training as the ultimate self-improvement project. As a trainee, you will likely be working alongside a number of pharmacy students, which affords you the opportunity to determine if you'd like to one day work with other students, residents, graduate students, or fellows to help them in their career development. If you find out that's not your thing, no worries. At least you haven't committed to a full-time employment position in academia if that field "doesn't do it for you."

Some say that a pharmacy residency is such a concentrated postgraduate experience that it equates to 3 years of experience. Building upon that concept, it would be virtually impossible for you to have the variety of experiences you get in a PGY-1 pharmacy residency (e.g., critical care, general medicine, pediatrics, oncology, infectious disease, ambulatory care, administration, medication therapy management, and medication safety surveillance) without changing jobs multiple times. We know that being a managed care pharmacist was not your career goal when you were 6 years old, but it may be your dream now. If you already know your career destination, postgraduate training may be something you've known to be your next step for quite some time. The same can be said of a fellowship. In order to receive the experience in research during a fellowship, you would need to work on several different projects, often with different principal investigators, over a series of years to gain the equivalent experience, guidance, and personal growth. Through the multitude of diversity that postgraduate training provides, the ability to see what interests you most, including specialty areas, teaching experiences, and styles of learning, can be explored. You also broaden your experience in different practice, business, or research models, and thus open your eyes to a bigger pharmacy world than you experience as a student.

Another reason for postgraduate training is to increase your marketability, especially in today's pharmacist job market. With the market for positions tightening, often a reasonable choice for employment is to consider additional training. Training in a pharmacy residency or fellowship assists the pharmacist in being more competitive as an applicant. Even more opportunities may be opened to you if you complete additional training beyond a PGY-1 residency.

> "Residency training allows you to keep all doors open as the market becomes more and more competitive for adequately trained pharmacists."
>
> *Morgan H. – Pharmacy Student, Tennessee*

Undoubtedly, postgraduate training allows you to distinguish yourself from others who may not have had such extensive training. Daniel M. Ashby, Senior Director at Johns Hopkins Hospital, stated, "The best way to acquire the knowledge, skills and abilities for clinical practice is through the completion of a postgraduate training program."

Perhaps you have heard the adage that it takes 10,000 hours to develop expertise in a field. Although that target will not be within reach by the conclusion of your training, it will put you much closer. Expertise is often developed by reiteration of skills that postgraduate training allows. Unlike in your pharmacy school rotations, the ability to have increased repetitions in research, writing, teaching, and presentations is a common reason to seek and complete additional postgraduate training. With the supervision of preceptors, the expertise in all of these areas can also be developed even more quickly due to the number of opportunities for feedback. Feedback builds confidence in your abilities; at other times provides you with a reality check if you grossly overestimate your knowledge or approach to problem solving. And, it allows for you to recognize the effectiveness of your decision-making skills and judgment.

To put the importance of feedback into perspective, think about it this way—you will not be receiving grades on your performance on a regular basis out there in the real world. In a permanent position, your manager may take the "no news is good news" approach to give you feedback on your performance. If you hear from the manager apart from your yearly performance review, there could be something wrong. However, postgraduate training not only gives you continuous feedback but also allows you to compare your evaluation of your own performance with that of your mentor or preceptor. That ability to ensure you have a realistic impression of your performance, and to "check yourself before you wreck yourself," is critical to your success. Patients will not be giving you a grade on your ability to assess blood pressure, or the caring or professional attitude you did or did not display when you saw them at the pharmacy yesterday. Most notably, assessment is a core element of residency training. Accredited residencies allow the resident opportunities for self-reflection that often are not fostered through other means. Unfortunately, new practitioners can easily develop an unrealistic view of themselves in the world of no news is good news. The opportunity for you to get input from so many individuals and learn how to better reflect on your own performance sets the postgraduate experience apart from a permanent position.

The networking you conduct during pharmacy training makes lifelong connections between you and preceptors, coresidents, other fellows or graduate students, and past graduates of the program. Mentoring both informally and formally occurs during this time. The mentoring may be an arranged relationship (e.g., an assigned advisor) or may be selected by the trainee. There are strengths and weaknesses to both arrangements; however, having a mentor is the important aspect. As a student, you may already find yourself under the wing of an upper-level pharmacy student, resident, or faculty member. Multiply these relationships by 10. Connections built during postgraduate training mean you will have an extensive "phone a friend" list to call on, for assistance with a difficult patient case, advice or recommendation for a potential career move, help getting your foot in the door to being involved in professional organizations, and many more situations you may encounter in the future.

As a pharmacy student, you likely have been successful by tackling one task or assignment at a time. Consider those days numbered – in postgraduate training, you learn more what it is like to be a preceptor, practitioner, or researcher, for whom time management skills and multitasking are imperative (see Chapter 4). Communication development occurs often in postgraduate training. You must learn to master the ability to influence others through persuasive yet evidence-grounded approaches. A meek, overly aggressive, or vague call to a physician to convert a drug to one that is covered by a patient's insurance provider may be met with resistance, while a tactful, diplomatic, and informative tone may result in immediate agreement. Rather than being competitive and individualistic in the classroom, you transition to a need for collaboration during pharmacy residency or fellowship. In order to accomplish everything that needs to be done for patients or research, you have to rely on others to assist you in accomplishing your goals. As you collaborate with other healthcare givers, researchers, or institutional administrators, being able to speak their language and react to their verbal and nonverbal cues must come from repetition and reinforcement. That's what postgraduate training is all about—repetition and reinforcement.

Leadership skill development is essential to residency training. You may not have an innate ability to speak the language of an administrator, understand how department budgets are managed, or know how to conduct strategic planning to match your unit's activities to your own mission and goals. Yet, you will always have a manager, supervisor, or administrator that will be guiding your work, and will speak and think in terms differently like those. Knowing how to speak their lingo and understanding how to devise a win-win situation when you wish to expand your medication therapy management services to a new population can certainly impact the outcome of your project. Unfortunately, in Doctor of Pharmacy curricula, leadership training may be sought out only by those who are seeking a career as a director of pharmacy, district pharmacy manager, or pharmacy owner. Recognizing these factors, leadership skill development does not come optional, especially in accredited pharmacy residency programs. It is built into the residency accreditation standards for development of the future of the profession. Residents are often looked at as the future of pharmacy leadership, so development of skills in leading groups, understanding team dynamics, and bringing people together are essential postgraduate pharmacy skills.

The challenges that come along with training, sometimes referred to by preceptors as character-building experiences, create situations where residents have to think critically, provide insight, and explain their decision making. These might be interacting with a challenging attending physician, meeting multiple difficult deadlines, or being provided with constructive feedback. Additional character-building activities such as special events like a residency banquet, a reception to celebrate the receipt of a research grant, and other activities can be unique to the training experience. Other things to expect in a residency year, including common activities and learning experiences, will be discussed at a later point in this book (Chapter 4).

WHY DO INSTITUTIONS SUPPORT RESIDENCY TRAINING?

Training needs to be mutually beneficial—a two-way street. With all of the benefits for residents, the institution must derive some value from conducting postgraduate training. As a trainee in the system, you can guarantee you are providing value to the institution.[1] This comes in the way of potential expansion of clinical pharmacy services beyond what can be offered by the preceptors. Clinical coverage of patients on more units or services than would have clinical coverage may be a benefit. Or perhaps the ability to do an additional research project or develop a business plan for a new service is another way that the institution may benefit. Residents often serve on committees, support quality improvement and medication use projects, and complete other innovative activities that your preceptor only wishes she/he had some time to complete.

Your preceptors also benefit from the challenge of working with postgraduate pharmacy residents or fellows. You raise the level of teaching of preceptors by challenging them to think about things differently or assist in innovation for solutions to difficult problems. The more you can contribute, the more time the preceptor has to focus on other tasks that might go undone, including research, teaching, or submitting a poster abstract about a medication safety improvement project just concluded.

Pharmacy residents also bring new fresh ideas and experiences from their different home institutions to their new location. Pharmacy is not a cookie cutter profession, so there are a variety of programs or models used to deliver patient care. Residents who had student rotations in a different hospital or clinic may be able to share ideas and stimulate new ways of thinking about practice in their new environment. Residents often come immediately from a year of Doctor of Pharmacy Advanced Pharmacy Practice Experiences (APPE). During that year, the pharmacy students have opportunity to interact with many institutions and pharmacists. This can lead to sharing of information and innovation for the new institution. There is also an infusion of energy and excitement about the profession of pharmacy that emanates from postgraduate programs.

If a gap exists between clinical specialists and generalist pharmacists or between the management team and the rest of the staff, the pharmacy residents can help bridge that gap since they are often associated closely with both groups. Also, the pharmacy residency program can be an effective recruiting tool for the organization as pharmacy residents often stay on to work at their place of training if there is a position available following completion of their program. Similarly, a fellowship or graduate program is a very effective method for a college of pharmacy to create a future faculty member. Finally, institutions that provide postgraduate training are organizations that appreciate learning, innovation, and providing for the future of the profession. Postgraduate training allows for these aspects of a department or academic unit to be explored.

THE NATIONAL CASE FOR RESIDENCY TRAINING

> "I was unaware of the significant push for the requirement of pharmacy residency training by 2020. This is an encouragement for pharmacy students unsure about the decision to pursue a residency."
>
> *Brittany W. – Pharmacy Student, Tennessee*

Pharmacy residency training has become an important credential for pharmacy practice and is supported as an entry-level credential by several national organizations. ASHP, in its policy statement 0701, asserts that by 2020 the completion of an ASHP-accredited PGY-1 residency should be completed by all new graduates who provide direct patient care.[2] ACCP has a position paper that was written to also support the completion of a pharmacy residency by 2020 for new graduates.[3] The Accreditation Council for Pharmacy Education (ACPE) in guideline 6.2 of the accreditation standards indicates that colleges of pharmacy should through collaboration "support the development and enhancement of postgraduate education, postgraduate accredited residency and fellowship training, and combined degree options."[4] The American Association of Colleges of Pharmacy has statements in support of Community Pharmacy Residency programs and the value derived from these programs, and has entire policies, resources, and tools for the conduct of fellowship and graduate degree programs.[5] All of these statements lead one to believe that postgraduate training and especially pharmacy residencies are going to grow in the future.

IS THE DECISION TO COMPLETE POSTGRADUATE TRAINING RIGHT FOR YOU?

Why, though, should YOU complete a residency or other postgraduate training? The decision to pursue postgraduate training is a very personal, important issue for you and your career development. A thought process can lead you to think "how can you not do it?" Discuss potential career options with a mentor you trust, someone who knows you, understands your perspectives, and has had experiences they can draw

> "[After reading this chapter], my reasons for choosing to pursue a residency were reaffirmed!"
>
> *Brad S.   Pharmacy Student, Pennsylvania*

on to assist you in your decision making. Then, evaluate your conclusions in what your plan is and confirm your thought processes are correct. Remember, the next 40 years of your career are yours and your happiness will affect the happiness of those special to you over that time.

Chapter Takeaways

▶ Undertaking postgraduate training is a very personal decision.

▶ Reasons for pursuing additional training are widely varied, but they all build upon the refinement of your professional knowledge, skills, abilities, and attitudes.

▶ Pharmacy professional organizations have outlined goals to establish pharmacy residencies as foundational for all pharmacy graduates involved in direct patient care by 2020.

ROLE FOR THE MENTOR

Discuss career paths and the roles residencies, fellowships, and graduate degree training can prepare the student for.

Provide examples of the personal benefits of postgraduate training.

Address common concerns about the pursuit of postgraduate training and possible corresponding solutions.

References

1. Smith KM, et al. Value of conducting pharmacy residency training—The organizational perspective. Pharmacotherapy. 2010;30:490–510e.

2. American Society of Health-System Pharmacy Policy Statement (0701). http://www.ashp.org/DocLibrary/BestPractices/EducationPositions.aspx. Accessed March 16, 2012.

3. Murphy JE, Nappi JM, Bosso JA. American College of Clinical Pharmacy's vision of the future: Postgraduate pharmacy residency training as a prerequisite for direct patient care practice. Pharmacotherapy. 2006;26:722–733.

4. Accreditation Council for Pharmacy Education. Accreditation Standards and Guidelines for the Professional Program in Pharmacy Leading to the Doctor of Pharmacy Degree. https://www.acpe-accredit.org/pdf/acpe_revised_pharmd_standards_adopted_jan152006.pdf. Accessed March 16, 2012.

5. Pharmacy Residency Resources. American Association of Colleges of Pharmacy. http://www.aacp.org/resources/education/Pages/PharmacyResidencyResources.aspx. Accessed March 16, 2012.

Who's in Charge? The Role of Accreditation in Postgraduate Pharmacy Training 3

Mary M. Hess and Kelly M. Smith

You often hear the word accreditation in many contexts, from degree programs to hospitals to colleges and universities. The word usually sparks a sense of urgency or concern in an administrator's voice, too, so it must be fairly important. While you undoubtedly don't lose sleep over accreditation or wondering how it fits into your life, it is of importance to you as a student, trainee, future preceptor or practice leader, and even patient. Let's dig a bit deeper into the concept.

THE ABCs OF ACCREDITATION

Accreditation is much like a final grade in a pharmacy course—an external assessment of performance as applied to predetermined criteria or standards. Without accreditation, it becomes difficult to understand the quality or performance of a hospital beyond the marketing, public relations, and external face the organization wears in the community. If your mother developed a life-threatening medical condition, you would want her to receive the best care possible and would likely search for unbiased measures of the care she could expect, rather than selecting a hospital based on its catchy marketing slogan. Relying upon the role of unbiased experts to examine the organization, its commitment to quality, and how patients fare, seems to be a much more prudent thing to do. That's where accreditation comes in. Most industries, and in our case the broad profession of health care, have expected standards that need to be maintained to ensure the best quality of care. In health care, we look to experts in accreditation to provide that outside source of information about an organization.

In the context of pharmacy in the United States, accreditation affects hospitals, universities, colleges of pharmacy, and workforce training (including residencies, fellowships, and technician training) programs, and it's even an emerging concept in community pharmacies, given the collaboration with

American Pharmacists Association (APhA) and the National Association of Boards of Pharmacy (NABP).[1] The Joint Commission (TJC) accredits hospitals and health systems to ensure "safe and effective care of the highest quality and value," and the National Committee for Quality Assurance accredits health plans, health and wellness programs, disease management programs, and behavioral healthcare organizations.[2,3] Colleges and universities are accredited by regional organizations (e.g., Southern Associations of Colleges and Schools Commission on Colleges) to grant academic degrees at higher education institutions.[4] Specific to pharmacy, the ACPE is an acronym you will continue to hear throughout your career in the United States, as that organization accredits Doctor of Pharmacy and pharmacy continuing education providers.[5] ACPE accredits Doctor of Pharmacy programs to ensure the school or college is providing quality education to you as a student to make you knowledgeable and prepared to be a competent pharmacist. This process protects you as a "customer," as you are investing a significant amount of time and years in your life to your profession, and you certainly want some assurance that those investments will pay off. Given that pharmacy licensure in the United States is predicated upon your graduation from an ACPE-accredited PharmD program (and even additional examinations for foreign institution graduates), accreditation is more important to you than you might realize. Your ability to qualify for certain federally sponsored financial aid packages is even dependent on your school or college of pharmacy being accredited.

Pharmacy residencies, fellowships, and technician training programs also have accreditation processes through American Society of Health-System Pharmacists (ASHP) and American College of Clinical Pharmacy (ACCP). Contrary to TJC's accreditation of hospitals, an achievement that has direct ties to the organization's ability to provide care and receive payment by third parties, workforce training programs have a voluntary or optional accreditation process. There is no federal mandate or underlying funding requirement tied to each program's accreditation status. However, there are benefits to receiving accreditation, both to the sponsoring organization and to you as the trainee. Because residencies comprise the overwhelming majority of pharmacy workforce training programs affiliated with accreditation, this chapter focuses on that process and its implications. See Chapter 24 for information about fellowship programs.

TO BE (ACCREDITED) OR NOT TO BE, THAT IS THE QUESTION

While pharmacy residency accreditation is optional in the United States, most programs participate in the process. The fundamental tenet of accreditation is an external appraisal of the program to ensure it meets the profession's standards, as well as to identify ways in which the program can improve. Residency accreditation provides for just that, as it measures how well and to what degree a site meets our profession's expectations. It also provides a forum for peers to discuss examples of methods and measures to improve and evaluate postgraduate level pharmacy training. It's these peer review and networking elements of accreditation that programs often find to be of greatest value.

Financial benefits flow to many programs that conduct accredited Postgraduate Year One (PGY-1) programs. Hospitals or health systems that conduct accredited PGY-1 training are eligible for federal funds to underwrite the program's cost, much like medical residencies are funded. This funding model is reliant upon the extent to which the institution provides care to Medicare patients, making most community, managed care, or Veterans Affairs (VA)-hosted PGY-1 programs ineligible for the funding. However, internal funding may also be tied to accreditation. Think about this in the context of renting a car. Is the rental company likely to give you the keys if you don't have a driver's license? Even though the car rental salesman wasn't in the car with you during your driving test, the fact that you possess a driver's license shows them that the state deemed you competent to drive. A similar concept applies to residency accreditation. Imagine the car rental salesman to be the chief executive officer of a pharmacy benefit manager or district manager of a chain pharmacy. Would that individual agree to fund a residency program that does not seek accreditation? It would be difficult to justify such an investment without knowing the money is well worth it.

Programs that are accredited by ASHP, or have applied to become accredited, are eligible to take advantage of several recruiting benefits. The first is a listing of the program in ASHP's Online Residency Directory, the only official listing of residency programs in the United States.[6] Second, a program that is in the accreditation pipeline, or is already accredited, is eligible to participate in the National Residency Matching Program. The match is a requirement for already accredited programs, and is optional for programs just beginning their first year of training, but who have indicated their intent to seek accreditation (pre-candidate). Both of these features provide a recruiting advantage to the program, as they are now part of the mainstream of the more than 1000 programs already in the loop. As a potential applicant, you can easily locate the list of programs in the match, as well as learn more about them through the online directory. Since there is no national, comprehensive database or reporting body that monitors both accredited and unaccredited pharmacy residencies, you'll have to do your homework if you want to know the total number of pharmacy residency programs at any given time. ACCP does provide a broader listing of postgraduate training options, but a program must opt in for inclusion in that directory, and can only be included if it is offered by a member of ACCP.[7]

Some within our profession might view unaccredited postgraduate training programs negatively, as they lack uniformity or required oversight. How our healthcare colleagues perceive us could be negatively influenced if we cannot agree to a minimum level of credentials necessary for practice, much less a training model that allows accreditation to be voluntary. Our efforts to gain the support of policymakers and third-party payers to assume a greater role in healthcare provision may be further diminished if we accept the possibility of unaccredited training as a suitable credential. While this is a philosophical dilemma, it does merit your consideration.

Despite these internal and external advantages of accreditation, some residency program directors (RPDs) do not seek accreditation for their programs. The accreditation process is rigorous, it requires substantial documentation and routine self-assessment, and there are annual fees to maintain accreditation. Some sites may not feel confident in their ability to meet the accreditation standards, particularly if they are just starting up, and they may therefore wait to seek accreditation until they have conducted the program for a number of years. There are yet others who do not wish to adhere to a training model that does not fit their own vision of training, yet those numbers have diminished greatly over the past 10 to 15 years. While unaccredited programs may provide a rich training environment for the resident, they lack an external measure of the quality or adherence to profession-wide standards of training.

WHO ACCREDITS PHARMACY RESIDENCY PROGRAMS?

ASHP has led the accreditation of postgraduate pharmacy training programs since 1962 (see Chapter 1). The modern accreditation process is overseen by ASHP's Commission on Credentialing (COC), a member committee whose purview also includes technician training programs. The COC leads the development of accreditation standards that are endorsed by the profession, creates regulations for the accreditation process, and recommends accreditation decisions to ASHP's Board of Directors, who act on COC recommendations. The administrative unit within ASHP that facilitates accreditation operations is the Accreditation Services Division, which is composed of ASHP staff employees, many of whom are former residency program directors and preceptors.

While ASHP administers residency accreditation, membership on the COC and the development of residency standards are conducted in concert with several other professional organizations, including American Academy of Colleges of Pharmacy (AACP), ACCP, Academy of Managed Care Pharmacy (AMCP), and APhA. If you were to participate in a COC meeting, you would find that the majority of its members are RPDs or preceptors who represent various practice backgrounds. The COC is also made up of a resident, a Dean from a college or school of pharmacy, and a public member. Such broad perspectives are sought in the members, each of whom is appointed by the ASHP Board of Directors. Members of the COC frequently serve as accreditation site surveyors and are responsible for reviewing all reports submitted by the survey team and respective institution before having discussion and recommending an accreditation status.

Given how quickly the profession changes, the COC continually monitors the practice of pharmacy and health care in general to determine when the residency standards warrant a revision. The standards are written to inspire individual practitioners and pharmacy leaders to design the *optimal* practice environment, services, and patient outcomes.[8] As a result, these optimal standards may stretch the program to achieve more. This is a critical distinction from most accreditation standards, like those of TJC and ACPE, which are designed for a minimum level of achievement. The COC has positioned the accreditation standards to push all of us to do more, and to not be complacent with our current roles or practice models. Thus, it's highly unlikely that any residency program will emerge "unscathed" from a residency accreditation visit. They will hear compliments about what they are doing well, but they will also be prompted to do more for patients, the profession, and the residents themselves.

THE ACCREDITATION HOW TO GUIDE

Learning how to decipher accreditation terms such as pre-candidate, conditional accreditation, on-site survey, and partial compliance may make you long to attend another pharmacokinetics lecture; however, the process a residency program takes to become accredited is sequential, and understanding the steps can help you become a savvy "consumer." Figure 3-1 highlights the key steps a program undergoes when obtaining initial residency accreditation, while Table 3-1 defines the formal accreditation status terms.

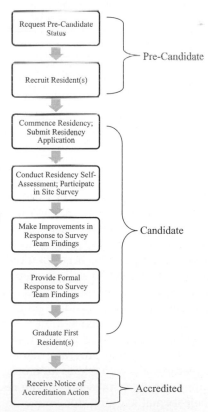

Figure 3-1: Program Steps to Obtain Initial Accreditation

TABLE 3-1 • Residency Accreditation Status Possibilities[9]

Accreditation Term	Definition
Pre-candidate	A program that has submitted a completed application indicating intent to seek "candidate" status
Candidate	A program that has a resident(s) in training, has applied to ASHP for accreditation, and is awaiting the official site survey, review, and evaluation by the COC
Preliminary accreditation	A status that may be granted to a program by ASHP, upon a recommendation by a site survey team following completion of the document review and site survey, indicative of a high likelihood that the COC will recommend accreditation
Accreditation	A program that has met set requirements and has been reviewed and evaluated through an official process (document review, site survey, and review and evaluation by the COC). An approved program is in an "ASHP-accredited" status
Conditional accreditation	A program that is not in substantial compliance with the applicable accreditation standard, as usually evidenced by the degree of severity of noncompliance and partial compliance findings. Programs must remedy identified problem areas and may undergo subsequent on-site surveys

ASHP, American Society of Health-System Pharmacists; COC, Commission on Credentialing.

The accreditation process begins well *after* the program is merely a glimmer in the RPD's eye, as a site must be poised to or already in the process of conducting training. Programs may choose to begin the process just prior to recruiting their first resident (pre-candidate) or once a resident has been secured (candidate)—the choice of when to apply for accreditation is not indicative of a program's quality or preparedness. When a site is prepared to formally recruit its first resident and intends to seek candidate status, the RPD may apply for status with ASHP as a *pre-candidate*. Pre-candidate programs gain access to participation in the upcoming residency match and the residency showcase at the ASHP Midyear Clinical Meeting, are listed in ASHP's online residency directory, and can gain access to the online program management tool ResiTrak® (see Chapter 4). These features are valuable to an emerging program, as they are able to effectively announce their presence on the residency stage, as well as to begin building their formal learning documents in ResiTrak®. If you are a resident in a new program that has filed its application for accreditation, the

> "Until I went through accreditation this year as a resident, I had no idea how much work and thought goes into organizing and running a residency. I have so much more respect for residency program directors everywhere."
>
> *Tiffany S. – Pharmacy Resident, Ohio*

program is considered to be in *candidate* status. Once in a candidate status, the program is fully functional. During this candidacy year, the program director is charged with conducting a self-assessment of the program (using a pre-survey questionnaire), during which the RPD and preceptors assess the extent of their adherence to more than 130 elements of the residency accreditation standard.[10]

Adherence to each element is measured according to a scale of compliance: noncompliance, partial compliance, and (full) compliance. Beyond this self-grading, the program must assemble a host of materials that provide evidence of the site's commitment to quality improvement, its organizational chart, its policy and procedures, evidence of the qualifications of its preceptors and program directors, and key examples of the residency evaluation process, among other important documents.

If you train during a program's candidacy year, you can expect that an accreditation team will visit your site during your ninth to twelfth month of the residency in order to validate your program's adherence to the residency accreditation standard, a process commonly referred to as a site survey or on-site visit. This timing is important, as the evaluation process is reliant upon a sufficient amount of time for the program to have demonstrated its training and guidance of you, which can best be measured near the conclusion of your training. If it occurs too early in the year, your RPD and preceptors will not have had the opportunity to demonstrate their ability to meet all elements of the residency standard.

> "When the [accreditation] site surveyors interviewed me, I thought they were going to grill me about all the things that are wrong with the residency. Instead, it was a good conversation about my residency experience and what I thought of it. They just wanted my opinion about how things were going and if I was getting a good experience."
>
> *Tiffany S. – Pharmacy Resident, Ohio*

The on-site visit will be conducted by a lead surveyor, either an ASHP accreditation employee or contract employee surveyor, as well as a guest surveyor for each program being reviewed. If your site has created two new programs in cardiology and oncology, for instance, the survey team will likely consist of one lead surveyor, one cardiology surveyor, and one oncology surveyor. The guest surveyors are generally directors of similar residency programs, and they may also be members of the COC. These features are important to maintain the peer review element of the process. The team will spend several days on-site reviewing the materials provided by your program and measuring them against the accreditation standard.

Beyond reviewing paperwork, the team will meet with organization leadership, pharmacists and technicians, physicians, nurses and others who interact with pharmacy residents, and, of course, with you, the pharmacy resident.

These meetings are conducted to verify the paperwork matches the insight each person interviewed provides about the institution, its policies and procedures, its commitment to care, and the actual nature of the residency program and pharmacy department. The survey team will also share their ideas for improvement or innovation, as well as commend the site for its notable practices and ideas that can be shared with other programs in the country.

At the conclusion of the site visit, the survey team will provide a verbal report of its findings to you, your preceptors and pharmacists, and other interested parties. For each element of the residency standard, your program will receive a compliance rating using the same compliance measures (e.g., partially compliant) as your program used in its self-assessment. The surveyors may also give consultative suggestions, which are "bonus" ideas about methods to improve the residency beyond what is required by the standard. The team may also convey *preliminary accreditation* to the program, should they believe it meets a substantial number of elements of the residency standard.

Usually within 30 to 45 days of the survey team's departure, the program will receive a formal, written report of the survey team findings and will be instructed to provide a formal, written response to areas of noncompliance or partial compliance. The RPD must provide an action plan and supporting documentation to explain what and how the program will correct the deficient standards. For example, if a program is found to be partially compliant in resident self-evaluations, the RPD should provide examples of completed resident self-evaluations conducted at the conclusion of each rotation. This entire documentation and reporting process will span up to 6 months, and perhaps longer.

The survey team's formal findings, as well as the program's response, are next presented to the COC for consideration. On the basis of the nature and extent of areas of lesser or noncompliance, the COC will recommend an *accreditation* status (i.e., no accreditation, accreditation) and length of accreditation for the program to the ASHP Board of Directors. A program that is fully compliant with the majority of the standard is likely to receive accreditation for 6 years, known as full-cycle accreditation; these programs are generally very well designed. The COC may also designate a shorter duration of accreditation, usually 1 or 3 years, based on the overall compliance level of the program with the standard. Programs that receive less than a full-cycle accreditation must work to remedy the areas to which they are less than fully compliant, and provide a written report of those improvements prior to their accreditation expiration. The COC will then review the new report along with the previous documents and recommend a new accreditation status and duration, often to complete the sum of the initial and extended accreditation up to a total of 6 years (e.g., initial accreditation, 3 years; continued accreditation, 3 more years). The self-assessment, on-site survey and written report process will recur every 6 years for programs that seek to maintain their accreditation beyond the initial total of 6 years. Once the ASHP Board of Directors takes action on the COC's recommendations, the program's final accreditation status will be granted retroactive to the date of the original application for accreditation. Thus, it is important for the RPD to make an application prior to or early during your residency year, so that you will have the opportunity to be considered a graduate of an accredited program. The residency is technically not eligible for full accreditation until at least one resident has successfully completed the residency program, much like a new college of pharmacy cannot be fully accredited by ACPE until it has graduated its first PharmD class.

Previously accredited programs may receive a finding of conditional accreditation, an unfavorable status indicating considerable problems with the residency and a significant number of partially or noncompliant elements that jeopardize the program's ongoing accreditation. For such a finding, the COC may authorize an additional, focused site survey to assess critical elements of concern, and then revise its accreditation recommendation accordingly given the team's findings. Conditional accreditation status allows the program to continue to operate as it addresses its deficiencies, also allowing you as a resident to complete an accredited program. If the program does not adequately address the noncompliance or partial compliance issues, the COC may choose to withhold accreditation. Once a program has its accreditation withheld, any subsequent residency graduates will be considered to have completed an unaccredited residency program. Fortunately, conditional accreditation is not common, as ASHP and Accreditation Services will offer a number of development tools to the site to enable it to demonstrate sufficient improvement and subsequent adherence to the standard.

HOW CAN YOU BECOME INVOLVED?

Residents in programs that are undergoing initial or reaccreditation have a unique role and perspective in the accreditation process. While the extent of your involvement depends on the guidance provided by your RPD, the survey team will encourage you to participate as much as the site will allow, recognizing the unique learning experience the survey process provides to you. This experience provides an excellent foundation for you in the future as you become a preceptor and perhaps RPD.

Beyond being interviewed by the surveyors during the on-site interview, you should seek opportunities to participate in the self-assessment process, from assembling written materials to providing feedback and suggestions for the program structure before the site visit.

"Though helping with accreditation added to my workload this year, I learned so much about the inner workings of a residency; plus I finally found out why we have to do all those ResiTrak® evaluations."

Tiffany S. – Pharmacy Resident, Ohio

As you can imagine, accreditation visits are stressful for your RPD and preceptors, as their methods and structure of training and precepting are being closely evaluated. As a resident, you can learn much from observing the nature of those interactions and how your role models respond. Yet, temper your observations with the realization of the significant personal and professional investment, the site, your RPD, and preceptors have made in the program, which is truly focused on you and your success.

ACCREDITATION...WHAT'S IN IT FOR ME?

Accreditation indicates that the practice site is suitable to facilitate the program being offered, that there are sufficient preceptors and program leadership, and that the program is evaluated on a routine basis. You should feel confident that the program is designed to meet the intent of the standard, will be delivered in such a way as to foster learning and skill development, and that the organization is committed (through both fiscal and human resources) to the success of the residency, and in turn you. Beyond those feel-good measures, there are some more objective indicators of the impact of residency accreditation.

For you to be eligible to apply to an accredited Postgraduate Year Two (PGY-2) program, you must have completed an ASHP-accredited PGY-1 program. Your credentials will be validated during the PGY-2 match process, and if they cannot be verified, you will not be matched with a program, even if that program includes an early commitment recruitment option. You may petition the director of ASHP's Accreditation Services Division to be granted an exception to participate in the PGY-2 match; however, your petition is likely to be approved only if you have substantial practice experience that is deemed equivalent to an approved PGY-1 residency experience (e.g., 5-year experience in an advanced practice setting).

Some employers already require residency training as a criterion for employment. In many cases, the requirement extends to accredited residency program completion, and the prospective employee will need to produce the residency certificate as proof of completing an accredited program. While this may be indicative of the philosophical value one organization places on accreditation, in other settings, the requirement may represent a step in the privileging and credentialing process necessary for you to be hired as a pharmacist, or for you to assume advanced roles in the organization (e.g., collaborative practice, prescribing). Other employers provide financial incentives based on your credentials, which may include residency training and, in some cases, specifically accredited residency training.

Your pursuit of specialty credentials may be affected by residency accreditation. Candidate eligibility for accreditation by the Board of Pharmacy Specialties (BPS) includes a specified amount of time spent in practice or completion of a residency.[11] Beginning in 2013, the residency credential must be obtained from an accredited program. This means that, if you complete a nonaccredited pharmacy practice PGY-1 residency, you will not be allowed to take the

Board Certification Pharmacotherapy Specialist exam until you have worked for an additional 2 years in a clinical setting after your residency. Meanwhile, your PharmD classmate who completed an accredited residency program in the same year as you would be eligible for the examination immediately after his residency concluded. This new requirement applies to all BPS specialties, with the exception of nuclear pharmacy.

CONSIDERING ACCREDITATION WHEN SELECTING A PROGRAM

The motivations for a site to pursue accreditation, the meaning of accreditation, and how accreditation may affect your professional career are all elements for you to keep in mind when you search for a residency program. However, there are some other points to consider. Remember that there may be relatively fewer PGY-2 programs that are accredited, since they universally lack sources of federal funding for their conduct. And, a lack of accreditation does not signal that the program lacks a sufficient quality—it may simply mean the program has yet to pursue or places a different value on accreditation.

You are likely to encounter residency programs that are not yet accredited, but may be in the process of or soon expect to pursue accreditation. Both pre-candidate and candidate programs have retroactively afforded the same rights and privileges of an accredited program, yet only if the program becomes accredited upon a timely application. Many residents pursuing residency training wouldn't have it any other way, though, as they are passionate about helping to build a new program, and thus they are specifically pursuing new programs. Still other candidates may not have pursued residency training until the conclusion of the residency match, and thus are now beginning their search process when many new programs are jumping into the mix. Despite the uncertainty, also recall that the COC is committed to ensure quality training experiences are provided to residents, and ASHP will provide developmental support to the site to minimize the likelihood that a radical accreditation action must be taken while a resident is in training at the site.

If residency accreditation is important to you, you should follow the adage *caveat emptor* (buyer beware). Check the program's status in the ASHP online residency directory. Ask the director, preceptor, and residents about the program's accreditation status. When is the program's next site survey? What was the accreditation length granted during the last program's cycle? What were the major areas of improvement found during the last site survey? It is wise for you to review the corresponding residency accreditation standard, so that you will understand what a program is expected to provide to you as a resident, and how the patient care services should be delivered.[8] For currently unaccredited programs, ask about their intent to seek accreditation, and specifically when they will submit an application. If they fail to apply prior to the conclusion of your residency, any changes in accreditation status (i.e., becoming accredited) would not apply to you.

THE BOTTOM LINE

> "It's okay to not know what type of post-graduate training you are interested in prior to rotations. To help figure out your interests, get a variety of experiences, including attending residency showcases prior to your P4 year."
>
> *Anokhi S. – Pharmacy Resident, Pennsylvania*

Although you may never be directly involved in the process, you are a consumer of the accreditation process through your pursuit of a college degree, pharmacist licensure, postgraduate training, and even your receipt of health care. Understanding the process for pharmacy training programs, and the accreditation options available, can help you best find a residency program that meets your professional needs.

Chapter Takeaways

▶ Accreditation for pharmacy residencies, fellowships, and technician training programs is a voluntary process in the United States.

▶ ASHP conducts pharmacy residency and technician training accreditation under the auspices of its Commission on Credentialing, a membership body composed of program directors and representatives from several pharmacy organizations.

▶ The duration of residency accreditation cannot exceed 6 years.

▶ Accreditation can influence your qualifications for PGY-2 residencies, specialty credentials (e.g., BPS examinations), and some employment positions. As a residency applicant, you should consider the value you place in accreditation, and then seek programs that match your values.

ROLE FOR THE MENTOR

Discuss the value you place on accreditation of postgraduate pharmacy training.

Share the experiences with residency accreditation that you have had.

Describe the role you predict accreditation will have for postgraduate pharmacy training in the future.

FREQUENTLY ASKED QUESTIONS

Q: **Why aren't all pharmacy residency programs accredited?**
A: Accreditation will not be granted until at least one individual has completed the program. Part of the accreditation assessment involves

evaluation of delivery of the program, which can only be done once a resident is in place. Accreditation is not mandatory; thus, all sponsoring organizations have an option of whether to accredit their program or not. There are financial incentives that may benefit some, but not all, organizations that obtain accreditation. Accreditation reflects a commitment to quality improvement of the program at all times, which requires the investment of human and financial resources, as well as an organizational commitment to the philosophy, purpose, and value of accredited residency training.

Q: If I am the first resident in a program, does that mean I miss out on being in an accredited program?

A: The timing is critical. Once accreditation is granted, all residents who completed the program after the original application was submitted will be considered to have completed an accredited residency. If the program does not apply for accreditation prior to the completion of your residency year (and subsequently become accredited), the program you completed will be considered unaccredited.

Q: What should I do if a program tells me they are going to seek accreditation and then don't?

A: Unfortunately, there is no organization that can enforce the program's intent to apply. However, such an occurrence would reflect poorly on the program and would likely make recruitment of subsequent residents difficult. Remember not to burn any professional bridges by reacting unprofessionally should this unfortunate situation occur.

One proactive approach you may wish to take is to request that the RPD insert comments regarding the program's intent to apply for accreditation in your residency offer letter (employment offer).

Q: What should I do if I have significant concerns about the quality of my accredited residency program?

A: First, have a discussion with your program director or a trusted mentor involved in the program. Be open minded during this discussion as the situation could just be that your expectations and that of the program are different. Ask open-ended questions regarding your concerns and why the program is designed as it is. The program preceptors may share the same concerns and are already working to make changes, or your inquiry may prod them to consider different approaches. However, realize that program changes can take time, and personal preferences or non-substantive adjustments may not be priorities for the program to make immediately.

Following your internal discussion, if you have significant concerns that need to be addressed and the leadership of the program or the sponsoring organization will not address them, you may wish to submit a complaint to ASHP. However, you should not make this decision lightly, as you will be accountable for your submission. ASHP will follow up with you, they may have discussions with your program leadership, and the COC will be made aware of your complaint.

References

1. American Pharmacists Association. Community Pharmacy Accreditation: Frequently Asked Questions. http://www.pharmacist.com/AM/Template.cfm?Section=Home2&CONTENTID=27248&TEMPLATE=/CM/ContentDisplay.cfm. Accessed March 18, 2012.

2. The Joint Commission. http://www.jointcommission.org. Accessed March 18, 2012.

3. The National Committee for Quality Assurance. http://www.ncqa.org/tabid/675/Default.aspx. Accessed March 18, 2012.

4. Southern Associations of Colleges and Schools Commission on Colleges. http://sacscoc.org. Accessed March 18, 2012.

5. Accreditation Council for Pharmacy Education. https://www.acpe-accredit.org. Accessed March 18, 2012.

6. ASHP Online Residency Directory. http://accred.ashp.org/aps/pages/directory/residency-ProgramSearch.aspx. Accessed February 25, 2012.

7. American College of Clinical Pharmacy Directory of Residencies, Fellowships, and Graduate Programs. http://www.accp.com/resandfel/index.aspx. Accessed March 18, 2012.

8. ASHP Residency Accreditation Regulations and Standards. http://www.ashp.org/menu/Accreditation/ResidencyAccreditation.aspx. Accessed March 18, 2012.

9. ASHP Regulations on Accreditation of Pharmacy Residencies. http://www.ashp.org/DocLibrary/Accreditation/ASD-Accreditation-Regulations-Residencies.aspx. Accessed March 18, 2012.

10. DeCoske MA, Bush PW, Teeters JL. Preparing for pharmacy residency accreditation surveys. Am J Health Syst Pharm. 2010;67:469–475.

11. Board of Pharmacy Specialties. http://www.bpsweb.org. Accessed March 18, 2012.

A Day in the Life: What to Expect as a Pharmacy Resident 4

Maria C. Pruchnicki and Marialice S. Bennett

Congratulations! You have made the decision to be a pharmacy resident. Residency is a time filled with learning and transitions—continuing as a trainee but beginning your professional career as a pharmacist. You will still receive formal evaluations based on the accreditation standards of your program, but also start to rely on self-evaluation and making corrections based on your own internal criteria. You will be taking greater responsibility for patients, and be making the decisions related to their best care. The day-to-day schedule is your path forward, a main determinant in how you advance toward the desired outcomes of your program. Knowing what to expect and understanding the rhythm of your residency are important first steps in preparing yourself for the adventure. This chapter gives you a glimpse of a resident's "day in the life" duties and responsibilities.

> "This chapter is very informative to pharmacy students interested in obtaining a residency and indicates the commitment that it takes to complete a residency successfully."
>
> *Adebayo O. – Pharmacy Student, Kentucky*

PATIENT CARE SERVICES

Postgraduate Year One (PGY-1) pharmacy residency programs place priority on direct patient care across broad populations, and experience in pharmacy operations to accelerate development of a high-level and engaged pharmacy workforce.[1] Postgraduate Year Two (PGY-2) programs build upon the competencies of PGY-1 graduates in specialized areas, particularly in complex patient management and clinical leadership.[2] In both years, a majority of your time and attention is focused on direct patient care. Services are provided in a variety of healthcare settings, including inpatient, ambulatory care, managed care, and community care arenas; your ideal program may have a particular focus on one or another. Though the specifics of the day undoubtedly differ between inpatient and outpatient rotations, the general roles of the pharmacy resident are similar and can be captured in the descriptions below.

Rounding

In inpatient residencies, "rounding" has very little to do with bumping numbers up or down to make them easier to work with. As you know from IPPE/APPE rotations, medical rounds are clinical meetings. The cases of patients assigned to a hospital service or unit are reviewed and discussed by the healthcare team. They are often inter- or multidisciplinary, and can be used for both patient care and teaching purposes. In fact, bedside rounds are considered the prototypic teaching method in medical education.[3] Rounds can take several forms—for example "working rounds," "attending rounds," and "grand rounds" as described in Table 4-1. Patient care rounds require you to evaluate for new and ongoing health problems, medication adjustments or selection, laboratory monitoring, and overall update on the patient's clinical condition. Discharge and follow-up planning are also discussed, and often are coordinated by a patient case manager. The team pharmacist should have input on

TABLE 4-1 • Types of Rounds Encountered in Residencies

Type	Description
Patient Care Rounds	
Pre-rounds	Reviews of medical data/chart by individual provider; may visit the patient alone, to identify any salient or new events in their clinical course
Working rounds	Review of patients with other members of the healthcare team, including resident physicians and interns, nurses, and others. Allows team members to catch up on patient events and information (or provide a "pass-off" from one shift to the next), practice oral presentations, and develop plans to discuss during attending rounds
Attending rounds	Formal meetings of the healthcare team, led by the attending physician; used to discuss and finalize the diagnostic and therapeutic plans
Walking rounds	Rounds conducted while walking through the medical ward, or at the patient's bedside. Team often interacts with patient and/or family members, to gather information or to explain the management plan
Chart rounds	Rounds conducted in conference using the patient list or medical chart (or electronic medical record) to discuss differential diagnoses and possible management plans. These are also sometimes called "table rounds" and may occur in combination with time at the bedside
Teaching Rounds	
Case/chart rounds	Group meetings that may include providers outside of patient's healthcare team; often multidisciplinary in nature. Purpose is to teach clinical information/reasoning skills for broader application
Grand rounds	Formal, scheduled presentation of a patient case or cases with the intent to teach new information and demonstrate clinical reasoning skills. Often planned to highlight current or interesting clinical problems and open to a larger audience than chart rounds

medication changes needed during the transition of care, and should assist in discharge counseling.

Teaching rounds usually use patient scenarios and cases to introduce new knowledge or application of information. Discipline-specific rounds may include aspects of care or education that are particularly relevant to one type of provider or specialist, and may occur outside of normal medical rounds. Also, the day may encompass a combination of rounding types (pre rounding, working rounds with preceptor, then walking rounds with team).

Patient Appointments

Pharmacy residents who train in outpatient settings provide patient education and medication therapy management services in a variety of practice models. Health–system-based ambulatory programs are a natural extension of hospital-based services and are common sites for pharmacy residencies. However, community and stand-alone ambulatory services may also provide rich training environments. In a single day (or over the course of a week), residents may participate in physician-based appointments, provide add-on pharmacy services to physician visits, or have a dedicated pharmacy schedule for patients. Services can include general practice (e.g., pharmacotherapy clinic or medication therapy management appointments) or specialty services (e.g., anticoagulation management, smoking cessation, or diabetes management). Depending on the training site, pharmacists may work collaboratively with physicians, physician assistants, and nurse prescribers on-site, or may work under a protocol with a supervising physician or medical director's oversight. Collaborative practice agreements, where a pharmacy provider is able to provide specific patient care functions (e.g., medication titration or monitoring) for individuals under a supervising provider, are also quite common. Ideally, ambulatory and community pharmacy residencies would offer a variety of models for you to enhance your training and patient care experience. In primary care, the patient-centered medical home model emphasizes the collaborative practice of healthcare teams and uses informational technologies to provide innovative practice experiences.[4]

Clinical Consultations

Consult services related to focused areas of expertise are often utilized to assist providers or the healthcare team in care of individual patients. Consult services are appropriate for any patient with a complicated medical course, multiple or significant comorbidities, or specialized care needs. Consult services are traditionally hospital-based but are also becoming more available in outpatient settings. Consultations may be related to a particular area of medical practice (e.g., infectious disease, cardiology, and nephrology) or for patients requiring specific medication, nutrition, or other care support (e.g., pharmacokinetic monitoring, total parenteral nutrition, or renal replacement therapy). The consult provider typically reviews the case with input from other providers and staff, the medical record, and the patient, and perhaps the patient's family.

> "Tables 4-1 and 4-2 give very detailed description of terminology not known to every student before starting rotations."
>
> *Adebayo O. – Pharmacy Student, Kentucky*

They provide recommendations with documentation of the consult events, and may also participate in team and family meetings in appropriate circumstances. Pharmacy residents may participate as team members for medicine subspecialties (see Chapter 20), special patient populations (see Chapter 21), or other widely available pharmacy-specific consult services performing tasks as described in Table 4-2.

TABLE 4-2 • Common Pharmacy-Specific Services

Type	Description
"Consult" Services	
Antibiotic stewardship	Recommending and monitoring antibiotic therapy for patients; assesses for appropriate IV (intravenous) to PO (oral) conversions
Antithrombotic therapy (warfarin, heparin and LMWH, direct thrombin inhibitors)	Providing medication education, INR monitoring and dose adjustment, medication assistance programs, and adverse event monitoring for newer anticoagulants and other antithrombotic agents
Clinical pharmacology	Assisting in challenging cases of complicated drug dosing, drug interactions, adverse events, and interpretation of new genetic tests
Diabetes	Assessment and intervention on diabetes self-management during inpatient hospitalization, per clinical recommendations
Drug information	Researching and formulating response for providers and patients; may be for individuals or population-based clinic problems, using appropriate references and medical literature
Home health	Assisting in the transition of care for patients receiving IV medications who will be discharged and receive services through home health, including appropriateness of medication therapy for the outpatient setting and recommending a monitoring plan (laboratory work)
Medicare drug benefit	Educating eligible Medicare beneficiaries about the available Prescription Drug Programs and Medicare Advantage Prescription Drugs
Medication dosing (Pharmacotherapy)	Pharmacokinetic dosing (aminoglycosides, vancomycin, warfarin, heparin, argatroban, digoxin, and others). Also may include renal dosing of any medication. Assessment for IV to PO conversions
Medication therapy management	Provide collaborative pharmaceutical care via an integrated practice model

TABLE 4-2 • Common Pharmacy-Specific Services (*continued*)

Type	Description
Nutrition support	Ordering and monitoring parenteral and enteral nutrition
Pain management	Ordering and monitoring acute pain management modalities, including IV, PO, and intraspinal infusions. May also refer to outpatient pain management services focusing on malignancy and nonmalignant chronic pain
Solid organ transplant	Medication education and clinical pharmacokinetic monitoring; assisting patients with medication adherence and managing adverse effects
Toxicology	Advising providers on clinical management of drug overdose and toxicologic emergencies
Other Services	
High fall risk medication review	Reviewing medication therapy for any patient deemed to be at high fall risk
Medication reconciliation/ discharge	Leading or participating in formal process of collecting and maintaining a complete/accurate list of a patient's current medications and comparing that list to the physician's orders at admission, transfer, or discharge
Pharmacist vaccination program	Reviewing patients for indications and contraindications for influenza and pneumococcal vaccinations (the pharmacist may order these vaccines for appropriate patients)

Pharmacy Operations

Understanding and improving the medication use system for pharmacy organizations is an important role for pharmacists, especially with today's emphasis on medication safety and the need to optimize patient outcomes through rational use of drug products (i.e., evidence-based practice). Pharmacy operations encompass the coordination of pharmacy personnel and services to support the healthcare system or pharmacy and include developing and maintaining drug formularies, establishing protocols for medication use, dispensing and facilitating access to drug products and managing drug shortages, and medication reconciliation and record-keeping. Pharmacist credentialing (e.g., academic degrees, licensure and relicensure, and advanced certificates and training), pharmacy licensing, and health system accreditation standards (e.g., The Joint Commission) are also important areas the pharmacy resident must understand. Management rotations can be structured as a dedicated "block" or as ongoing, longitudinal experiences. Specialty or combined PGY-2 residencies in pharmacy leadership and administration (see Chapter 22) and advanced degrees like the MBA or masters programs (see Chapter 25) are also available.

Clinical informatics is an emerging area of pharmacy operations and refers to the integration of information technology/computer science with healthcare practice. PGY-1 residents develop competence as they interface with electronic health records, automation, and clinical support tools in every day patient care duties; it is also a recognized area of specialty practice (see Chapter 22). Becoming familiar with operational strategies for advancing and managing pharmacy informatics during administrative rotation(s) can enhance clinical skills and can be an area for residents to develop innovative research and project management experience. As a resident, you may have the option to choose rotations to enhance your exposure to informatics standards and near-horizon technologies. Management of information through communication and collaboration will be the clinical skills of highest value in our professional future, and will aid the transition of pharmacy from a dispensing to a service-oriented profession.

Dispensing

Distribution and dispensing services are important components of the medication use process, and the activity most traditionally associated with pharmacy as a profession. Today's pharmacists and pharmacists in training must not only be accurate and experienced in dispensing functions but also understand distribution technology and automation, the role of pharmacy technicians in preparing and delivering drug products, and quality improvement initiatives in promoting rational medication use and medication safety. No doubt, you will participate in dispensing roles through your clinical rotations, and serve as cross coverage or backup for other pharmacists during the workday. After your clinical orientation, you will typically also have residency staffing expectations with distribution/dispensing duties for evenings, weekends, and holidays. Staffing requirements should be defined in the residency contract and would typically include a prespecified cycle (e.g., cover every third or fourth weekend) and a number of major and minor holidays (e.g., cover two of three winter holidays: Thanksgiving, Christmas, or New Year's; and two of three summer holidays: Memorial Day, July 4th, or Labor Day). In the past, residents sometimes had the opportunity to "moonlight" by providing overtime or staff coverage to supplement their residency salary; however, consideration of resident duty hours may often preclude this in today's residency programs. As a residency candidate, you should evaluate how much and what type of dispensing experience is available in each of the programs you are considering, as well as staffing expectations and opportunities. This will help ensure a good fit with your selected program, taking into account your prior experience and individual goals.

On-Call Responsibilities

On-call programs may be used to extend coverage of the pharmacy department or clinic beyond regular operating hours, provide extra support for specialized services, and mobilize a rapid and dedicated response for medical emergencies (e.g., code blue response). In your residency, you should expect to train in and participate in one or more on-call programs, first with supervision and then with increasing independence. On-call cases should be reviewed and discussed just as your other clinical learning opportunities. As a residency candidate, ask for specifics for each residency program you are considering. Special training may be required (e.g., Basic and Advanced Cardiac Life Support certification); costs you are responsible for as well as accommodations for off-site training should be discussed. Multisite residency programs may have different expectations for residents at different training sites, depending on their variety of services. Time on call may also vary depending on the number of residents or staffing changes from year to year.

POPULATION-BASED CARE

In addition to the care of individual patients, pharmacy residency programs also require and provide training in various aspects of population-based clinical management. This includes quality improvement efforts in the medication use process, adverse events reporting and clinical rules development, and drug information resources and services.

Medication Use Evaluations

Sometimes called MUEs, these are tools employed to promote the systematic improvement in medication-related performance in a health system or pharmacy. MUEs can be narrowly focused, concentrating on a specific drug and/or disease state, or broadly designed to encompass a therapeutic class or indication. Different institutions will likely have their own process for determining when an MUE may be needed, as well as some criteria to guide the process, but some information is also available in the literature.[5] In addition to learning about the quality improvement process, you may want to consider an MUE as the foundation for your major residency project (you will hear more about the residency project later in this chapter). MUEs can be easily accomplished in the limited time frame of a residency year because they typically rely on data that is already available in medical or pharmacy records, and can address a very specific clinical question or problem. Depending on the uniqueness of the question and the strength of the study design and available data, they are also potentially publishable.

Drug Information

Despite the multitude of online, accessible databases for medication and disease information, drug information services remain a mainstay of clinical pharmacy practice in all patient settings. New drug approvals, publication of updated therapeutic guidelines and landmark clinical trials, and conflicting information on safety and usefulness of medication strategies require a critical and practiced approach to interpret and prioritize medication information and to guide clinical decision making. Communicating this information effectively to the ultimate user (e.g., providers and patients) is as important as answering the question itself. Practice in formulating drug information responses is often emphasized in IPPE and APPE rotations; as a resident, you will find that unprompted use of drug information resources including primary literature sources to inform patient care activities is an expectation your preceptors will have of you. Proactively collecting, synthesizing, and communicating results on significant clinical issues enhances your practice relationships and the perceived value of pharmacists as members of the healthcare team. When addressing formulary issues or developing a therapeutic protocol, drug information services can contribute to population-based medication management.

Adverse Drug Event Reporting and Management

Medication safety is rightfully considered the purview of pharmacy professionals. National programs such as the Institute for Safe Medication Practices and MedWatch, the FDA Safety Information and Adverse Events Reporting Program, highlight the dramatic effort that is needed to safeguard patients from unintended and preventable adverse medication effects. Residents can expect that pharmacists at their institutions are key members of medication safety committees, help develop protocols and clinical pathways as strategies to preempt medication problems, and constantly monitor for and report medication errors. Health systems often have dedicated medication safety pharmacists to coordinate the pharmacy components of medication safety and regulatory compliance; you should seek out exposure and interaction with these individuals during your training. Participating in adverse event reporting via institution-specific protocols, familiarity with the voluntary MedWatch system (details at www.fda.gov), and training to reduce human errors are all important aspects of this practice area. Drug counterfeiting and dealing with drug shortages and alternative (perhaps unfamiliar) therapies are other well-publicized issues related to medication safety. Depending on the program, you may get this exposure during a drug information or administrative rotation, or it may be more longitudinal in nature.

EDUCATION

You are already aware that pharmacy knowledge changes rapidly and that there is always more to learn. To put it bluntly, the half-life of medical information is short and what you know with certainty today could be out of date or inadequate tomorrow. Ongoing professional development is a need of all pharmacists, and you will start in your residency. Think it through: guidelines will (hopefully) be revised, eagerly awaited clinical trials may be published (and others stopped early due to unexpected results), and you will discover that not all clinical questions have an evidence-based answer. Each day will provide a new opportunity to learn something about pharmacy practice that you did not even imagine you needed to know. Residency year is a time to advance your learning skills and begin lifelong habits as your future education will be nearly all self-directed. This means you must know the resources available to you and practice making the most of them.

Your development as a practitioner can take many forms, and should include some individual strategies as well as participation in more formal training programs. Active learning through projects and teamwork is also a great way to become proficient at something new. The next section describes opportunities that you should definitely look to take advantage of.

Staff Development and In-Services

Training via workshops or continuing education is probably your most familiar way to learn, as it mimics the didactic environment of a classroom or case conference. The objectives and learning outcomes are usually predefined, and they are often delivered by national or local experts in the topic area. Webinars are increasingly available and a popular choice, since they minimize travel away from your site. Continuing education credit toward pharmacy license renewal may be provided (a bonus) and can be an incentive to encourage regular attendance. Yes—as a resident you may need to worry about continuing education, depending on in which state you are licensed. In larger health systems, pharmacy departments may offer an ongoing clinical series; these can be directed toward the resident audience in particular (resident education session) or be open to all pharmacy practitioners (generalist/specialist education series). Pharmacy or medical grand rounds are excellent forums to learn about cutting-edge practice issues. For residencies based in stand-alone clinics or pharmacies, it is usually necessary to collaborate with other disciplines or partner with other residencies or a college/school of pharmacy to deliver a substantial ongoing program. Keeping the schedule with dates/times and topics in your residency calendar is a good way to keep programs on your radar and protect development time. Some residency programs require that you deliver a continuing education or formal topic lecture at least once during the year, to develop the necessary teaching skills and fine tune presentation abilities. Though it can seem a little daunting up front, these are excellent ways to learn about new topics and practice active learning techniques. A preceptor mentor is often assigned to help you get started and provide feedback after the presentation. If one is not assigned, you may want to ask a preceptor or other colleague to give you this feedback.

Journal Club

Evaluation and application of the medical literature is an important skill in patient and population-based care, and a cornerstone of evidence-based practice. As a student, you were introduced to clinical literature evaluation and had some practice in IPPE/APPE rotations. Of course, the best way to get *really* good at it is to continue to practice—a lot. It also helps if you can observe others who are doing it. Thus, the residency journal club is a prototypic professional development activity. Organized journal clubs can focus on clinical/applied science or many other aspects of residency training (e.g., education, practice management, and impact of pharmacist services). Again, residents usually get the chance to both participate in and lead discussions through the year. As the administrative requirements are minimal—you only need a scheduled day and time plus space to meet—residents could consider organizing an informal journal club if your residency does not offer one.

An early and related challenge you will face as a resident will be to develop a systematic approach to stay abreast of the incoming tide of current research and key articles published in your fields of interest. Journal watch services are excellent resources, consisting of regular and concise summaries of recently published clinical articles in a particular field. They are often accompanied by insightful commentary summarizing key points and clinical perspective, and allow for a relatively quick review of multiple publications (compared to a journal club that provides extensive and detailed review for one study at a time). Journal watch summaries are delivered directly to your mailbox or email inbox; they can be provided through your institution or by an individual subscription. A complementary strategy is to meet with fellow residents or other colleagues regularly (e.g., every week or two) and quickly walk through a table of contents from a recent issue of a high impact journal in your field. You can skim through an article or two, and pick out any that merit more extensive review. This provides a broad overview of current research, and can assist in identifying articles for journal club activities.

Professional organizations and special forum email list services (list-servs) can also alert you to clinical controversies and broader perspectives on recent publications, and to augment and inform your practice. List-servs are a good way to network with a larger number of colleagues, and can be useful (as one example) in learning about clinical problems that are not well described in the literature.

Precepting and Classroom Teaching

Residency programs at all levels include goals and objectives related to clinical teaching and precepting; specific recommendations for teaching development in residency programs have been further described in primary literature.[6] Many (but not all) programs provide direct instruction and opportunities to practice foundational skills in classroom teaching. This is probably most common in programs sponsored by or affiliated with colleges/schools of pharmacy. Enrollment in teaching certificate programs and formal preceptor development offerings have increased in recent years. These are sometimes considered "extra" programs a resident could choose to participate in, while for others they are required experiences. Availability and program expectations may be one criterion you use as a residency candidate use to distinguish between your preferred residency programs. In some institutions, teaching responsibilities or teaching assignments can contribute toward the staffing requirement, or be an option to develop your individual interests. An elective rotation with a faculty member in a pharmacy school is a good way to learn about the range of academic responsibilities. Teaching development programs and academia rotations should include the opportunity to create a formal teaching portfolio (often helpful in your job searches). Residents who are interested in pursuing academic positions or clinical practice in a teaching institution should strongly consider selecting a residency with a teaching component.

SERVICE RESPONSIBILITIES

Committee Service

Health systems, academic institutions, and professional and business organizations rely on committees or teams of individuals to maintain and advance key functions. Committees are created to focus on both ongoing duties (standing committees) and special projects (*ad hoc* committees). The service provided may be discipline-specific (e.g., a pharmacy practice model committee) or multidisciplinary in nature (e.g., Institutional Review Board [IRB]). The size of the committee depends on its overall purpose, responsibilities, and workload, but could range from 5 to 20 or more individuals. Many programs include committee service as an ongoing or limited function of residents, as it will enhance your group working skills, and expand your understanding of pharmacy and health system operations. Advantages of committee involvement include promoting team and leadership abilities, improving persuasive communication skills and conflict resolution. You will also gain experience with parliamentary procedure and how to effectively conduct meetings. Committee assignments can be individualized to participants' interests and provide unique opportunities outside the day-to-day work responsibilities.

As a resident, you will likely participate in the Pharmacy and Therapeutics (P&T) Committee, which oversees policies and decisions on all matters related to medication use in the health organization. This is the formal connection between the pharmacy department and medical personnel. Committees related to P&T (or designated subcommittees of P&T) may include those related to drug formulary, medication safety, and antibiotic stewardship. Quality improvement committees in specific areas of medical practice (e.g., critical care and pediatrics), strategic planning, or accreditation committees, and human resources committees may also be good resident experiences. It is usually preferable to have an ongoing participation in at least one committee or working group through the year. Attending a wider variety of committee meetings as a one-time guest or by accompanying rotation preceptors is another option.

Organization Involvement

Residency programs seek candidates who have actively participated in and demonstrated leadership in student pharmacy organizations. Showing involvement in organizations that align with the mission of residency programs you are applying to is an indicator of your commitment. For example, if you are interested in hospital pharmacy, involvement in American Society of Health-System Pharmacists (ASHP) would be a good fit. If you are interested in a community residency in an independent pharmacy, then NCPA would be a good fit. All residents should also expect to participate as members of professional organizations during their residency year. Membership in organizations like ASHP, ACCP, APhA, and AACP is a good way to begin learning about professional advocacy and enhancing your personal growth. Educational programming and resources are usually available in a variety of formats. As a trainee, membership fees are very affordable. Attending annual or midyear meetings is critical to broaden your professional perspective and stay connected within the relatively small world of pharmacy. As a resident, you should plan on attending one or more meetings in addition to the regional ASHP residency conferences. Residency showcases at meetings are one strategy to recruit future candidates to your program, and may be a required service of residents to your program. Travel expenses may be funded as part of your residency program; be sure to ask about expectations and support for travel to national meetings at the interview.

As a resident, you should also consider other ways to participate in professional organizations at either a regional or national level. Membership in special interest groups, contributing to a project or publication, and even holding resident leadership positions can be a good way to learn more about the group's structure and purpose. It can accelerate leadership development, increase networking opportunities, and enhance your professional visibility. Opportunities exist that are geared specifically to residents and other postgraduate trainees. For example, a standing committee of ACCP is the National Resident Advisory Committee, whose purpose is to inform the development of new services and programs for postgraduate members of ACCP. The committee is appointed by the organization's leadership, following a call for applications in spring each year. ASHP offers the Live Resident Visit Program each autumn, a 1-day visit to ASHP headquarters in Bethesda, Maryland.[7] Residents learn more about ASHP's history and program, as well as ways to gain from membership including opportunities for active involvement in the New Practitioners' Forum. More information about the New Practitioners Forum is available on the ASHP Web site.

One word of caution—it may seem advantageous to load up your residency schedule with education and service opportunities, or to pursue leadership positions in high-visibility arenas. They certainly *can* be very rewarding, but you must be sure they also support (rather than distract from) your commitment to the residency program you have selected. Being highly visible within a national organization will not be a substitute for earning the residency certificate, and having the support of your program director and preceptors. Be sure to discuss your interests in organizational service (and even plan your involvement) with your residency program director (RPD) in the first months of residency, *at the latest*. It is even better to begin this discussion during interviews to find a program that best fits your needs.

RESEARCH/PROJECT MANAGEMENT

Project management skills are an expected outcome for PGY-1 pharmacy residents, and additional research skills are required for PGY-2 trainees. Though residents typically have a variety of small and larger projects during the training year, they usually focus on one major project to fulfill program requirements related to clinical inquiry and presentation skills.

Major Project

One of the major challenges for residents is to complete the major project within the limited time frame of the residency year, especially if the project requires IRB approval that ensures the protection and appropriate inclusion of study participants. While this is a necessary step in conducting research projects, it can also be time consuming. The type of IRB approval needed is also relevant as some types of projects will be exempt from board review (but still require an application outlining the research purpose and methods), while others can be reviewed in an expedited (i.e., accelerated) process. Projects that include patient interventions or more than minimal risks (either actual or potential risks) to the study participants will require a full IRB application. This includes full board review and discussion, which can delay the start of a residency project by many weeks or months. Many (and probably most) institutions and health systems currently require IRB training for those leading and/or contributing to research studies.

Some residencies will allow or require you to participate in a formal research education series with established time lines, others will rely on individual mentorship from the RPD or certain preceptors to support the major project. Some programs offer a dedicated month for the major project, but important pearls for all residents are to (1) begin early—planning should begin in the first month of residency and (2) be focused—stay realistic in your choice of project and ask for input from others. Prospective studies with multiple phases or follow-ups may seem appealing but are nearly impossible to plan and implement in time to meet important milestones. Retrospective data sources, surveys, and smaller pilot projects are usually much more feasible.

> "Instead of listing 'project' on my to-do-list, I found it helpful to break it down into smaller sections so that I had specific and achievable tasks to complete."
>
> *Liz E. – Pharmacy Resident, Wisconsin*

Areas of competency necessary for a successful clinical researcher are literature evaluation, scientific thinking and creativity, developing research behaviors, communication skills, technical proficiency, and research ethics and integrity.[8] In choosing your residency, look for different activities that may help you acquire these skills, some of which are listed in Table 4-3. Having a project mentor or mentors with research experience and access to a biostatistician for data analysis are important and can mean the difference between an optimal and an unsatisfactory outcome. For any program, it is a good idea to ask about project process and support during your residency interview. You may also want more information on how projects are selected, the amount and type of input you can expect from the RPD and preceptors, and how your own preferences weigh in project selection.

TABLE 4-3 • Developing Research Skills in a Pharmacy Residency

Skill	Activities
Literature tracking and evaluation	• Attending a review of clinical literature evaluation skills • Performing a literature search for background of major project • Completing small writing projects: e.g., mini-review, case report • Leading and participating in journal club/journal watch activities • Preparing seminar or lecture on topic of interest; researching drug information questions at pharmacy site
Critical scientific thinking and creativity	• Leading and participating in journal club activities • Reviewing and discussing previous residents' research/major projects (with preceptors and other residents) • Reviewing abstracts and manuscripts (with preceptors) • Preparing and presenting research project to peer group (with preceptors and other residents)
Behavioral development	• Attending research training sessions • Writing and participating in development of research protocols (at pharmacy site) • Writing and submitting IRB applications • Participating in site-specific or multisite research projects: e.g., demonstration projects
Communication skills	• Communicating with peers and coordinating activities as administrative resident • Preparing and presenting research project to peer group (with preceptors and other residents) • Teaching assignments: lecture, laboratory, and case discussions • Practice sessions for presentations (with preceptors and peer group) • Participating in poster and podium sessions to disseminate your own research findings
Technical proficiency	• Attending a primer/review on research methods and statistics • Attending seminars on research tools: e.g., databases and codebooks, statistical software • Consulting with research faculty in research development or outcomes analysis for existing projects (with preceptors) • Preparing and implementing an original, independent research project (with preceptors)
Research ethics and integrity	• Attending training on IRB history and requirements • Writing and submitting IRB application for major project • Protecting patient information for daily practice and research project (HIPAA)

Adapted from Pruchnicki MC, Rodis JL, Beatty SJ, et al. Practice-based research network as a research training model for community/ambulatory pharmacy residents. J Am Pharm Assoc. 2008;48:191–202.

Regional Resident Conference

ASHP sponsors regional pharmacy residency conferences in the spring of each year to provide each resident with an appropriate forum to present their project results. Some residency programs (e.g., Managed Care or PGY-2) may have residents present their work in alternative venues, such as regional or national meetings of their particular area of focus. Residency sites will assist their residents in preparing for the podium or poster presentation sessions, usually beginning in the winter months. Thus, you will need to have data collection completed or almost completed around February. A final written report of the completed project in manuscript style is needed to earn the residency certificate, and some programs also expect that it should be submitted for publication in an appropriate journal.

Although important for all residents, those whose career aspirations include specialty areas of pharmacy practice and education, full- or part-time academic appointments, or precepting pharmacy residents should consider the residency project as a critical factor in their PGY-1 and PGY-2 training.

RELATIONSHIPS WITH RESIDENCY PROGRAM PERSONNEL

To this point, we have described all the things that you will *do* as a resident. It is equally important to consider the interactions and relationships that will get you through to the end of your training. The program personnel who will guide you through your residency experience include the RPD, preceptors and mentors, and your fellow residents. Along with your personal support network, they will be the most important source of information, encouragement, guidance, and friendship to assist you.

Residency Program Director

The RPD is the individual who is ultimately responsible for your residency experience. Typically, she will coordinate the residency orientation, set and monitor your residency schedule, develop your individualized plan, and provide mentorship and administrative support to the preceptors responsible for your training. She ensures the quality and time lines of your evaluations and often provides career counseling and professional advice. You should know she is usually your first point of contact when personal commitments or crises intersect with professional responsibilities. For program oversight, she will also be responsible for residency accreditation, fiscal matters, and annual recruitment.

Preceptors

Preceptors are the guides and instructors who deliver the individual learning experiences that comprise your program. They develop the learning experience and facilitate your progress through the rotation. They determine the activities that will allow each resident to meet the assigned goals and objectives and serve as a role model and coach. They provide direct instruction and supervise your day-to-day activities/patient interactions. They coordinate your formative self-evaluation and provide informal and formal evaluations. Your preceptors will complete the program's summative evaluations and review your progress with the RPD. In addition to patient care rotations, you may have an assigned primary preceptor for the residency project (or teaching) who will serve as your main contact or coordinator for the year.

Fellow Residents

The size and composition of your residency class can be an important consideration, especially if you are looking at larger programs with multiple residents or multiple sites. In addition to providing moral support and friendship through the year, these folks will be a professional resource (fortunately) and maybe an occasional source of frustration (unfortunately). Your scheduled orientation and informal social opportunities are an excellent start to establish a group dynamic and identify individual goals and strengths. Planning for travel, residency meetings and presentations, and service activities may be accomplished most efficiently when coordinated as the larger group. Responsibilities can be rotated by month (e.g., administrative resident) or as specific assigned duties (e.g., communications liaison). Some programs may have a "chief resident" who oversees specific administrative responsibilities of the residency class. This can be a formal designation (sometimes with an added stipend) or informal position.

Working in Teams

This chapter would not be complete without a few words on teamwork and establishing effective relationships as a pharmacy resident. There is simply no way to have a good residency experience if you neglect this aspect of your training. You will be busier than you can even imagine, and will rely more on your personal and professional teams than you realize. So take some time up front to plan, and consider what system will help you with time management (hint: you *must* have a calendar) and communication (e.g., a smart phone or pager is a good idea).

> "If you don't keep a calendar now, start keeping one once you start residency. My calendar has been my lifeline when it comes to keeping track of meetings, due dates, project deadlines, and presentations. It is a must-have for a resident."
>
> *Tiffany S. – Pharmacy Resident, Ohio*

If you will spend time traveling to clinical or teaching sites, be sure to take that into account in planning your day and consider if you will have access to clinic records via the Internet and/or electronic access to needed resources when off-site. Have a frank discussion with family, friends, and significant others regarding your work schedule and time you will need outside of the business day for work or projects. What you will protect as personal time is also critical. You may need to practice some negotiation skills here!

Managing yourself is hard work. Working with and managing multiple teams for a variety of purposes can be *really* hard. For many residents, a major struggle is first to understand the *timing* needed to meet milestones and deadlines, and then to take appropriate action to address (or ideally prevent) missteps along the way. As a resident, everything you do will be reviewed and scrutinized since activity without feedback and reflection may not really advance your learning. Some time lines will be flexible but many deadlines will be outside of your control and not open to the influence of your personal preferences or circumstances. In other words, ASHP will not adjust its poster presentation abstract submission deadlines to accommodate the long-planned timing of your wedding (as just one example). If you want to make "last-minute" adjustments to a grant proposal, classroom lecture, or podium presentation, you will need to do this at least two, three, or five days in advance of the actual due date since there may be two, three or seven people on your team who need to approve the new version or change. This clearly puts a whole new priority on planning, clear communication, and accountability to others. If you experience a failure along the way (which is likely), it is important to acknowledge the error in an open and timely manner, apologize to those affected, and work to prevent it from happening again.

Finally, a word about feedback. In interviews, we hear from nearly every residency candidate how much they value feedback and yet it is often a source of frustration or despair during residency when it is overwhelming in quantity, emanates from too many sources, or is too vague to inform corrective action. Having a too-busy or distracted preceptor, multiple preceptors who don't communicate well, or too many ongoing projects can be obvious problems. Sometimes the difficulty comes from trying to decide what feedback must be acted on and when you have the final word. Poor self-evaluation skills can also leave the resident unsure of their next step. Being honest and direct with preceptors and having an attitude for self-improvement are helpful strategies to keep in mind. A few more practical feedback tips are (1) engage in it frequently—incorporate formative discussions into daily interactions with your preceptor and (2) keep it focused—identify one example of strength and one area to improve for the objective being evaluated. And remember— you are working to become an independent practitioner. Sometimes the most appropriate feedback of all is the question "what do you want to do?"

DAILY ACTIVITIES

At this point in your reading, you should have a pretty good idea of what you are getting into in terms of the variety and scope of your residency activities. What is possibly (probably) still muddy is *how* you can get it all done. Though there are standards for program outcomes, there is (fortunately) more than one right way to deliver a residency program. This offers you flexibility in program structure and plenty of ways to individualize your training. Program elements that you should investigate include the residency orientation (including length and type of training), rotation structure (whether block

Acute Care Residency

	Mon	Tue	Wed	Thu	Fri	Sat/Sun
AM	Patient care activities	Patient care activities	Patient care activities	Patient care activities	Patient care activities	
PM	P& T meetings/ practice management	Teaching	Project time	Ambulatory clinic	Resident education	Staff (every third weekend)

Community/Ambulatory Care Residency

	Mon	Tue	Wed	Thu	Fri	Sat
AM	Patient care/clinic	Teaching or longitudinal elective	Patient care activities	Teaching/ teaching assistant meetings	Patient care activities	Staff (every second Saturday or every third weekend)
PM	Patient care/clinic	Project time	Patient care activities	Committee meetings/ practice management	Resident education	

Figure 4-1: Sample of Resident Schedule by Week

rotations versus longitudinal), and timing and number of learning experiences (what are the required versus elective opportunities). Find out the preferred or required date by which you must have completed the requirements for your state pharmacy license (you can ask about this during the interview). Residencies may have resources to facilitate the application process and tips on when/how to schedule any needed examinations. Summative evaluations in an ASHP accredited program consist of a preceptor evaluation of the resident, resident self-evaluation, and resident evaluations of the preceptor and learning experience. They are typically scheduled at the end of block rotations and at least quarterly for longitudinal experiences. Some examples of rotation schedules are found in Figure 4-1, while Figure 4-2 shows an actual "day in the life" of a 2011–2012 pharmacy resident at our institution.

Residency candidates should consider the options and which program structure is optimal for them. Blocks with a different learning experience scheduled for each calendar month allow you to focus on one area of learning at a time; however, some activities like teaching or project management are best delivered over an extended period. Longitudinal structures may require the resident to focus on time management skills and being able to prioritize daily activities. Since the timing of clinical duties, meetings, and educational opportunities can often overlap, you will need to be able to discern which are most important at a given time and how to make the right choices (in consultation with your preceptors and RPD). One resident testimonial from an ASHP blog describes it this way:

This starts to create a bit of a balancing act—'how much of A will I miss if I do B' and 'what will I have to give up to attend C?' You start to have to be in multiple places at once and eventually it starts to feel as though

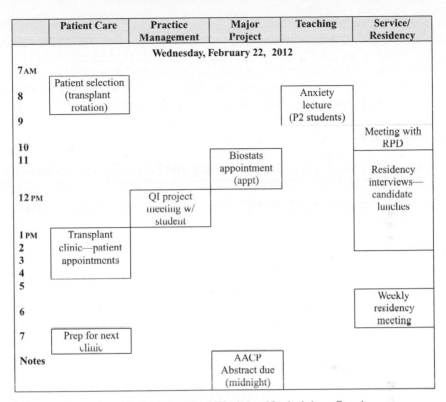

	Patient Care	Practice Management	Major Project	Teaching	Service/ Residency
			Wednesday, February 22, 2012		
7 AM					
8	Patient selection (transplant rotation)			Anxiety lecture (P2 students)	
9					
10					Meeting with RPD
11			Biostats appointment (appt)		Residency interviews— candidate lunches
12 PM		QI project meeting w/ student			
1 PM	Transplant clinic—patient appointments				
2					
3					
4					
5					
6					Weekly residency meeting
7	Prep for next clinic				
Notes			AACP Abstract due (midnight)		

Figure 4-2: **Example of Actual Resident Workday (Ambulatory Care)**

you are not very successful at being at any of those places. I have learned to 'hypertask' as a resident—this term refers to a higher form of evolved multi-tasking which supposedly makes one the epitome of efficiency. However, I am starting to suspect that 'hypertasking' is really code for doing a bunch of things at once and not doing any of them terribly well.[9]

Clearly, this description is far from our ideal (and should make you more than a little nervous as you read it, suggesting it is not possible to do your work as a resident properly), but it does highlight the judgment that a resident must use in prioritizing and completing their extensive task list. Up until now you may have put forth 100% effort toward each student project and assignment, all deemed important to your success. And no doubt this strategy has worked well: you have likely developed good time management skills and have been effective in your efforts (otherwise you would not be in the position to choose and commit to a residency). But it might be better to consider the products of your residency and future professional work from a slightly different perspective. Competence rather than perfection is often the desired and realistic standard, and more productive. With our residents, we have this discussion early in the year. A helpful analogy is deciding between "boxes and bows." When you are "packaging" your work in residency, consider what can simply be placed in a box for delivery or for later use, and which efforts truly need the fancier "wrapping and bows." Extra time and detailed effort are helpful to highlight unique work and special projects, but time lines and efficiency may be more meaningful in completing routine duties. Practicing this critical assessment can be the key to honing your time management skills, and actually help you minimize the type of "hypertasking" described in the blog. Learning to set and address priorities appropriately is part of your transition from effective student to responsible resident practitioner.

SUMMARY

Residency training is a demanding but rewarding experience. Understanding the key duties and responsibilities of a resident's schedule can help prepare you for a strong start and successful year.

Chapter Takeaways

▶ Residents should expect their training to include patient care activities, practice management experiences, research, and teaching components.

▶ Continuous professional development is critical in forming lifelong learning habits and keeping residents' knowledge base and skills up to date.

▶ Institutional and organizational service experiences can enhance your residency year experience—be sure to plan for them.

▶ Managing multiple priorities and longitudinal projects can be very challenging. Get started early, develop realistic time lines, and break things down into smaller steps.

▶ Invest in developing successful relationships with your residency year "team" and enhance your professional network.

ROLE FOR THE MENTOR

Help incoming residents understand their program's schedule and expectations; this is best done early in the year.

Guide residents in considering and weighing opportunities, so their individualized residency plan reflects their interests, builds on areas of strength, and maximizes the learning opportunities.

Guide residents in developing a systematic process to maintain a contemporary knowledge base and expand depth and breadth of understanding as a lifelong learner.

Provide guidance and ongoing support as residents build skills in self-directed professional development, project management, and team behaviors.

Encourage the resident to relax and enjoy their year—it will go by quickly!

References

1. Accreditation Standards for PGY-1 Pharmacy Residencies. American Society of Health-System Pharmacists. http://www.ashp.org/menu/Accreditation/ResidencyAccreditation.aspx. Approved September 23, 2005; glossary revised September 23, 2010. Accessed February 10, 2012.

2. Accreditation Standards for PGY-2 Pharmacy Residencies. American Society of Health-System Pharmacists. http://www.ashp.org/menu/Accreditation/ResidencyAccreditation.aspx. Approved September 23, 2005; glossary revised September 23, 2010. Accessed February 10, 2012.

3. Linfors EW, Neelon FA. The case for bedside rounds. N Engl J Med. 1980;303:1230–1233.

4. NCQA Patient Centered Medical Home. National Committee for Quality Assurance. http://www.ncqa.org/tabid/631/default.aspx. Accessed February 21, 2012.

5. American Society of Health-System Pharmacists. ASHP guidelines on medication-use evaluation. Am J Health-Syst Pharm. 1996;53:1953–1955.

6. Lee M, et al. Final report and recommendations of the 2002 AACP Task Force on the Role of Colleges and Schools in Residency Training. Am J Pharm Educ. 2004:68(1), Article S2. doi: 10.5688/aj6801S2.

7. ASHP Live Resident Visit Program. American Society of Health-System Pharmacists. http://www.ashp.org/menu/MemberCenter/SectionsForums/NPF/Programs/ResidentVisit.aspx. Accessed February 24, 2012.

8. DiPiro JT, American College of Clinical Pharmacy, American Society of Health-System Pharmacists. Encyclopedia of Clinical Pharmacy. New York: M. Dekker; 2003.

9. Van Devender E. A day in the life of a pharmacy resident. ASHP Connect. American Society of Health-System Pharmacists. http://connect.ashp.org/blogs/viewblogs/?BlogKey=4209d135-64bf-4e9d-abe3-c8b5087dc48a. Published October 21, 2011. Accessed January 27, 2012.

II

How to Program Your GPS

- *April Miller Quidley and P. Brandon Bookstaver*

INTRODUCTION

So, now you're sold. You've learned what residency training is, and now you just *have* to get there! Selecting a program, putting together an application, interviewing, and the match all seem like wandering through the jungle with no water, no food, and no map. That's where this section comes in. Use it as a map to your residency training destination. Here you'll find the details on exactly *how* you use your awesome expertise, skills, and abilities to get matched up with the residency program you want.

You'll start with figuring out what really makes the "best" residency program for you, then figure out what you should do to be the best residency candidate you can be. From there, get advice on the nuts and bolts of it all, from applying, interviewing, and matching. There's also lots of extra material along the way. Be sure to see the checklists to help you assess programs (Table 5-2) and yourself (Table 6-1), sample curriculum vitae (CV) (Figures 7-1 through 7-3), illustrations on how to (and not to) dress at professional meetings (Figures 8-2 and 8-3), and sample letters of intent (Figures 9-1 through 9-3). Things wrap up with some advice on interviewing, mastering the match, and working with mentors. There's also a guide to getting settled in at your destination—the residency program that fits you perfectly.

Selecting the Ideal Residency Program 5

Beth Bryles Phillips

There are over 950 Postgraduate Year One (PGY-1) residency programs in the United States.[1] With so many residencies to choose from, it can be exciting, yet overwhelming, to determine which is best for you. Each program carries a unique set of characteristics, including but not limited to structure, preceptors, patient population, and practice model. Variations in these characteristics allow you, the prospective resident, to select programs that fit with your professional and personal goals. The purpose of this chapter is to describe various residency program characteristics to aid in your search for the ideal residency program and determine the best "fit" for you.

SELF-ASSESSMENT

> "Don't base your opinions on what others say about a certain program. Do your own research and seek out interactions with residents and preceptors to get your own sense of the program. Trust your gut, good or bad!"
>
> *Kathryn E. – Pharmacy Student, Arizona*

To select the ideal residency program, you will need to identify residency program characteristics best suited for your interests and career goals. The first step is completing a self-assessment to determine what you want and what appeals to your interests. Why do you want to pursue residency training? Being able to clearly articulate your reasons for completing residency training will not only help you now but will also help you later on in the interview process. What are your career goals? In answering this question, start with the end in mind and think about your future career goals. Begin by asking yourself these questions:

- What type of position do I ultimately want?
- Where do I see myself in 5 years, 10 years, and beyond?
- Am I primarily interested in patient care and clinical practice?

- Do I want to engage in teaching? If so, what kind of teaching? Do I want experience with small group/one-on-one teaching, large group/didactic teaching, or a combination of both? Do I prefer teaching pharmacy students, primarily other healthcare professionals, or a combination?
- Would I thrive in an environment where research and scholarship are expected?
- Is direct patient care my passion? Or do I prefer improving medication use and outcomes through population-based interventions?
- Do I want face-to-face interaction with my patients or is the critical care environment with less direct patient interaction more exciting?

To further define your clinical interests and attributes, think about what have been your favorite aspects and professional challenges in pharmacy so far. Think about your courses in school, IPPE and APPE, organizations, and work experiences. What aspects of the profession have you found most and least rewarding? For this part of the self-assessment, it is important to conduct a realistic self-evaluation of your strengths, limitations, and past accomplishments.

Your career goals and interests will help you decide what type of PGY-1 residency to pursue or you may also choose from a number of combined PGY-1 and Postgraduate Year Two (PGY-2) programs. Once you have determined this, it is really about considering program characteristics and finding programs that match your personality interests. You should consider program size and whether you like working with large or small groups of people. Also, in what aspects or specialties within pharmacy would you like to gain more experience? The types of patients an institution has can be important. If you have a wide variety of interests, consider programs that provide a wide range of medical and pharmacy services to a diverse patient population. If teaching and working with pharmacy students is important to you, consider looking for programs that offer these opportunities. Reflect on your learning style. Do you thrive in a high-pressure environment or would you prefer a more laid back atmosphere? Hopefully this list will get you started thinking about program characteristics.

INSTITUTION CHARACTERISTICS

Institution Type

Traditionally, PGY-1 pharmacy residency programs (previously known as pharmacy practice, clinical, and general residencies) have been offered in hospitals. Changes in the American Society of Health-System Pharmacists (ASHP) 2007 PGY-1 pharmacy residency standards allowed greater flexibility in conducting programs at other sites.[2] Although the majority (approximately 95%) of PGY-1 pharmacy residency programs are still conducted in hospitals, more programs are being offered at nonhospital sites, such as ambulatory clinics or home infusion companies.[3] PGY-1 managed care residencies are conducted in health plans, pharmacy benefit management companies, and other managed care organizations. As the name implies, PGY-1 community pharmacy residencies are conducted in community pharmacies and are commonly cosponsored by colleges of pharmacy. Hospitals offering residency programs can be placed into basic categories, including academic medical centers, community teaching hospitals, community hospitals, managed care hospitals, and Veterans Affairs (VA) or other government medical centers. The third section of this book provides more information on different types of residency programs.

Academic medical centers generally have a three-part mission of patient care, education, and research, for the greater good of society. They are affiliated with medical schools and often colleges of pharmacy, as well as other healthcare professional schools and programs. These affiliations can lead to trainees from a variety of disciplines practicing and learning in the medical center at any given time. Patient care services are often provided by multidisciplinary teams and characterized by patient care rounds, in which a team of healthcare professionals and trainees (e.g., medical and pharmacy residents; medical, pharmacy, and nursing students; and social work) is led by an attending physician (senior physician who has completed all training) or fellow (physician completing additional training after residency). Patient care services are often highly specialized, providing for a number of diverse rotation opportunities for residents. Academic medical centers also generally have the largest number of available residency preceptors and a high preceptor to resident ratio. Because of the presence of these students and trainees, a focus is placed on education and teaching. It may seem that there are education and teaching opportunities everywhere you look, from teaching during medical rounds, in-service presentations during nursing meetings, one-on-one teaching with pharmacy students, grand rounds lectures, didactic lectures in a college of pharmacy, and conferences. Many academic medical centers engage in cutting-edge research. Most, if not all, of the attending physicians practicing in these institutions are faculty members within the affiliated college of medicine. As such, many of them are responsible for obtaining grant funding, conducting research, and publishing papers in the medical literature. These factors create opportunities for involvement in research and collaboration. A residency in an academic medical center may appeal to you if you are interested in specializing in a particular area of pharmacy practice, working in large multidisciplinary teams, working with students and trainees in pharmacy and other disciplines, and engaging in teaching or research.

The focus of community hospitals is to serve their surrounding communities. The primary mission emphasizes patient care, although education or research may also be included, especially in the case of community teaching hospitals. Community teaching hospitals share some similarities to academic medical centers with respect to patient care, teaching, and research activities, but these are typically conducted on a much smaller scale. Students and residents from medicine, pharmacy, and other disciplines may train in the hospital. Multidisciplinary rounds, when present, are usually limited to specific areas of the hospital (e.g., internal medicine floors). Teaching of other healthcare professionals and students may occur during rounds, grand rounds, and in-service presentations in this setting. For nonteaching hospitals, physicians typically do not hold formal rounds. Pharmacy residents may interact one-on-one with the physicians discussing drug therapy goals and making recommendations for optimal drug therapy. There are generally greater numbers of general internal medicine patients, and less specialized care, in community hospitals compared to academic medical centers. Additionally, there are often fewer numbers of preceptors and pharmacy residents and a lower preceptor to resident ratio.[4] Pharmacy practice in community hospitals is frequently more independent as opposed to working in a structured, formal multidisciplinary team. This independence may lead to greater responsibility for drug therapy management on the part of the clinical pharmacist. In the teaching and non-teaching community hospitals, community service programs such as diabetes education classes, brown bag medication reviews, and medication-related presentations to the lay public are common. A residency in a community hospital may appeal to you if you are interested in more one-on-one interaction with a smaller number of preceptors.

Hospitals that are part of a managed care organization share many aspects with community hospitals, but the focus is on serving its members rather than the community as a whole. The mission is also the provision of patient care, with specific interest in improving patient care outcomes, wellness, and health prevention. A strength of many managed care organizations is the integral role pharmacists play in safe and efficacious use of medications, including development of drug therapy protocols and organizational practice guidelines, drug utilization reviews, and disease management programs. Common teaching opportunities may include education of healthcare professionals, patient/member education classes, and some experiential teaching of pharmacy students. A PGY-1 in this type of hospital may appeal to you if you are interested in a broad-based experience within a managed care setting.

The primary mission of VA medical centers is to provide patient care to men and women veterans. Many also include education and research in their mission statement. The VA system as a whole is the largest single provider of pharmacy residency training. It is not uncommon for a VA medical center to be physically located in close proximity to academic medical centers or within the same hospital complex. These residency programs may share several similar patient care, teaching, and research opportunities with academic medical centers, but to a lesser extent. Medical rounds are often multidisciplinary and include multiple students and residents of various disciplines. Faculty attending physicians affiliated with a college of medicine also engage in obtaining grants, conducting research, and publishing in the medical literature. A strength of VA medical centers is the degree to which clinical pharmacists are involved in the medication use process. Medication administration with bar code technology and centralized prescription dispensing allow clinical pharmacists to focus more time on direct patient care activities. Credentialed clinical pharmacists have prescriptive authority to order medications and laboratory tests to manage and monitor drug therapy. Residents participate in these activities as well, under the direction of their preceptor. Clinical pharmacists are also responsible for designing and implementing drug-related policies and managing medication use, such as developing institutional guidelines for formulary agents, evaluating requests for nonformulary medications and management of drug shortages. It should be noted that automation and managing medication use are employed and conducted in other hospitals as well. The difference in VA hospitals is the extent and consistency with which these are used system wide and by all clinical pharmacists. The prescriptive authority within the VA allows clinical pharmacists to practice in a more independent manner compared to other settings. While the veteran population does represent both genders and all ages, middle aged and older male veterans make up a majority of patients receiving care within the VA system. A VA residency may appeal to you if you would like to gain experience managing drug therapy in a unique patient population.

Some PGY-1 pharmacy residency programs are conducted in nonhospital sites, such as an ambulatory clinic or a home healthcare agency (e.g., home infusion company). The sites offering these programs are diverse and generally do not adhere to a particular model. To meet the residency standards, programs must provide a variety of patient populations and disease states for resident learning. You may choose to complete a PGY-1 residency in an ambulatory or home infusion company if you have specific interests in one of these areas.

PGY-1 managed care pharmacy residencies are conducted in health plans, benefit management companies, or managed care organizations. Residencies in these sites may choose to follow the PGY-1 pharmacy (as described above) or the PGY-1 managed care pharmacy residency standards. The main difference between these programs is the focus on population-based care with activities such as formulary management, medication use management strategies; and pharmacy benefit design rather than the care of individual, specific patients in managed care residencies. Programs conducted in managed care hospitals most often follow the PGY-1 pharmacy residency standards due to their focus on direct patient care.

PGY-1 community pharmacy residencies are conducted in chain, grocery store, or independent pharmacies. The main differences between these types of sites are the level of corporate structure and entrepreneurial opportunities. Chain pharmacies and large grocery store chain pharmacies incorporate more managerial and corporate aspects to the learning experiences. Many independent pharmacies and local chains often have a less complex business model and structure. Additionally, as a resident, you may have the opportunity to frequently work side-by-side or directly with the owner of the pharmacy or company.

Institution Size

Hospital size is often measured by the number of beds, or the number of patients who could be admitted at any one time. One thing to keep in mind is that hospitals are typically licensed for a larger number of beds than they actually utilize at one time, and the average census is a more accurate reflection of hospital size. For example, a 500-bed hospital may only run an average census of 350 patients. The size of a hospital is not necessarily limited by its type or affiliation. For example, academic medical centers may be medium-sized (e.g., 300 to 500 beds) or very large (e.g., more than 1000 beds). Small hospitals generally have less than 100 beds. Very small hospitals of less than 50 beds are often located in rural areas and rarely sponsor residency programs, although some programs may offer rotations in rural settings. As you may suspect, larger hospitals (i.e., 500 beds or more) are more likely to house a greater diversity of disease states and patient complexity, including patients with lots of comorbid diseases This has the potential to enhance residency training opportunities by exposing you to more complex patients and clinical situations. However, remember that several other key factors are important in determining the right fit for you.

For pharmacy residencies at nonhospital sites, managed care pharmacy and community pharmacy residencies, institution size may be measured by number of annual patient visits, number of covered lives, annual patient service days, or daily prescription volume.

Patient Population

The demographics, ethnicity, and socioeconomic status of the patients receiving care at a particular institution make up the patient population. The patient population really has little effect on learning opportunities. Where it can make a difference is the type of experiences you may receive. Differences in medication use and adverse effects may arise due to variations in cultural norms and attitudes related to medications. Institutions serving patients with limited access to preventative health and primary care services may have a greater complexity of patient care needs compared to patients at other institutions. Managing drug therapy for certain disease states is dependent on the patient population, and patient education needs will also vary. For example, the approach to educating a patient with a medical degree on warfarin therapy will be different from educating a patient with an eighth grade education or a Spanish-speaking patient. Some institutions have a particular priority for patient needs, such as a safety net hospital serving primarily uninsured patients. However, many institutions will serve a diverse patient population and have a mixture of patient care needs. When searching for the ideal residency, consider the type of patient population you enjoy most. Understanding the patient population will also provide you with insight as to the type of learning opportunities and experiences available.

Scope of Service

The term scope of service, as it relates to pharmacy practice, is the number, type, intensity, and complexity of pharmacy services provided at the institution. It is an important factor for the future pharmacy resident to consider. Information on a particular department's scope of pharmacy services can often be found on the institution's department of pharmacy Web site and through interactions with the program at meetings or interviews.

Institution size and patient population play a role in determining scope of services. For example, a 500-bed hospital may specialize in the care of cardiac, obstetric, and orthopedic patients, but may also have general internal medicine, general surgery, pediatric, and oncology patient care services. The pharmacy department in this hospital is unlikely to have as many clinical pharmacy programs and direct patient care activities in oncology patients as a hospital that specializes in this area. Consider these factors and your particular areas of interest while evaluating residency programs.

Another important factor to consider is the commitment of the pharmacy department for advancing the practice of pharmacy within the institution. There are several elements you can evaluate to help you gauge the practice environment. Look at the extent to which the pharmacy department is taking advantage of collaborative practice within their institution, or development of Pharmacy and Therapeutics (P&T) Committee protocols allowing clinical pharmacists to manage various aspects of drug therapy. Most hospital and ambulatory pharmacy departments have basic protocols in place for changing intravenous medications to the oral route in appropriate patients ("IV to PO switch"), pharmacokinetic dosing of vancomycin, and outpatient anticoagulation management. Determine what services the pharmacy department has beyond these, and whether they are planning or developing new programs to expand clinical pharmacy services. Departments should also be continually making improvements in existing services. Look for evidence that pharmacists are an integral part of the healthcare team. Some clues may include preceptors receiving pages from physicians or other providers regarding recommendations for drug therapy, documentation of formal notes in the medical record, and serving on patient care-related committees.

The same general principles of scope of services apply to community and managed care residencies. One key factor to consider for community residencies is the pharmacy practice laws in the state where the program is located. States with broader pharmacy practice laws and those allowing collaborative practice are more likely to have and support greater depth and complexity of patient care services within the community pharmacy.

PROGRAM CHARACTERISTICS

Program Size

The number of PGY-1 residents in a program varies greatly between programs and institutions. Small programs may have 1 to 2 residents, and large programs may have 15 or more PGY-1 residents. Because of high demand and nationwide efforts to increase the capacity of residency training programs, the number of PGY-1 residents in various programs will likely continue to grow. Many institutions also have PGY-2 residency training programs, further increasing the total number of residents at a particular site. Residents in small programs may experience more one-on-one interactions with the program director and preceptors and greater flexibility in scheduling rotations or events, such as grand rounds presentations. Residents in large programs have a bigger pool of colleagues with whom to foster relationships and support, and often have more choices for required and elective experiences due to the size of the program. However, a larger group of residents can reduce the flexibility of scheduling rotations. When searching for your ideal residency program, consider whether you prefer working in larger or smaller groups and the advantages associated with each.

Rotations and Programs Offered

The number and type of rotations offered in a residency program are dependent on the number of preceptors in the program and the scope of services. Most programs have a number of required and elective experiences. The required rotations and experiences should be a reflection of the program's strengths. Some programs in large institutions with a wide scope of services may utilize "selective" rotations, which permit the resident to choose from a number of experiences within a broad category. For example, a program with a critical care requirement may allow the resident to choose from experiences in the medical intensive care unit (MICU), surgical ICU (SICU), cardiovascular ICU (CVICU), or neurosurgery ICU. Institution size may dictate the number of rotations to some degree, but a more important factor is the number and structure of pharmacy services provided and number of preceptors.

Over and above core and elective rotations, there will be other required activities the resident must complete to graduate from the program. Most residencies require residents to develop their speaking and literature evaluation skills through presentations. Residents may be required to give specific presentations throughout the year. Some examples include grand rounds, seminar, continuing education presentations, journal clubs, patient case discussions, and presentation of residency research at the regional residency conference. Most PGY-1 residencies utilize block (e.g., monthly) rotations with some longitudinal experiences. Acute care rotations in the hospital typically are scheduled in blocks, while ambulatory care rotations, residency research project, or management projects are often conducted longitudinally. Information regarding required activities can be found on the program's Web site.

A staffing component is a requirement of most PGY-1 residency programs. However, what "staffing" looks like in each program can be quite variable. The type of staffing may include clinical staffing, operational staffing, or a combination of both. Examples of clinical staffing may include weekend coverage of the pharmacokinetic service, monitoring and ordering of total parenteral nutrition (TPN), drug information, or other services. Operational staffing often includes activities such as order processing and verification. The frequency of staffing also differs between programs. Most programs require staffing on average of one to two times per month. A few, but not many, may include some compensatory ("comp") time for these weekends worked. Residents in some programs complete staffing requirements during the week or weeknight. The advantage here is that it may free up some time on the weekend, but it can also require you to work long hours in a single day and take you away from rotation activities. Most residents report a number of benefits from staffing experiences such as improving time management skills, promoting clinical independence and confidence, and familiarity with drug products. Many programs will provide information about the staffing requirement on their Web site. The optimal amount and frequency of staffing is a personal choice. Discuss staffing experiences with current residents in the program and determine the level of support and training they receive.

Some programs also utilize a resident on-call program. These are most commonly found in programs with a large number of residents due to the manpower and resources needed to provide such a program. As with staffing, the amount required, type of on-call program, and number of calls received vary between programs. The resident may take in-house call, meaning the resident stays at the hospital overnight and usually for 24 hours, or at-home call, where the resident receives calls by pager at-home after leaving the hospital at the end of the day. Often, the residents take ownership and cover the service entirely. In most programs, the amount and complexity of calls differs from night to night, as does the amount of sleep the resident receives. Many residents cite development of clinical competence and confidence as a result of on-call experiences. A residency with an on-call program may appeal to you if you are looking for experiences that will challenge you to grow clinically in a fast paced environment.

In addition to rotations, residencies may offer other programs to their residents. Examples include various teaching and publishing opportunities, health fairs and immunization programs, medical mission trips, professional organization experiences, graduate certificate programs, chief resident program, and other off-site elective experiences. One such program gaining popularity in recent years is a teaching certificate program, in which residents participate in a series of lectures and discussions on teaching-related topics and create a teaching portfolio.[5] This particular program may appeal to you if you would like to pursue a full-time or adjunct faculty position during your career.

Affiliations

Some residency programs are affiliated with a college of pharmacy. The type of affiliation may vary widely between institutions but may include college of pharmacy full-time, part-time, or adjunct (also called volunteer) faculty as preceptors; college of pharmacy sponsorship of program; or an agreement between the college of pharmacy and hospital to educate a specified number of IPPE or APPE students. Programs that are affiliated with a college of pharmacy generally offer more teaching and formal learning opportunities. For example, programs affiliated with a college of pharmacy may offer a teaching certificate program for pharmacy residents. A majority of hospitals offering residency programs also teach APPE students, whether they are affiliated with a college of pharmacy or not. Programs with a formal college of pharmacy affiliation may offer a greater number and variety of teaching opportunities, such as facilitation of laboratory or recitation courses. There also may be additional opportunity for involvement within the college itself, such as participation in health fairs, college of pharmacy admission interviews, committee involvement, and administration of structured examinations. If you are interested in teaching or precepting pharmacy students, be sure to look for a residency program with a college of pharmacy affiliation.

Training Environment

The training environment is probably one of the most critical factors in determining your experience as a future resident. Several factors contribute to the training environment. You will be able to find some characteristics related to the training environment, such as institution size and rotations offered, in your early search for residency programs through printed recruiting materials, program Web sites, and residency directory information. However, the bulk of the information will be obtained during your face-to-face discussion with representatives of the program, such as the residency program director (RPD), preceptors, and residents, during the residency showcase and interview. Critical information including preceptorship, mentoring, commitment of the program to residency training, and overall resident opportunities will take more investigation on your part to determine if a particular residency is the right place for you.

A residency program should have sufficient numbers of preceptors dedicated to residency training to deliver the program. For many programs, a list of preceptors can be found on the program Web site. While the optimal numbers will be different for every program, there are certain elements for which you should look. Find out how many preceptors you will be interacting with on a frequent basis and determine whether you think you will be able to learn from them. In order to keep up with contemporary drug therapy and maintain current skills, preceptors should practice in the area for which they take residents. Sometimes, preceptors take residents in more than one area or rotation. This practice is most effective when the preceptor practices or is actively engaged in these areas. Examples include an internal medicine preceptor who also precepts the residency research project, a faculty preceptor who takes residents on clinical rotations and also precepts an academic rotation, or a clinical pharmacist who precepts the drug information rotation and the medication use evaluation. What should be kept to a minimum or avoided altogether is a preceptor taking residents on multiple clinical rotations at the same time or in multiple areas for which they do not practice. Ask the program how many nonpharmacist preceptors are utilized in the program. While other health professionals, commonly physicians, can offer great value in precepting rotations, a clinical pharmacist should be coprecepting or monitoring the experience in some way to ensure that the resident is gaining experience in critical evaluation of drug therapy. Nonpharmacist preceptor rotations should be limited in number and offered to residents toward the end of their training experience.

Preceptors are your role models for the future practice of pharmacy. It is likely you will adopt elements of practice as you were trained. Practice models may vary between institutions and even between rotations within an institution. However, look for the presence of key elements such as critical evaluation of drug therapy, patient assessment, recommendation and implementation of a drug therapy plan, and documentation of patient care activities in the medical record. Also look for preceptors who are engaged professionally. Preceptors who are active members and hold leadership positions within the institution and professional organizations are able to pass on their knowledge of issues facing the pharmacy profession to their residents. These preceptors are also more likely to look for and be aware of opportunities for resident involvement within the profession. Look for preceptors who serve on drug-policy making bodies within the institution, such as the P&T Committee and its subcommittees. Also look for preceptors who are active in local, regional, and national professional societies, such as those who hold elected office or who have been appointed to committees and task forces. This information is dynamic and may not necessarily be listed in the preceptor information on the Web site. You may need to do a preliminary search using the Internet instead. You could follow up by engaging in a discussion about professional organization involvement during the residency showcase or interview. Look for preceptors who keep up with changes in the profession and practice area. Preceptors who regularly contribute to the medical/pharmacy literature or give presentations at national meetings and conferences are not only keeping current with cutting-edge practice but are also demonstrating that they are respected among their peers. Some key elements to note are preceptors with board certification in their area of expertise, certifications, and additional training related to the practice area. Achieving certification or other status among the profession often goes beyond passing the exam. Candidates for these certifications usually must establish a certain level of expertise and minimum number of hours prior to eligibility, as well as complete continuing education from approved sources on a regular basis.

One of the most important factors that will determine your future growth and overall success in the residency is the precepting style, which includes such elements as frequency of interaction between the RPD/preceptors and resident, amount and type of feedback provided, preceptor commitment, mentorship, and guidance. In any given program, various precepting styles will be present. The key is to determine if the preceptors as a whole are committed to training residents and whether you could learn and work well with the preceptors you meet. Find out how much time the program director and preceptors spend with the residents. Not only will this amount vary between programs, but the optimal amount and frequency of interaction will depend on your needs as well. Ask yourself how much feedback you desire about the job you are doing. Some people prefer to work more independently after orientation and training with occasional meetings. Some prefer formal meetings to discuss progress, while others thrive on "on the fly" interaction as issues arise. By talking with current residents, you can get an idea if the feedback provided helps residents develop into competent and confident practitioners, educators, and scholars. Ask about the RPD's philosophy, as well as those of the main preceptors, on training individual residents. Also ask about the types of opportunities the residents have taken advantage of in past years and determine whether the RPD is continually looking for those opportunities for each resident.

In each program, you should see evidence that the program and department are committed to residents by providing them with resources to be effective. At a minimum, residents should have a desk, computer, and access to drug information resources. You should be able to tell that rotations and activities are designed in such a way to help your learning and not just provide a service to the institution. Most pharmacy/patient care-related activities will have some value in resident learning. The difference is that the program committed to residency training will take the time to evaluate each activity and develop it in such a way to optimize learning. For example, the department should have enough individuals to provide pharmacy services in a way that gives residents time to learn. They should be adequately staffed so that workload issues are not hindering patient care or training. As a resident you should receive training in the areas you are working, and adequate feedback on your performance. Ask the residents and preceptors what types of orientation and training are provided for incoming residents and how often feedback occurs. Find out if residents are encouraged to become involved in professional organizations and attend professional meetings and how often this occurs. Most programs provide some support to attend at least one professional meeting, often the ASHP Midyear Clinical Meeting. However, sometimes they are unable to provide financial support or support for more than one meeting.

Salary and Benefits

Residents are typically paid approximately one-half to one-third of a practicing clinical pharmacist salary. Salaries do vary from program to program, often based on the regional cost of living in which they are located. Most programs also offer 2 weeks of vacation, sick time (variable), and health insurance. The salary and benefits are often listed in residency directories and the program Web site. Although it may be tempting to compare salaries between programs, the differences generally are small especially when averaged over 12 months. If the salary seems unusually high, further investigation may be warranted. A better strategy is to find the program with the best "fit" for your needs and interests.

Accreditation

Pharmacy residencies are accredited by ASHP, and it is the only organization granting accreditation for these programs. The accreditation process is voluntary, and programs are evaluated for quality against a set of established optimal standards.[6] All residents completing an accredited pharmacy residency program must meet a uniform set of outcomes, goals, and objectives. These are essentially the same for all residency programs with some variations for additional elective outcomes, goals, and objectives. What differs between programs is the activities and rotations the resident completes to meet these requirements.

Residents graduating from an accredited residency training program can be assured of the quality and rigors of their chosen program. While you may gain good experience in a nonaccredited residency, the program will lack peer review of program content. The profession is moving progressively toward accredited training programs, and greater opportunities are available to graduates of these programs. Some of these opportunities include the ability to apply for and complete an accredited PGY-2 residency program and eligibility for Board of Pharmaceutical Specialties certification. For example, graduates of accredited PGY-1 residencies are eligible for Board Certified Pharmacotherapy Specialist (BCPS) certification upon completion of the residency as compared to graduates of unaccredited programs who must practice for 2 more years before meeting eligibility criteria.[6] Additionally, graduates of accredited programs are eligible to serve as preceptors or program directors of accredited PGY-1 programs in 1 and 3 years, respectively, compared to 3 and 5 years, respectively, for graduates of unaccredited programs.[7] More details on accreditation can be found in Chapter 3.

RESIDENCY RESOURCES

The key places to find information regarding specific residency programs are the residency directories available through ASHP and American College of Clinical Pharmacy (ACCP), and the individual program Web sites (Table 5-1). In each of the residency directories, you can search programs by location and type. A good way to start is to narrow your search to a particular geographic location. Once you have identified programs you are interested in, you can broaden your search to find similar programs.

The ASHP residency directory is an online resource listing information on accredited programs and those seeking accreditation.[3] The information included in this directory includes the program name, address, type, and

---

TABLE 5-1 • Selected Residency Resources

ASHP Online Residency Directory. Available at: http://accred.ashp.org/aps/pages/directory/residencyProgramSearch.aspx

American College of Clinical Pharmacy (ACCP) Directory of Residencies, Fellowships and Graduate Programs. Online version available at: http://www.accp.com/resandfel/search.aspx

American Pharmacists Association (APhA) Community Residency Locator. Available at: http://www.pharmacist.com/ResidencyLocator/ResidencyLocator.asp

Academy of Managed Care Pharmacy. This Web site contains separate database information on accredited managed care residencies, accredited residencies in the managed care environment, and nonaccredited residencies. Available at: http://www.amcp.org/Residencies/

accreditation status; names and contact information for the RPD, residency coordinator (if applicable), and director of pharmacy; residency length, number of positions, application deadline, benefits, starting date, and salary; program Web site; and a narrative description of the program and institution. You can search by program type, name, or location. The directory also includes an interactive map for easy location of individual programs. While the program's name, type, and accreditation status are kept current by ASHP, the other details listed in the directory cannot be easily updated by the program. Just keep in mind that information regarding salary, number of positions, and program contacts may be outdated.

The ACCP directory of residencies, fellowships and graduate programs is available both in print and online.[8] As the name implies, this directory contains information on research fellowships and other graduate programs in addition to residencies. The directory is open to programs posted by any ACCP member and includes both accredited and nonaccredited programs. Additionally, all information including program type and accreditation status is voluntarily reported and is not verified by ACCP. The information in this directory includes program name, type, length, contact information, Web site, number of positions, accreditation, and description. The salary, contact information, and program description in the ACCP listings are more likely to be current, since the ACCP member posting the information may update the details at any time. Additionally, the listing expires 1 year after the last update.

An additional resource for specific residencies is the program Web site. The amount and extent of the information and recruiting materials found on the Web site is variable, but most residencies provide information such as program description, photographs, required and elective rotations, preceptor information, current residents, past residents and positions accepted upon completion, the local community, salary, and benefits. Additionally, the program Web site is usually located within the larger institution Web site where detailed information about the practice site and institution can be found. The Web site is typically listed in the residency directory. It is a good idea to familiarize yourself with the Web site content prior to contacting the RPD with specific questions that can easily be found by reviewing the available information.

Other professional organizations also post information on residencies. The APhA lists PGY-1 community pharmacy residency programs, and the AMCP lists PGY-1 managed care residencies. However, updated information on all PGY-1 residency programs can be found in the ASHP residency directory.

MID-CAREER RESIDENCY OPPORTUNITIES

What if you are a practicing pharmacist who wishes to complete a residency? The good news is that there are more opportunities now than ever before. There are a significant number of pharmacists who make the decision to leave their current position to pursue a full-time residency position. The number of practicing pharmacists applying for PGY-1 residencies has increased steadily over the past 5 years, with over 250 interviewing for programs in 2012.[1] Motivated candidates with practice experience as licensed pharmacists and evidence of commitment to and advancement of the profession may have an advantage over other candidates in the application and interview process who lack practice experience.

Another option for practicing pharmacists is a nontraditional residency program available at some hospitals. Practicing pharmacists accepted into these programs complete the same requirements as other PGY-1 residents but over a longer period of time, generally 2 to 3 years. This type of program takes longer to complete because the resident is part-time and cycles between regular work responsibilities and resident rotations and activities. The salary is generally maintained at a level higher than a typical full-time resident salary because the nontraditional resident continues to work as a pharmacist throughout the duration of the program. If you are a practicing pharmacist with other personal commitments, this arrangement may appeal to you.

Nontraditional residency programs are generally open to pharmacists already employed by the institution. However, the length of employment required for program eligibility varies. To find information about nontraditional residencies, search program Web sites of institutions in your area. The available residency directories cannot be searched by nontraditional residency at this time. Another option, although likely incomplete, is to conduct an Internet search using the term "nontraditional pharmacy residency."

THE IDEAL PROGRAM AND "FIT"

Selecting the ideal program is all about finding the right "fit." There are many great programs out there, each with its own set of distinct features. After carefully evaluating all of the programs you have selected, consider your own professional goals and personal priorities. Table 5-2 provides an example of how you can compare and contrast unique program characteristics. Additionally, a blank table is available in the Appendix 1. The ideal program must be a good "fit" for both the candidate and the residency program. From your point of view, you want a program that will help you achieve your goals and pursue your interests. Consider these questions when determining program fit. How did you feel when you talked to the program? Were you excited about the opportunities discussed? Would this program help you achieve your goals? Does the precepting style match the way you like to learn? How would you fit with the organizational culture? Could you see yourself working in that institution? Overall, what is your "gut feeling" about the program? From the program's perspective, good fit means that the program strengths, qualities, and opportunities match the candidate's your career goals, interests, and achievements.

TABLE 5-2 • Example Comparison of Residency Program Characteristics

Characteristic	Where Can I Find It?	How Important Is This Characteristic to Me? (1 [low] to 5 [high])	Example: University Medical Center (UMC)	Example: Regional Medical Center (RMC)
		Institution		
Type (e.g., academic, community, VA)	Web site	5	Academic	Community Hospital
Institution size (# beds/average census, # annual patient visits, daily prescription volume, etc.)	Directory, Web site	3	500 beds/ average 350	800 beds/ average 650
Location (e.g., urban, rural, local)	Directory	3	Urban	Local
Complexity and diversity of patient population	Web site, showcase	5	+++	++
Scope of services	Web site			
Automated dispensing devices	Showcase	2	++	+++
Chart documentation	Showcase	5	+++	+
Code response	Showcase	3	+++	+
Collaborative practice/ prescriptive authority	Showcase	5	+++	+
Electronic medical record/ computerized prescriber order entry	Showcase	4	+++	+
Pharmacokinetics/ anticoagulation consult services	Showcase	3	+++	++
Other				
		Program		
Accredited	Directory	5	Yes	Yes
Affiliations	Web site	4	+++	+
College of Pharmacy				
Program Size	Directory			
# PGY-1 residents	Directory	3	10	5
# PGY-1 + PGY-2 residents	Directory, Web site	2	20	6
Preceptor: Resident ratio	Showcase	2	+	++

TABLE 5-2 • Example Comparison of Residency Program Characteristics (*continued*)

Characteristic	Where Can I Find It?	How Important Is This Characteristic to Me? (1 [low] to 5 [high])	Example: University Medical Center (UMC)	Example: Regional Medical Center (RMC)
PGY 2 Program in area of interest	Web site	3	Critical care, infectious disease	No
Rotations and programs	Web site			
Rotations in areas of interest	Web site, showcase	4	+++	++
On-call program	Web site, showcase	1	++	No
Advanced cardiac life support certification	Web site, showcase	1	Yes	No
Teaching certificate program	Web site	4	++	+
Graduate certificate	Web site	4	No	No
Off-site elective rotations	Web site	1	Yes	No
Staffing	Web site, showcase	2	+	+
Teaching opportunities	Web site			
Experiential (precepting)	Web site, showcase	4	++	+
Facilitation/ laboratory instruction	Web site, showcase	3	+	No
Didactic	Web site, showcase	2	No	No
In-services/other	Showcase	3	+	++
Scholarship opportunities				
Poster presentation	Showcase	3	+	?
Grand rounds/CE presentation	Web site, showcase	3	+	+
Publications	Showcase, Pubmed	3	?	No/?
Other				
Professional organization involvement	Web site, showcase			
Meeting attendance	Showcase	3	+	+
Other opportunities			No	++

(continued)

TABLE 5-2 • Example Comparison of Residency Program Characteristics (*continued*)

Characteristic	Where Can I Find It?	How Important Is This Charac- teristic to Me? (1 [low] to 5 [high])	Example: University Medical Center (UMC)	Example: Regional Medical Center (RMC)
		Training Environment		
RPD				
RPD Board certified	Web site	4	Yes	Yes
Local/regional/ national offices and appointments	Web site, Internet	4	+	+++
Track record of presentations at meeting and publications in literature	Pubmed, Web site	4	+	++
Faculty appointment	Web site	5	+	+
Frequency of RPD meetings	Showcase	4	+	++
Preceptors				
% board certified	Web site	3	+++	+
Local/regional/ national offices and appointments	Web site, Internet	3	++	+
Track record of presentations at meeting and publications in literature	Pubmed, Web site	3	+	+
% faculty appointment	Web site	3	+++	+
Precepting style	Showcase	5	+	++
Positions taken by former residents	Web site, showcase	4	Mostly PGY-2s	Clinical staff, PGY-2

How to Use TABLE 5-2

Column 1—Characteristic: Specific characteristics have been listed and categorized as discussed in the chapter. There is also space at the bottom of each category to write in characteristics that are important to you.

Column 2—Location of information: This column tells you where to look to find the characteristic for each program. In some cases, more than one place is recommended. In many cases, preliminary information can be found in a residency directory or on their Web site. However, detailed information can be determined only after talking to representatives of the program, such as the RPD/preceptors/ residents at the residency showcase.

Column 3—Importance of characteristic: This column provides a place to rank the importance of each characteristic to you. For example, if the institution type, complexity of patient population, and teaching certificate are important to you, these characteristics should be ranked as a four or five out of five.

Columns 4 and 5—Specific program information: The next several columns provide examples of how to list specific programs for comparison. Two examples have been provided for you in the table.

Chapter Takeaways

▶ Each residency program has its own distinct mix of characteristics. All accredited programs must meet the same set of residency standards and learning outcomes. The opportunities and the way in which the program is designed (e.g., structure, practice model, patient population, and training environment) make each program unique.

▶ Complete a self-assessment to determine your goals and interests and what program characteristics are important to you.

▶ Consider institution characteristics, program characteristics, and the training environment when evaluating programs. Use Table 5-1 to compare and contrast programs of interest.

▶ Use the available residency directories to identify programs, obtain their Web site address, and contact information.

▶ The programs you pursue should match your goals, interests, and needs. The ideal residency program is a good fit for both candidate and program.

ROLE FOR THE MENTOR

After sharing your career goals and interests, a mentor can suggest program types that may be a good fit, recommend specific programs, and assist in narrowing the seemingly never-ending choices for programs.

A mentor can also give you more insight into the information programs provide and help you develop questions to ask that give you more specific information about a program.

FREQUENTLY ASKED QUESTIONS

Q: Where can I find the best residency program?

A: There are many great residency programs available from which to choose. The best program is the one with a good "fit," meaning the program meets your needs and interests and you have the desired strengths and characteristics from the program's perspective. This is an individual decision and the same set of programs will not be a good fit for all residency candidates.

Q: Where should I look to find detailed information about each program I am considering?

A: A good place to start is one of the available online residency directories. The ASHP Online Residency Directory keeps updated information regarding accreditation status of each program. The ACCP Directory of Residencies, Fellowships and Graduate Programs allows programs to update information such as description and salary information as needed. Once you have identified programs of interest, more detailed information can be found on the program Web site listed in the residency directory.

Q: To how many programs should I submit applications?

A: The optimal number of applications to submit will vary for each candidate. Factors to consider include the number of interviews you will be able to complete if offered, geographic location of the programs and travel time and cost required for interviews, competitiveness of your chosen programs, time off needed from your APPEs for interviews, and the number of interviews you think you will need to secure a residency position. Your own regional location or desired location may also dictate how many applications to submit. If you are located in an area with a large number of applicants compared to residency positions, you may need to apply to more programs than if you are located in an area with fewer residency applicants. Most RPDs and preceptors would recommend that you apply to more than one program. Whether you apply to four or ten programs is a personal choice you will have to make and one in which a mentor can help you decide.

Q: I am geographically limited. Should I apply to every program in my area to increase the likelihood of obtaining a residency position?

A: It is generally best to determine which programs in your area may offer the best "fit" for you related to your career goals and interests and pursue those programs. Most often, the programs in your area will likely be attractive to a wide range of candidates and may not be suited for all residency applicants. For example, a PGY-1 residency offered in a VA medical center and one offered in a pediatric hospital likely would not be the best "fit" for the same type of candidate. If a candidate applies to every program in the area, programs often wonder what it is about their program that appeals to the candidate.

Q: How can I find out if a program is accredited and in good standing?

A: The ASHP online directory provides updated information regarding accreditation status of each program. Only accredited programs or those seeking accreditation are listed in the directory.

Q: I talked to a new program at the ASHP Midyear Residency Showcase that is not currently accredited but has applied for accreditation. Should I consider applying to this program?

A: New programs can offer great opportunities for self-motivated residents with good communication and people skills who are interested in developing and refining existing services. All programs applying for accreditation are evaluated against the same set of optimal residency standards during an on-site survey. Almost every program has some areas they are working to improve. New programs usually have a greater number of citations and areas of improvement than some of the existing programs, if nothing else, because they are new and do not have the benefit of a number of years to develop optimal practices. Residencies demonstrating a commitment to residency training and providing evidence of program and service changes in response to the accreditation survey report are likely to become accredited. Programs with significant patient safety and residency training concerns may not be granted accreditation, and none of their residents receive the benefit of completing an ASHP-accredited residency. To protect yourself, you should ask questions of the program to determine their level of commitment to the process. Does the program seem aware of the process and procedures related to accreditation? Completing the process of accreditation takes a tremendous amount of work and effort on the part of the program. If a program is unaware of the procedures involved, this may be a sign that they are not prepared to meet the standards. Has the program already completed the on-site accreditation survey? If so, what are some of the changes the program has made in response to the report? When does the program expect to find out whether they have been granted accreditation?

References

1. ASHP Resident Matching Program. Summary of programs and positions offered and filled by program type for the 2012 Match. http://www.natmatch.com/ashprmp/stats/2012progstats.htm. Accessed September 4, 2012.

2. ASHP Accreditation Standard for Postgraduate Year One (PGY-1) Pharmacy Residency Programs. http://www.ashp.org/DocLibrary/Accreditation/ASD-PGY-1-Standard.aspx. Accessed February 8, 2012.

3. ASHP Online Residency Directory http://accred.ashp.org/aps/pages/directory/residency ProgramSearch.aspx. Accessed April 2, 2012.

4. Paciullo CA, Moranville MP, Suffoletta TJ. Pharmacy practice residency program in community hospitals. Am J Health Syst Pharm. 2009;66:536–539.

5. Romanelli F, Smith KM, Brandt BF. Teaching residents how to teach: A scholarship of teaching and learning certificate program (STLC) for pharmacy residents. Am J Pharm Educ. 2005; 69:126–132.

6. Residency Accreditation. http://www.ashp.org/menu/Accreditation/ResidencyAccreditation.aspx. Accessed February 13, 2012.

7. Board of Pharmaceutical Specialties 2011 Candidate's Guide. http://www.bpsweb.org/pdfs/CandidatesGuide.pdf. Accessed February 15, 2012.

8. American College of Clinical Pharmacy. 2012 Directory of residencies, fellowships, and graduate programs. Lenexa, KS: American College of Clinical Pharmacy; 2011.

The "Ideal" Residency Candidate 6

John A. Armitstead and Suzanne Turner

Now that you are familiar with residency programs and excited about pursuing postgraduate training, it's time to begin thinking about the qualities that residency programs look for in resident candidates. In many ways, looking like the "ideal" residency candidate is about marketing yourself. But, before you think about marketing, it's time to develop a great product: You!

CHARACTERISTICS OF THE "IDEAL" RESIDENCY CANDIDATE

The Plan

The first key aspect of preparing for residency training is that you should have a plan to demonstrate that you are the ideal residency candidate. The plan for your residency training and the rest of your professional career should start well before the residency application materials are prepared. In essence, you should consider what you can do early in your pharmacy school career as a pre-residency candidate to develop skills and qualities that will prepare you for residency training. Keep in mind that rather than participating in activities for your application, you should thoughtfully consider spending your time engaged in activities that interest you and will prepare you for the residency training and career that lies ahead. Remember that we don't plan to fail in our lives (and residency applications), but often we fail to plan.

> "Do all you can during pharmacy school to be the ideal candidate to the residency programs which you are applying."
>
> *Matthew W., Pharmacy Student, Michigan*

Pharmacy residency programs will evaluate applications in a number of ways, but the core areas are experiential training, professional organization involvement, leadership activities, community service, academic performance, scholarly activities, professional work experiences, other employment experience, and overall communication skills. Ideal candidates will excel in all of these categories.

Experiential Training

When evaluating a candidate for a residency program, experiential training is a strong area of interest. Although many colleges of pharmacy have similar Introductory Pharmacy Practice Experience (IPPE) and Advanced Pharmacy Practice Experience (APPE) rotation requirements, the ideal residency candidate will maximize these experiences. Experiences in community, ambulatory care, and acute care pharmacy practices sites are all valuable for pharmacy students to prepare them for the rigors of postgraduate training.

> "Be sure to leave a good impression during your student rotations! Many residency sites will reflect back on your performance as a rotation student when considering you for a residency position!"
>
> *Huda-Marie K. – Pharmacy Student, Illinois*

Students who are planning to apply for a residency program need to choose their elective rotations wisely. Prior work or volunteer activities can give you a head start by providing exposure to lots of practice areas. If you have already been exposed to multiple practice areas, you will be able to choose elective rotations that will match the type of residency program(s) you are considering. For example, if you are certain that a Postgraduate Year One (PGY-1) residency in acute care is your only interest, you should not complete all your electives in the community setting.

Rotations in unique practice settings such as academia, professional organizations, or research will give you a well-rounded experience. Opportunities to complete one of these unique rotations that compliment your postgraduate training interests should be taken. Nonpatient care rotations, when carefully selected, can add to the overall experience of the applicant. Be careful not to simply take "the easy" rotation, and be prepared to demonstrate or explain what was accomplished on the nonpatient care rotation (projects, presentations, etc.).

Completing all of your rotations in one setting has its advantages and disadvantages. Rotations are a time for students to be exposed to how pharmacy is practiced, not only in a variety of settings but also within different institutions and with different practitioners. If possible, complete rotations at more than one institution or in varied settings. Experiencing pharmacy practice in a teaching hospital compared with a community hospital or ambulatory care in the VA system compared to a non-VA system can provide you with a valuable insight on the type of residency program that will best fit your practice interests.

Residency candidates who have all of their rotations in the same institution have the advantage of being familiar with the institution's computer system, formulary, and policies throughout the year. Rather than learning every month where the restroom is and where you can buy coffee, your time can be spent diving in to patient care on your rotations. You will spend less time learning how to find patient data and more time focusing on patient specific pharmacotherapy. In addition, at a single site, your preceptors may be able to communicate with one another and help you develop your strengths and improve on weaknesses from rotation to rotation. If you remain at a single site, make an effort to work with different preceptors. Interactions with new preceptors, observing different practice settings and preceptor styles, as well as hearing about their career experiences will provide you with a diversity of experiences.

Keep in mind that no matter what the IPPE and APPE rotations are, the key is making the most of the learning experience. Take advantage of opportunities to see new things, make presentations, or work on extra projects. The ideal candidate will go above and beyond the expectations of the preceptor. These experiences look great on your CV, but more importantly are experiences that help prepare you for the challenges you will see in residency training.

Professional Organization Involvement

Candidates who are well prepared for residency training are well rounded in their professional organization involvement. The experiences of being involved in organizations and exposure to the practice of pharmacy are both equally important. It is difficult to exceed in all these areas while maintaining a heavy course load, but these types of involvement help develop time management skills and provide opportunities for leadership.

> "Leadership experiences are key to not only getting an interview, but also answering the interview questions themselves! When asked behavioral interview questions, I had many examples from my leadership experiences."
>
> *Meg C. – Pharmacy Student, South Carolina*

Becoming a member of different pharmacy organizations is a must for the pharmacy student interested in a residency. Membership in pharmacy organizations should begin early in your pharmacy school career, not 1 month before applying for a residency program. The ideal residency candidate will take their professional organization involvement beyond that of just membership. After joining an organization, take the next step! Try taking on an informal leadership role such as volunteering to lead an activity, such as a local Residency Showcase or a Brown Bag Program. These activities are the perfect stepping stone to formal leadership positions.

Consider becoming involved with organizations outside your college. Many organizations, including ACCP, ASHP, and APhA, create a number of opportunities for students to be involved on the national level. Many state pharmacy organizations do this as well.

Memberships in honorary professional organizations such as Rho Chi or Phi Lambda Sigma are also characteristics of the ideal residency candidate. While you cannot apply for membership in these organizations, becoming a leader academically or within organizations is essential to being invited, and residency programs will recognize this.

Another important part of being involved with professional organizations is attending professional organization conferences. Exposure to the profession on a state and/or national level can best be acquired at these meetings. These experiences will help you see the world of pharmacy beyond your college "bubble" and begin to see what real pharmacists do to increase their knowledge and network with colleagues. You may also find a number of great opportunities for networking at these meetings.

Leadership Activities

Beyond membership, being a leader in activities and organizations will help you develop skills and demonstrate that you are an ideal residency candidate. Getting involved as a member in multiple professional organizations and narrowing down leadership activities to a few organizations is a common approach. Find an organization that matches your personal values and get involved. It's important to continue to stay active in other organizations; however, being a leader and active member in a few organizations is a better choice than being a nonactive member of numerous organizations.

Holding a leadership position teaches you responsibility, time management, team building, and working skills. It also helps you develop strategies to deal with conflict and learn important skills in negotiation and compromise. Your leadership experiences will also give you a repertoire of experiences to draw from during your interviews. Have a specific example of a time when you held a leadership role in mind when you head into residency interviews. Know what your responsibilities were, how you dealt with conflict, and what you did to help motivate group members to accomplish a goal.

In addition to formal leadership positions in professional organizations, the ideal resident candidate will exemplify leadership through participation in activities such as serving as a class representative or as a mentor to underclassmen. These types of activities help teach you the importance of advocating for others and putting the needs of others first.

Leadership roles outside pharmacy organizations should be included in your CV as well as your pharmacy experiences. Many excellent candidates have gained leadership skills during their undergraduate years in social or academic organizations.

Community Service and Extracurricular Activities

Many pharmacy professional organizations participate in community service activities and your involvement can be a rewarding experience that prepares you for residency training. Although many candidates focus their volunteer efforts on the healthcare setting, there are also nonpharmacy extracurricular activities and service experiences that can enhance your application.

The key factor in any extracurricular activity is showing a sustained contribution to the community or organization. Participating in several community service projects within a short period of time is not as impressive as one or two long-term commitments with sustained contribution of the candidates' time and energy. Medical mission trips, serving as a role model in boys' or girls' clubs or tutoring, are some common examples of extracurricular activities seen in resident candidates.

Academic Performance

Just like your applications to college and pharmacy school, your academic performance (aka "grades") is an important part of the evaluation process. Pharmacy school is difficult, and completing the Doctor of Pharmacy degree is an achievement. But, when it comes to residency programs grade point average (GPA) or whether you are enrolled in a Pass/Fail program will be evaluated.

Although the GPA alone is not the only measure, as a general guide, many programs require having a GPA of 3.0 (4.0 scale) or better as a minimum standard. Outstanding applicants will have a 3.5 GPA or higher, but once again this is only one piece of the application for predicting success. Programs may also consider your class rank to help give an idea what your GPA means. Keep in mind if your GPA is lower than this, that you will have opportunities to explain your academic performance, and that programs will take other factors into account. For example, maybe you had a bad semester due to personal issues. If this is the case, this can be explained in your application. Be prepared to answer questions on the subject during your interview.

As a tip from one preceptor, always be able to identify and justify weak performances in certain course work, such as that C or D grade in microbiology. The preceptor interviewers may ask about the tough times and look for how well the situation is defended, sidestepped, or eloquently explained.

In many programs, the reputation of the college of pharmacy may be a factor in assessing the caliber of the potential residency applicant. Some examples include rating schools by the comprehensive nature of the education and setting, US News and World Report rankings, and referencing NAPLEX examinations pass rates of the colleges. Although it may be thought to be unfair by some to categorize applicants in this manner, the rigor of the program (known or perceived) can potentially be a factor in the candidates' status as well as predicted success in the postgraduate program.

In the past several years, there has been a rapid rise in the number of pharmacy schools.[1] While these programs are accredited by ACPE and have been established at excellent universities with strong reputations, the college of pharmacy may not have a long list of successful graduates to demonstrate their skills and abilities. These colleges of pharmacy have a wealth of new experiences to offer resident candidates; just be prepared to discuss these things in an on-site interview.

Scholarly Activities

Scholarly activities are a significant differentiating factor in assessing how well candidates can perform in residency training. Scholarly success can indicate whether or not the applicant is able to discover and investigate pharmacy practice opportunities and potentially rise to high or established levels of excellence.

For the purpose of this section, let us define scholarly activities as both oral and written presentations and written and electronic publications. This can include abstract and poster presentations and articles in newsletters or peer-reviewed journals. Scholarly activities generally go above and beyond academic performance and are usually associated with long-term high performance in pharmacy practice. For resident candidates, evidence of scholarly activity is a strong differentiator of candidate qualifications. Scholarly activities usually indicate excellent skills in time management, research, writing, communication excellence, and often teamwork. These skills are all essential and will be built upon during a residency program.

Research is a high-level scholarly activity that may be a challenge to attain, but should be pursued.

Research can encompass everything from small independent projects to large collaborative research investigations. Examples include anything from a contained medication use evaluation to some experience with a large clinical trial. For ideas about research, investigate opportunities with a mentor, participate in college of pharmacy-sponsored independent studies, and investigate honors programs. Sharing findings from your research experiences will be great opportunities for both presentation and publication. Resident applicants should have a number of presentations to their peers at the college of pharmacy and from APPE rotations, but this serves only as baseline for all applicants. Evidence of reaching beyond typical audiences and settings is advisable and demonstrated by outstanding applicants. In essence, think "good, better, best" in regard to "local, state, and national" presentations. Seek out opportunities to do "extra" presentations and to be involved in organizations in this way.

> "Try to gain research experience in an area of pharmacy you are interested in! When working on a project, you are also able to develop a relationship with a clinical pharmacist who can serve as a mentor as you begin to apply for residency."
>
> *Meg C. – Pharmacy Student, South Carolina*

Similarly, poster presentations are valuable and usually offer more mobile and smaller individual audiences for presenting than formal oral presentations. They are a common way that research findings can be presented. As a presenter, you prepare a poster on your project or some other topic and are immediately available for questions and dialogue with those interested in the topic. The similar theme of local, state, and national "value" applies to poster presentations, but a poster presentation can help set you apart.

Publications are truly an outstanding characteristic of a residency candidate. Although this may be a challenge to have a publication, high-performing candidates should "stretch their limits" and attempt to have at least one prior to their residency search. Publications are one of the strongest indicators that the applicant is able to seek and attain goals consistent with residency success. Once again, target "good, better, best" as you attempt to write something for publication, but consider pharmacy department newsletters, state pharmacy society newsletters, and rotation projects, as well as the "high bar" of a peer-reviewed national publication.

Honors and Awards

Honors and awards are an indication that your efforts have been recognized by others. They can be professional, academic, philanthropic, or humanistic. In most cases, we don't always intentionally seek honors and awards in daily life, but they are valued in assessing candidates. Make sure you highlight honors on your CV.

In other situations, you should explore the honors and awards opportunities that are available to you and seek them out. Seek the ones that set you apart from others and highlight your skills. Remember that it is hard to be awarded first prize in the race if you are not in the race! Some excellent examples include awards for clinical skills and patient counseling—The ACCP Clinical Pharmacy Challenge, APhA Patient Counseling Competition, and ASHP Clinical Skills Competition. Keep in mind that as you compete, the objective is not always winning. Participation in these competitions can help you in developing the intellect, performance, and team skills that you are learning in the process. Scholarships that you have received during pharmacy school can indicate that you have stood out from your classmates and attained distinction. Congratulations!

Professional Work Experiences

Ideal pharmacy residency candidates will have pharmacy internship experience in a professional work capacity. Professional work experiences, including an internship in an applicable field for more than 1 year, demonstrate a solid, advancing, and sustained pharmacy track record.

Candidates should preferably have professional work experience which indicates that they have been employed and earned some income as part of their career development. Residency programs look for work experience because demonstrating an

"I was surprised that some of the programs required letters of recommendation from employers. Make sure you have thought of other individuals, in addition to clinical preceptors and faculty, that are able to write positive letters for you."

Kathryn E. – Pharmacy Student, Arizona

employee commitment indicates that the candidate is able to meet job requirements and establish an employee–employer relationship.

Work experiences in the field of pharmacy will help you stand out from your peers. It is especially helpful, but not required, that your experiences be within the field you are interested in. For example, if you are interested in a PGY-1 pharmacy practice residency, health system pharmacy experience would be ideal. In the past several years, the job market for pharmacy positions has been quite difficult, and programs understand if you do not have relevant work experience.[2] If you are unable to establish a formal employment relationship, consider volunteering in a pharmacy without pay. Any experiences, even short informal experiences, in various practice areas of pharmacy can be important. Seeing the variety of job requirements and activities that a pharmacist provides will give insight into what will be expected of a resident. Ideally, start to participate in these work experiences early in your academic career, before you choose your advanced practice rotations.

Nonpharmacy Employment Experiences

Work experience, even if not related to pharmacy practice, is universally regarded as an important way of developing employability skills and business awareness. Other employment experiences can indicate that you have had an employee–employer relationship and can be considered a positive attribute in evaluating candidates. Working in the same environment for a long period of time may be of value in indicating high-quality applicants, as it can mean that candidate is committed and has solid employment performance. Outlining advancing responsibilities over time is also advantageous. Indicating that you contributed to your future career through service and performance as a member of the workforce is also viewed as another accomplishment in your life. Showcasing these experiences can be of value and also can be used as evidence of teamwork, problem solving, and related skills.

Communication Skills

At some point in your college career, you have probably had a professor or two who were brilliant in their field, well recognized, and the envy of all the other faculty. That same professor may also have not been the best at explaining difficult concepts to you. When you reflect back on this, the problem was mainly in their communication skills! Now, realize you don't want to be that person

"Pharmacy is a small world. Be conscious of your interactions with other members of the profession because you never know who could be interviewing you for your dream residency position."

Yelena A. – Pharmacy Resident, California

when it comes to your residency application. With that in mind, be on your best behavior when it comes to preparing written application materials and interacting with residency programs. Chapters 7 through 10 will help you avoid being "that guy" that no one understands.

The Fit

Before having characteristics of the "ideal" residency candidate, there is one more intangible quality that programs look for: Fit. This means that both the program and the candidate match well together. Each candidate is an individual and each program is different.

Unlike a professional matchmaker, National Matching Services can't screen candidates and programs, so as a candidate you should seek out programs that work well with your objectives and career goals.

> "Don't compare yourself to your peers or other candidates. Everyone has different personalities and career goals that will make you a better fit with certain programs over others."
>
> *Kathryn E. – Pharmacy Student, Arizona*

Finding the right fit primarily refers to the match between what the candidate is looking to gain from a residency program and whether or not that program can meet those expectations. For example, if a candidate states that his/her career goal is to work at a large teaching hospital and serve as adjunct faculty, a residency program at a small community hospital not affiliated with a college of pharmacy would not be a good fit. If a resident candidate wants to complete a Postgraduate Year Two (PGY-2) in pediatrics and eventually becomes a pediatrics specialist, a PGY-1 in a children's hospital would be an ideal fit.

Fit can also refer to the personality type of the candidate to that of the program design or primary preceptors. If a resident candidate states that he/she performs best in a well-structured environment and does not adapt to change easily, a newly established residency program may not be the best type of program for that candidate.

Lastly, fit can refer to the overall culture of the institution or pharmacy department to that of the candidate. Each pharmacy department has its own culture or "personality." A residency candidate who is intensely competitive may not be a good fit in a more relaxed pharmacy department where being personable and communicating well with others is more important than publishing lots of articles. These things are often found out later, during the interview

> "As a student, I kept track of every activity, leadership role, and award/recognition that I got in a spread sheet. When I went to type up my CV for the residency application process, it was all right there. I knew I didn't leave anything out or forget something important."
>
> *Leslie E. – Pharmacy Student, Washington*

TABLE 6-1 • Resident Candidate Self-Assessment Tool

Factor	Aspect	Self-Evaluation
Experiential training	Number of clinical experiences Acute care or ambulatory care experience Specialty populations, diverse experiences Experiences in the candidates stated area of interest Level of responsibility during experience	
Professional organization involvement	Membership in pharmacy organizations Attendance at state or national pharmacy conferences Leadership positions Accomplishments	
Leadership activities	Informal leadership roles in organizations Formal leadership roles in organizations	
Community service and extracurricular activities	Volunteer activities Community service Neighborhood activity Shadowing experiences	
Academic performance	Transcripts Overall GPA Trends in grades GPA in therapeutics/pharmacology courses Previous degrees NAPLEX pass rate of your college Reputation of college of pharmacy	
Scholarly activities	Participation in research or projects Presentation of a poster at a regional, state, or national meeting Publications	
Honors and awards	Membership in honorary societies Local, state, or national awards and honors Merit-based scholarships	
Professional work experience	Pharmacy: Community, health system Internship experience Length of employment Duties Accomplishments	
Other employment experience	Nonpharmacy employment Length of employment Duties Accomplishments	

TABLE 6-1 • Resident Candidate Self-Assessment Tool (*continued*)

Factor	Aspect		Self-Evaluation
Communication	Written—Letter of intent	Knowledge of specific program	
		Interest and enthusiasm in residency and residency/career match	
		Grammar, punctuation	
	Written—Essay of goals	Motivation for residency	
		Organized, style, logical flow of thoughts	
		Mature and open-minded goals	
	Verbal—Presentation	Professional, communicative	
	Verbal—Interview	Poised, thoughtful, insightful	
	Verbal—Informal	Conversational, warm, friendly, thankful	
	Written—Follow-up	Thank you note timely and sincere	

This table includes typical screening questions used by the interview selection committee when reviewing resident candidate application packets. A larger version for copying is available in the Appendix 2.

process. It can be helpful to research not only the qualifications of the program but also the "personality" of the program through speaking with faculty, preceptors, students, and representatives of the program at ASHP MCM.

Table 6-1 provides a checklist to evaluate where your strengths are and locate weaknesses that can be improved upon in order to become the ideal resident candidate.

CONCLUSION

"To be, rather than to seem." No, that's not the advice of a Jedi master, it's the North Carolina State motto (Don't worry, residencies won't quiz you on this!). But, it does describe the best way to become the "ideal" residency candidate. Don't focus on things just for your residency application.

Instead, focus your efforts on preparing yourself for residency training. Get involved in organizations, become a leader, be active in your community, study hard, take advantage of scholarship opportunities, and gain some work experience. Before you know it, you'll BE the "ideal" residency candidate.

Chapter Takeaways

▶ Preparing for residency training requires development and efforts in a wide variety of areas

▶ Take advantage of opportunities to be involved in organizations, participate in research, do optional projects or presentations to help you stand out from other candidates

▶ Focus on your own personal development to help figure out your interests and to prepare you for residency training

---

ROLE FOR THE MENTOR

Especially early in your pharmacy career, mentors can help identify professional opportunities in organizations, volunteering, or research

A mentor on a research or writing project will teach you the specifics of research and help you with poster presentations and publication

Mentors can provide advice areas where you need more experience or ways to get involved with activities that you need to make you a well-rounded candidate

---

FREQUENTLY ASKED QUESTIONS

Q: If my GPA is low, should I forget about applying to a residency?

A: Grades alone do not determine whether or not you will match with a residency program, but they are one factor. A general rule of thumb is if your GPA is less than 3.0, be prepared to identify the reasons for your relative lack of academic excellence. If these are well explained, this should not be the sole reason you do not get a residency.

Q: Will a great GPA guarantee me a residency position?

A: Most residency programs are looking for great team players who have demonstrated that they can be involved in a variety of activities, have good time management skills, and have a range of experiences. Grades matter, but don't spend all your time on getting a 4.0 and none on other activities.

Q: The job market is pretty tough right now, what if I am unable to find a job as a pharmacy intern in my area of interest?

A: Programs know that all candidates can't find jobs in the field prior to residency training. Any work experience can be valuable, so if you can find a job in a different field, you should pursue it. Likewise, consider volunteer opportunities. If you have an interest in health system pharmacy, but can't find a paying position, consider volunteering there. You never know where it might lead!

Q: Will being a member of lots of organizations assist in my application?

A: Evaluators often see candidates have a long list of professional organization memberships on their CVs without any activity listed. Rather than simply paying dues in lots of organizations, get involved in a few that meet your interests. Active involvement matters!

References

1. Accreditation Council for Pharmacy Education. Accredited Professional Programs of Colleges and Schools of Pharmacy. https://www.acpe-accredit.org/shared_info/programsSecure.asp. Accessed April 2, 2012.

2. Pharmacy Manpower Project. Aggregate Demand Index. http://www.pharmacymanpower.com/. Accessed April 2, 2012.

Curriculum Vitae Preparation 7

Melissa L. Theesfeld and Andrew P. Traynor

Curriculum vitae (CV). The words sound foreign, but it must be something you should know about since EVERY residency and postgraduate application is asking for one. The CV is really just your life story pared down to a manageable few pages. Okay . . . it's not really your ENTIRE life story since not everyone needs to know about your pet fish and your collection of autographs from the 1953 Wisconsin Badgers or 1962 Minnesota Golden Gophers Rose Bowl football teams. But a CV does highlight the important aspects of your education and career to potential residency program directors (RPDs) and employers.

The terms CV and resume are often used interchangeably, but they are very different documents. Resumes are traditionally one- or two-page documents that give a very brief synopsis of your education and employment history. Resumes do not typically include lengthy descriptions of accomplishments or participation and are often truncated to be applicable to the position you are seeking. On the other hand, CVs are generally much longer in length than resumes and include a complete history of your accomplishments. CVs for a recent pharmacy school graduate can be 3 to 6 pages long, but will eventually grow to be 10-, 15-, or 20-page documents as your career progresses. A CV is the perfect place to provide descriptions of educational and employment involvement and contributions. The use of CVs varies from country to country, but a good rule of thumb is that professional careers in the health sciences and academia require a CV. You have entered a profession where the use of CVs is the norm.

If CVs are so much longer than resumes and have so much detail, why would anyone who is looking to hire a resident or pharmacist even bother to read all of it? In reality, they might not read every detail, but they will want to be able to discern the types of rotations you've completed, your involvement in pharmacy school, and your past employment history. RPDs can be flooded with 10 to 15 times as many applications as there are actual resident spots, thus CVs are often used as the first way to pare down an overwhelming list of potential residents and determine who is invited for a residency interview. CVs are also used extensively in the residency interview process. An applicant's CV is the source of lots of information for an interviewer and should be an easy source of talking points for you.

You might be thinking to yourself right now that there's no way you have enough material to create a substantial CV. You may also be worried that you may not be strong enough in certain areas of your CV. We certainly don't condone including fictitious or embellished accomplishments (more on that later in the chapter), but if you stop for a minute and think about all of the things you've done in pharmacy school, we're pretty sure you'll come up with some great material for a CV. Don't stress too much about being everything to everyone on paper. Research in the area of CVs and employability scores shows that strengths in two of three areas (work experience, academic qualifications, and extracurricular activities) achieve similar employability scores as strengths in all three areas.[1] Thus, we encourage you to play up your strengths and not worry about making up for areas of potential weakness. That's why you're doing a residency, to grow and improve, right?

WHAT'S IN A CV?

By the time you are approaching residency, you should realize that there are lots of gray areas in pharmacy. Gone are the days of a majority of black and white answers. Diving into the gray is what a residency is all about. Similarly, there are lots of "gray" areas when it comes to creating CVs. Even the different categories of information included in CVs can vary greatly. When you are graduating from pharmacy school and applying for a residency or other positions, there are "must have" sections for your CV as outlined in Table 7-1. These sections are also described in more depth below in a possible order to be placed on your CV. Keep in mind that there is no correct placement for information, but that things should flow logically.

There is some room for tailoring the document to your experience and the program you are applying to; however, there are items outlined in Table 7-2 that should not be included in your CV. The text below and the FAQs section touch on some of the "gray" areas that generate questions for pharmacy school graduates and give you some things to think about. Keep in mind that there are no "right" answers when deciding what to include on your CV. You may need to modify the content of your CV for different job or residency applications.

TABLE 7-1 • **Strongly Suggested Sections to Include on a Resident Candidate CV**

Personal Information	Licensure & Certification
Education	Work Experience
IPPE/APPE Rotations	Leadership Experience
Honors & Awards	Service
Publications	Presentations
Organization Memberships	Meeting Attendance
References	

TABLE 7-2 · Items to Avoid on a CV

Date of Birth	Redundant or excessive descriptions
Social Security Number	Hobbies
Classes taken in Pharmacy School	High School Activities

Personal Information

The contact information that is listed in your CV is a KEY way through which potential residency programs have to get in touch with you. Therefore, it's imperative that you include contact information that is accurate. Leading with your personal information at the top of page 1 is vital so that it is easy to find. Include your full, formal name and mailing address where you reliably receive mail. A phone number where you are most readily contacted is also advisable. You may wish to include a daytime and evening phone number or your cell phone number if that's the only telephone you have. Be sure that your voice mail greeting is appropriate and professional; this is not the time to play your favorite hip hop song in the background. Also be sure to check your voice mail messages regularly.

In today's digital world, email is generally the preferred method of communication, so make sure the email address on your CV is valid and that you're actually checking that account. If you use an email address associated with your school of pharmacy, be sure that the email account will continue to be valid during your APPE rotations and after graduation so that you don't miss any important information. If you have concerns about your university email account, there are several free, Web-based email programs to choose from and you can then access your email anywhere. Remember to be professional when you are creating a free email account. While it may be difficult to create a unique account with your name included, don't resort to something so creative that it sounds unprofessional. Once you have submitted your residency application materials, it's imperative that you check your email account at least daily so that you are responding to any follow-up messages in a timely fashion. Whenever you submit your application to a program, make sure the RPDs email address is in your safe sender's list.

Licensure and Certifications

Information to include in this section will vary based on whether you are applying to Postgraduate Year One (PGY-1) or Postgraduate Year Two (PGY-2) programs. For PGY-1 programs, if applicable, provide intern licenses for states in which you hold a licensure or certificate. This will communicate the level of familiarity you have with practice in those states. For PGY-2 programs, include your state(s) of pharmacist licensure, along with license number, current status (active, expired, emeritus, etc.), and date of expiration (if active). You may also highlight certificates of completion for programs you may have participated in, such as immunization delivery, or certifications such as basic life support. Make sure to avoid the error of confusing something as a "certificate" versus a "certification." Certificates indicate completion of a course with a specific focus. A certification indicates mastery via an assessment process that is based on a set of standards established by a standard-setting body.

Education

Your CV should provide a very brief outline of the educational institutions you attended after high school. The name, location, area of study, degrees obtained/anticipated or areas of study (such as prepharmacy studies when undergraduate degrees are not obtained), and dates of such degrees/areas of study should be included here. If applying for a PGY-2 program, you may also include your PGY-1 residency program information in this section. The same information should be included for your PGY-1 residency, but should also include your RPD's name and the name of your residency project. Should you be applying for a PGY-2, you may wish to follow this section with a separate section of information related to your PGY-1 rotations, analogous to the Introductory Pharmacy Practice Experience (IPPE) and Advanced Pharmacy Practice Experience (APPE) rotations format discussed below. Alternatively, you may include residency training in its own section.

Work Experience

Work experience, in addition to educational experiences, is a great way to show that you have additional skills and awareness beyond the pharmacy school curriculum. By the time you are applying to residency, it is possible that you've held many positions from high school work all the way through college. While pharmacy experiences are likely to be the most relevant, don't automatically discard other experiences rooted in service industries or research that may introduce skills utilized in residency. Use your judgment on what or how many to include. Including 12 different service industry jobs may be a bit overwhelming. Work experience should include those experiences you apply for or where one receives a stipend. Volunteer work, because of the altruistic nature and philanthropy it represents, should be included in its own section.

Again, consistency is key. For each of your work experiences include the name and location of your employer, name of position held, and dates of employment. A common question to consider is whether or not to include a description of duties. Sometimes less is more on a CV. With many to look through in an application cycle, you have to consider what you want RPDs to focus on. Including descriptions of duties that are generally well known for the position (e.g., pharmacy intern or technician positions) held takes time to read and may be redundant. If you think that what you did or learned in the position is unique and stands out, you may wish to include a brief description. Using bullet points may be advisable to keep the description succinct. Alternatively, if the duty could be considered another position, you may wish to include it as another separate work experience with new position name.

Rotations

The Accreditation Council for Pharmacy Education (ACPE) requirements for IPPEs and APPEs, also known as rotations, have changed significantly in recent years. In addition, IPPEs and APPEs look very different from school to school. As you graduate from pharmacy school, it is important in your CV that you at least include the names of the rotations you've completed and where you completed them. Should you be applying for a PGY-2, including your PGY-1 rotations is advisable. You may also consider deleting student rotations from your CV should you be applying for a PGY-2.

A CV may include the names of the preceptors for each rotation. This could potentially work for or against you as a candidate. We know you've heard that pharmacy is a very small world. RPDs, interviewers, and potential employers may use their connections to get more information about you or gather perspectives about your performance while on their rotation. Think of how you can use these connections to your advantage and think about them with intention when you are doing rotations. Often, RPDs may know your preceptor just from the name of the site and type of rotation. Pharmacy is a small world! Again, consistency is critical. It may look awkward to a RPD if you have some preceptor names listed for some rotations and not all.

> "The pharmacy world is a small one. I realized this when an interviewer told me he was a classmate and co-resident of two of my preceptors and asked me what they would say about me if he talked to them!"
>
> *Vi D. – Pharmacy Student, Texas*

Another common CV concern is whether to include descriptions of what you did on each rotation. As you approach graduation, detailed information about your IPPE rotations is probably not necessary. However, descriptions of daily responsibilities, projects, patient cases, or journal clubs that you completed during your APPE year may directly pertain to the residency you're applying for. This information can also help demonstrate the rigor of your APPE rotations.

Leadership Experience

Roach and Belling defined leadership as "the process of influencing an organized group toward accomplishing its goals."[2] Where and when have you done this in your professional development? Cast a wide net in your consideration of what counts. Whether involving an elected, assigned, or voluntary role, RPDs want to see this practice so it can be furthered and applied in their organization and our profession. Consider situations where you have been an officer in pharmacy organizations, led a service initiative, or otherwise were responsible for organizing a group of individuals to get a job done. Casting this wider net of leadership, including a title that describes the leadership experience, organization it was affiliated with, and time frame for involvement will complete this section. If you think of situations where you did some, but not all of the parts of leadership, consider the situation as something to describe in the service section.

Honors and Awards

With not a lot of room for lengthy descriptions in a CV, we often depend on the reputation of honors and awards bestowed upon us to communicate the caliber of our work and efforts. With only a few exceptions (such as being Eagle Scout, for example), these honors and awards should be those gained since beginning of your college career. Scholarships, awards, and certificates of achievement should be named along with the recognizing organization and date it was bestowed to you.

Service

Service activities are often considered in one of two ways. While philanthropic activities of a volunteer nature in the community often come to mind first, activities for one's school, professional organizations, and workplaces that are volunteer in nature can also be considered service. For example, providing education on a disease state at a church, working at a soup kitchen, or mentoring a child is easy to categorize as service activities. Make sure to also think about things such as giving tours during pharmacy school interviews, sitting on panel discussions, or sitting on task forces and committees. Many service roles, while volunteer in nature, may also be considered leadership experiences by nature of the position held or work that you do. In these cases, it may be advisable to list these roles under a "Leadership Experience" section of your CV. Be careful to only list experiences and activities once, rather than in multiple sections of your CV.

Publications

While there are many elements of a CV RPDs expect to see, a list of publications an applicant has authored can be a distinguishing section.

> "Clinical research and poster presentations are great extra-curricular activities to complete during rotations. It looks great on a resume, and is a great talking-point at interviews."
>
> *Samantha P. – Pharmacy Student, Alabama*

Seeing any type of publication on the CV of an applicant is evidence to a RPD of your ability to communicate, process, and apply information, manage time and workload and work with others. You will do many projects during your residency and writing is likely to be a significant component of many of these projects. In addition, many programs expect that your residency project should be written in a way that makes it suitable for submission as a manuscript.

While you've learned about the weight that certain papers carry based on study design and journal they appear in, you'll want to broaden your horizons for what counts in this section. Ask yourself, "Has anybody seen this work I have written and potentially used it for some purpose?" The following categories include what may count as publications that you may think about including in your CV.

- Articles appearing in or submitted to national and state professional journals
- Published abstracts
- Articles in practice site or student organization newsletters, periodicals, or supplements that are related to healthcare topics
- Reports that pull together information to share with others such as formulary reports or topic reviews
- Audiovisual productions that communicate a message

Consistency in citing publications is vital to maintain flow and organization of your CV. Consider using a standard reference guide such as the *American Medical Association Manual of Style*. Should you have a variety of publications in several categories, you may wish to group similar things under a subheading that represents the article type.

Presentations

Presentations are another way of showing your ability to both process and apply knowledge as well as communicate to others. Determining which presentations to include can be a "gray" area, because you have potentially given a lot of presentations throughout the course of your pharmacy school career. Since you are now at the point of applying for postgraduate training or employment, it is probably time to pare down that list to only include significant presentations. You should always include invited presentations and presentations given outside of your required pharmacy school curriculum. Presentations delivered during APPEs are also relevant to your residency application. Again, be prepared to speak to anything you include on your CV. If you can't remember the main points of your presentation, it's probably best to leave it off of your CV. If you have participated in poster presentations that did not include a published abstract, you may wish to include that presentation in this section as well.

Organization Memberships

In addition to the achievement of specific learning objectives related to knowledge and skill, residency education also focuses on shaping attitudes and instilling professional pride. A great way to introduce your professional pride is via the professional, fraternal, and honorary organizations you have joined. In addition to professional associations, you may wish to include fraternity membership, honor societies, and civic or community groups. Feel free to expand beyond the realm of your profession, as you never know what can make a connection. However, if membership in an organization was short-lived or long ago and no longer relevant in your life, it may be best to avoid these.

Typically, the organization name and dates of membership are the only information included in this section. If you wish to showcase leadership positions and experiences, it is best to do this in a "Leadership Experiences" section.

Professional Meetings

Professional meetings are a great way to network and learn about current pharmacy issues as a candidate. If you have attended several meetings during pharmacy school, including a listing of them can help demonstrate your involvement and dedication to the profession. However, remember that anything on your CV is fair game during an interview. If you only attended a meeting because it was in a warm climate, you might not want to include it on your CV. Be sure that you can speak to at least one session or event you attended for each meeting.

References

One of two options exists for addressing references. The shortest is the line "Available upon request." The alternative is to list the names, positions, and contact information (address, phone, email) of your references. It is safest to use "Available upon request." You may wish to list certain people for certain positions you are applying for based on familiarity with practices or programs. If you choose to streamline the process and include your references up front, be sure that the people you have listed know that you are listing them and know what kind of position you're applying for. As their contact information can change, ensure that this is current. Regardless of whether you include this information in your CV or not, it is good to keep a list updated and ready to go should there be a reference request.

CV STYLE AND FORMATTING CONSIDERATIONS

If you asked to look at 10 different pharmacists' CVs, you will undoubtedly see 10 very different documents. There will be differences in formatting, layout, and content and none of them will be "wrong." While there's not one "right" way to create your CV, there are some definite do's and don'ts. Very little in the world of a pharmacist is black and white, and we mentioned earlier in the chapter how "gray" the creation of a CV can be. Patient care decisions are contingent upon a variety of factors, and the creation of your CV will also have you following a similar decision-making process. You do have a lot of latitude in how your CV looks and feels, but the items mentioned below are an absolute must!

Proofread Your CV carefully!

Your final CV document will probably be filled with names of preceptors, pharmacy rotation sites, and medications you've given presentations on. None of these names will be caught via the spell check function on your computer, so it's imperative that you carefully read your CV. RPDs are looking for candidates who are detail-oriented, and nothing will turn them off faster than a CV with typos. It's also especially embarrassing if you are applying for a residency at an institution where you've completed rotations and you spell a preceptor's name incorrectly. CV documents should always include full, formal names of institutions and individuals. In addition, your name and the names of preceptors should include their credentials. Be sure that the credentials you include are accurate for each individual. If you're not sure whether your critical care preceptor is BCPS-certified or not, ask first! You never want to shortchange the work that people have put into their careers; and on the other hand you don't want to incorrectly represent their accomplishments.

Another potentially error-prone aspect of CVs is all of the dates that are included in the document. You will have rotation dates, presentation dates, meeting attendance dates, dates of honors and awards you've received, and so on. Be sure to check all of the dates in your CV carefully so that they're accurate. You'll also need to make sure that items are listed in reverse chronological order (more on this later in the chapter).

> "Ask several mentors to read through your CV. Pick mentors with different backgrounds and experiences—they may offer different advice! For example, pick a professor at your pharmacy school, a clinical preceptor, and a pharmacy manager you work for."
>
> *Huda Marie K.   Pharmacy Student, Illinois*

Be Consistent

Nothing drives a detail-oriented, obsessive–compulsive pharmacist crazier than inconsistencies. The very nature of CVs makes them prone to individual differences, but we want to point out several areas where consistency helps make your CV more readable and appealing to the reader.

Proper punctuation is incredibly important in areas of written communication. It helps ensure your ideas and thoughts are conveyed to the reader (in this case, the person who is going to select you for a residency!) and makes it easier for the reader to understand the document. In a CV, consistency is key! If you choose to put periods at the end of your bulleted statements, be sure to use periods throughout your document. If you choose to put a colon after each subheading, make sure that those colons appear after every subheading. Consistency in spacing and justifications is also key. Whether you want one or two spaces after a bullet point, make sure it looks good and is consistent.

The font you use on your CV is the first thing potential employers see when they pick up the document. A professional CV is not the place to experiment with fancy fonts. It is also not a document that you want to use multiple fonts in. Pick an easy-to-read font (Times New Roman or Arial are always good) and use that same font throughout your CV. You will likely use different sizes of the font to emphasize headings and subheadings throughout the document, but there is no need to use more than one font. The font used for the main portions of your CV should be large enough to read easily, but not so big that it looks unprofessional. Font sizing is also dependent on the type of font used, so be sure to print out a copy of your CV and give it a test read before sending it to anyone. Times New Roman and Arial fonts in sizes 10 or 12 are good places to start. Some headings may be in a slightly larger font, but again remember that you don't want portions of your CV to overwhelm the page.

Along those same lines, keep the use of font "fanciness" to a minimum. Special effects such as bolding, italics, and underlining can be useful in differentiating important aspects of your CV, but they must be used judiciously. Too much use of the bold effect makes it difficult for a reader to decide what's really important. Similarly, underlining helps important headings stand out, but can be difficult to read when embedded in a paragraph.

Bullet points are a great tool to use in a CV. They can help delineate important information for the reader and help you, as a writer, limit the information presented to the most pertinent aspects. The bullet point formatting that you use should again be easy-to-read and professional. The CV that you use to apply to pharmacy residencies should not use smiley faces or other cutesy bullet point markers. Be careful! Word processing programs can sometimes automatically format bullet points in inconsistent or awkward ways. Keep things simple and professional (a solid black dot will suffice) and use the same marker throughout the document. There is no need to use a different bullet point marker in each different section of your CV.

Once you start writing, it will be tough to know when your CV is "long enough." There is no page number limit on a CV, but be cognizant of the fact that someone else is responsible for reading the document and understanding everything you have included. With this in mind, keep the formatting of your CV as easy-to-read as possible. There is no need to stretch out or space information to make the CV longer. It's a good idea to maintain 1-inch margins on all sides of your document so that there is adequate "white space" on each page. This helps make the CV attractive to look at and is also a place for interviewers to make notes. There is no need to use smaller margins just to make your CV a few pages shorter. Also, be sure that the margins that you use are the same on all of the pages in your CV document.

Make Your CV Easy to Read

Items within CVs are generally presented in reverse chronological order. This means that your most recent jobs, rotations, and accomplishments are listed first in each section. When you are updating your CV, keep in mind that the new information you are entering should likely go at the beginning of each section. Each section of your CV needs to maintain this reverse chronological format.

Many CVs will include a header and/or footer on pages after the first page of the document. You can consider including information such as your name, date of the CV, page number, or the words "Curriculum Vitae." Often this information is helpful to the reader if the document is very long or if the pages happen to get separated.

Headings and subheadings are a great way to make your CV easier to read. See the sample CVs provided with this chapter to get an idea of formatting.

However, within each of these headings are the opportunities for various subheadings. For example, presentations could be further subdivided into invited presentations, posters, and/or abstracts. Subheadings can help the reader focus on areas most pertinent to the job you are applying for or areas they are most interested in.

WHAT DOES A "GOOD" CV LOOK LIKE?

The definition of a "good" CV can vary widely from reader to reader. We hope that we have provided you with some general guidance in the previous sections and that you now understand where individual variations can come into play. Example CVs for a pharmacy student applying to residency can be found in Figures 7-1 and 7-2. Figure 7-3 provides a sample CV for a PGY-1 resident who is seeking a PGY-2 residency. Figure 7-1 also includes callout boxes to highlight things to consider when designing your CV and also things to avoid. You'll note the CVs are different with regard to formatting, but the overall look of them is appropriate, with a good balance of words and white space to increase readability. Information is presented logically and the use of bullet points directs the reader to what is most important.

UPDATE YOUR CV FREQUENTLY

Your CV is a document that you will use for the rest of your career. That means it's something you're going to have to live with for the next 30 to 40 years (or longer!), so it's important to make sure it's accurate and kept up-to-date. Starting early, even as early as your first year of pharmacy school, and updating often are key to success! It is a great idea to get in the habit of updating your CV on a regular basis. This strategy will help you remember important things to include on your CV and help eliminate the possibility that you forget to include items such as publications, awards or scholarships, and the names of your preceptors or supervisors. You're also more likely to forget important items if you're rushing to submit an updated CV before an application deadline.

> "Update your CV regularly! You never know when someone is going to ask for it."
>
> *John M. – Pharmacy Resident, Wisconsin*

During your first years of education, updating your CV at the end of each semester or quarter is advisable. As a student or resident, an easy thing to do is to update your CV at the end of each rotation. That way the rotation is fresh in your mind and it should be a quick process to include your responsibilities and accomplishments. After you graduate, there are fewer defined time periods in your life that make finding a good time to update your CV a bit more challenging. The timing for updates may depend on the nature of your work. It is advisable to update your CV at least once per year, so perhaps an important annual date can be your trigger (e.g.,

CAROLINE E. MOLNAR

While it helps the candidate's name stand out, this font is difficult to read and does not have the same feel as the rest of the document. Arial or Times New Roman fonts are easier to read.

1551 Bricktown Road
Mequon, WI 53121
Telephone: 618.555.9515
E-Mail: [phoxypharm@email.com]

It's good to use a web-based email program that is easily accessible, but this email address (albeit very clever) portrays a very unprofessional image.

Education

September 2008–present

Doctor of Pharmacy Candidate
(anticipated completion May 2012)
Great Lakes School of Pharmacy
Mequon, WI

September 2002–May 2006

Bachelor of Science
Biochemistry
University of Great Lakes College of
Letters and Science
Madison, WI

[August 1998–May 2002

High School Diploma
City High School
Wrightstown, WI]

You are getting ready to graduate from pharmacy school. It is no longer necessary to include information from your high school days. It's assumed that if you've made it through pharmacy school, you also survived high school.

[Professional Experience]

May 2010–August 2010

Pharmacy Intern II
Health First Hospital
Milwaukee, WI
Supervisor: Rick Johnson, RPh, CDE

In this CV, Professional Experience that is directly related to the field of pharmacy is listed separately from Additional Work Experience, which may not be pharmacy-related.

- Participated in daily rounds with pharmacists and physicians
- Attended monthly staff and P&T Committee meetings
- Completed a drug use evaluation
- Reviewed patients' medication profiles and made appropriate recommendations
- Verified prescription orders and medication carts

June 2006–April 2010

Study Coordinator
Drug Metabolism and Bioanalytical
Services
Special Laboratories, Inc.
Madison, WI
Supervisor: John Tockmann, PhD

- Composed experimental protocols, amendments, and reports
- Coordinated the delivery of all necessary supplies prior to study start and shipment of all samples at study conclusion
- Monitored progress of all study phases
- Communicated results to external and internal study personnel and study sponsors at pharmaceutical companies

A footer is not needed on the first page of your CV since this information is included at the top of this document. However, headers and/or footers on subsequent pages with your name, page number, etc. can be invaluable if the pages get separated.

[Caroline E. Molnar]

Figure 7-1:
An Example CV for a PGY-1 Resident Candidate. Note the Common Do's and Don'ts Provided.

Advanced Pharmacy Practice Experiences

May 2012	Outpatient Pharmacy St. Mary's Medical Center Milwaukee, WI • [To be completed]
April 2012	General Internal Medicine St. Mary's Medical Center Milwaukee, WI • To be completed
March 2012	Community Pharmacy Health Maintenance Pharmacy Cedarburg, WI • To be completed
February 2012	Veterinary Pharmacy The Pet Store Plus Pewaukee, WI • To be completed
January 2012	Surgical Critical Care Health First Hospital Milwaukee, WI • To be completed

November 2011	Academia
	University of Great Lakes School of
	  Pharmacy
	Madison, WI
	Preceptors: Rebecca Peters, PharmD,
	  BCPS and Kelly Driggers,

MS, [RPh]	• Led small- and large-group discussions
	  for second- and third-year pharmacy
	  students
	• Presented pharmacotherapy skills and
	  counseling pearls to second- and third-
	  year pharmacy students
	• Developed on-line drug quizzes for
	  third-year pharmacy students
	• Graded drug information papers, quizzes
	  and group and individual assignments

[October 2011	Infectious Disease
	Great VA Medical Center
	Milwaukee, WI
	Preceptor: Dick Waters, RPh]
	
	• Monitored patient antibiotic regimens
	  for progress and appropriateness
	• Discussed therapeutic decisions with
	  medical team members
	• Attended daily rounds with infectious
	  disease staff
	• Participated in weekly meetings and
	  teaching sessions with pathology and
	  microbiology staff

Annotations:

A reader can tell by looking at the date of this experience that it is still to be completed. It is redundant to include this unnecessary statement. This section could also benefit from subheadings to identify completed and pending rotations.

OOPS! Carefully double-check your formatting to be sure that items like these credentials aren't dangling into the next line of text inadvertently.

Always keep the entire description of your experience on the same page. This could get very confusing if the pages were out of order.

Figure 7-1: *(continued)*

September 2011

Nutrition
Great VA Medical Center
Milwaukee, WI
Preceptor: Julie Watson, PharmD, [BCPS, BCNP]

- [Completed daily TPN monitoring forms.
- Made recommendations to nutrition staff for TPN adjustments.
- Attended daily rounds with nutrition staff.]

Be sure you know your preceptors' actual credentials when including them in your CV. This preceptor may or may not have both board certifications, but in either case, the correct abbreviation of the nutrition certification is BCNSP.

August 2011

Neonatal Intensive Care Unit
St. Luke's Regional Medical Center
Marshfield, WI
Preceptor: Zane Taylor, PharmD

- ♥ [Monitored antibiotic levels and made recommendations for appropriate dose changes
- ♥ Counseled new mothers regarding appropriate medication administration
- ♥ Developed a medication administration calendar to provide [too] new mothers
- ♥ Compounded formulations for neonatal patients]

Be consistent with the use of punctuation in your bullet points. This section includes periods at the end of each statement, but the periods are not included in other sections. Either include them for all bullet points or remove them from all.

Check your grammar carefully to avoid mishaps like this.

July 2011

Diabetes Care Clinic
St. Luke's Health Clinic
Racine, WI
[Preceptor: Doug Walker, RPh and Sally Allen, PharmD, BCACP]

As mentioned earlier, keep the formatting of your bullet point icons consistent throughout your CV. In addition, keep them simple and professional. Cute or funny icons may be viewed as unprofessional.

[Introductory Pharmacy Practice Experiences]

Great VA Medical Center	June 2009
Basic Pharmacy	June 2010
St. Luke's [Revional] Medical Center	June 2011

What happened here? All of the other APPE rotations include brief descriptions except this one. For consistency, you should include a description for all rotations or eliminate it for all rotations

Additional Work Experience

June 2003–August 2003

Summer Intern
United States Department of Agriculture
    Forest Service
Forestry Lab
Wrightstown, WI

- [Investigated the effects of growth conditions on photosynthetic enzyme rates in oak trees
- Maintained a red oak tree line]

The formatting in this section is totally different than the previous sections. Make sure you are consistent throughout your document. Reverse chronological order is the standard for CVs, so your most recent accomplishments or events should be listed first in a section.

[May 2005–May 2006

Bartender
The Regal Beagle
Madison, WI]

Presentations

November 2011

Pharmaceutical Care–Patient Interview Techniques

- Presented to second-year pharmacy students at Great Lakes School of Pharmacy

Watch your spelling carefully! It's easy to gloss over simple errors.

Watch your page breaks!

While this job is part of your work history, it's not really relevant to the career you are now pursuing. It's probably best to remove entries that are not relevant to the pharmacy field.

Figure 7-1: (*continued*)

October 2011	*[Antibiotic-Lock Technique for IV Line Infections]*
	• Presentation to pharmacy staff and pharmacy students at Great VA Medical Center
August 2011	*Respiratory Syncytial Virus Prophylaxis in Neonates*
	• Case presentation to pharmacists and pharmacy students at St. Luke's Regional Medical Center

> Font effects such as italics and underlining can help identify important elements of your CV. Be judicious in using these effects as combining too many makes the text hard to read and may make it difficult for the reader to discern what's really important.

[Elective Coursework]

Herbals, Dietary Supplements, and Homeopathy	Summer 2011
Selected Topics in Pharmacy Practice-Infectious Diseases	Spring 2011
A Team Approach to Emergency Care	
Fluids and Electrolyte Therapy	Fall 2010
Radiopharmaceuticals	
Non-Prescription Medications	

> This section is not necessary in a CV. If you want to highlight pertinent coursework when applying for a job or residency, do so in a cover letter.

[Professional Organizations and Activities]

November 2005–present	Participated in Great Lakes School of Pharmacy PharmD Admissions Committee meetings regarding candidate interview and profile review processes
Sep. 2002–present	Great Lakes Student Pharmacist Association (GLSPA)
	• Participated in MEDIC and Operation Diabetes
	• Attended monthly meetings
Sept. 2002–present	Wisconsin Society of Pharmacists
	• Attended 2005 PSW Annual Meeting in Madison, WI
	• Attended 2005 Legislative Day in Madison, WI
[September] 2002–present	American Pharmacists Association (APhA)
September 2002–present	American Society of Health-System Pharmacists (ASHP)
	• Attended 2005 Midyear Clinical Meeting and Exhibition in Las Vegas, NV
April 2005	Provided tours of the Great Lakes School of Pharmacy during a campus-wide open house
September 2003–May 2004	Minority Affairs Program in Pharmacy (MAPP)
	• Attended monthly meetings

> This section contains a lot of good information. If you have leadership positions that you wish to highlight, you can also do so in a separate section entitled "Leadership Experience".

> We can't say it enough... consistency is key! There are three different ways of showing the September date in this section alone. Pick one and use it throughout all of the sections of your CV.

> WHOOPS! Watch your formatting carefully so that all of the margins line up appropriately.

> It's great that this applicant has so many service activities to include on her CV. However, this section is difficult to read and she's using lots of different date formats. This may be the ideal place to use subheading to delineate professional service from church and/or community service.

Honors and Awards

September 2010	Miller Memorial Scholarship
[May 2010]	School of Pharmacy Honor Roll
September 2009	Pharmacy Alumni Association Scholarship
January 2009	Great Lakes School of Pharmacy Honor Roll
September 2008	Pharmacy Alumni Association Scholarship

[Service Activities]

August 2010–present	Pharmacy Mentor
	• [Mentored incoming pharmacy students.]

> This is a great example of redundancy in a CV. It's evident from the title of the position that these are the responsibilities. In this case, there's no need to elaborate further.

Figure 7-1: *(continued)*

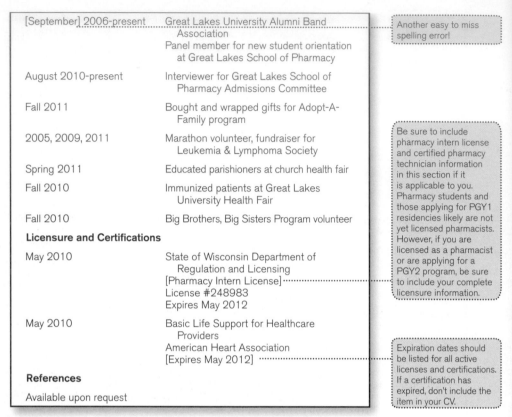

[September] 2006-present	Great Lakes University Alumni Band Association	*Another easy to miss spelling error!*
	Panel member for new student orientation at Great Lakes School of Pharmacy	
August 2010-present	Interviewer for Great Lakes School of Pharmacy Admissions Committee	
Fall 2011	Bought and wrapped gifts for Adopt-A-Family program	
2005, 2009, 2011	Marathon volunteer, fundraiser for Leukemia & Lymphoma Society	
Spring 2011	Educated parishioners at church health fair	
Fall 2010	Immunized patients at Great Lakes University Health Fair	
Fall 2010	Big Brothers, Big Sisters Program volunteer	

Be sure to include pharmacy intern license and certified pharmacy technician information in this section if it is applicable to you. Pharmacy students and those applying for PGY1 residencies likely are not yet licensed pharmacists. However, if you are licensed as a pharmacist or are applying for a PGY2 program, be sure to include your complete licensure information.

Licensure and Certifications

May 2010	State of Wisconsin Department of Regulation and Licensing [Pharmacy Intern License] License #248983 Expires May 2012
May 2010	Basic Life Support for Healthcare Providers American Heart Association [Expires May 2012]

Expiration dates should be listed for all active licenses and certifications. If a certification has expired, don't include the item in your CV.

References

Available upon request

Figure 7-1: (*continued*)

your birthday or Halloween). For people in positions where they deliver a lot of presentations or write many publications, a monthly or as the event happens update may be best to ensure one doesn't forget anything.

As the years pass by and a CV grows in length, you'll be faced with decisions about what to trim and what to keep in your CV. Getting in the habit of reflecting on what you've done and how it applies to the next step of your career/life is important to maintain brevity and focus of your CV. Looking down the road a bit, while certain elements should be carved in stone on your CV such as professional experiences, honors and awards, and publications; other topics will become less pertinent over time. For example, rotations as a student should be replaced by your residency rotations after you're done with residency education. After a couple of years of noninvolvement in service activities or membership in organizations, these may be removed as well.

USING YOUR CV–THE NEXT STEPS

It will take many drafts and reviews to get your CV to completion. Before attaching that CV to your residency application, you may wish to consider

JOHN R. BRIGGS

Current Address: 800 Williams St Apt. 2204
Columbia, SC 29201
Mobile Phone: (865) 555-8589
Email: JRBriggs@email.edu

Education

2008–Present	Lower South University College of Pharmacy Columbia, SC Doctorate of Pharmacy Anticipated Graduation May 2012
2006–2008	Lower South University Columbia, SC Pre-Pharmacy Coursework

Introductory Pharmacy Practice Experiences

June 2010	**Introductory Institutional** Practice 1st Hospital, Greenville, SC Preceptor: James Green, RPh
June 2009	**Introductory Community** Chain Pharmacy # 2399, Columbia, SC Preceptor: Donald Lopez, PharmD

Advanced Pharmacy Practice Experiences

Completed:

November 2011	**Ambulatory Care** Eastern South V.A. Medical Center, Columbia, SC Preceptor: Helen Adams, PharmD, CDE
October 2011	**Acute Care-Cardiology** Regional Cardiology, Columbia, SC Preceptor: Ron Baer, MSN, APRN, CCRN, NP-C, FNP-BC
September 2011	**Academic Pharmacy Elective** Lower South University Carolina College of Pharmacy, Columbia, SC Preceptor: Shirley Nelson, PharmD
August 2011	**Community Pharmacy** Special Clinic Pharmacy, Kahului, HI Preceptor: Matthew Carter, RPh
July 2011	**Acute Care-Psychiatry** Eastern South V.A. Medical Center, Columbia, SC Preceptor: Sarah King, PharmD, BCPS
May 2011	**Health Care Team: Drug Information** Southeast Health, Columbia, SC Preceptor: Virginia Turner, PharmD

To Be Completed:

April 2012	**Advanced Institutional** Southeast Health, Columbia, SC Preceptor: Edward Morgan, PharmD

Figure 7-2:
An Example CV for a PGY-1 Resident Candidate.

March 2012	**Acute Care- Pediatrics** Southeast Health, Columbia, SC Preceptor: Kenneth Rogerso, PharmD, BCPS
January 2012	**Acute Care-Infectious Disease** Eastern South V.A. Medical Center, Columbia, SC Preceptor: T. Perry Jones, PharmD, BCPS (AQ-ID)

Professional Experience

June 2006– Present	**Pharmacy Intern** ABC Pharmacy #7837 Columbia, SC Supervisor: Marcus Lopez, PharmD ABC Pharmacy # 7823 Greenville, SC Supervisor: Kevin Bailey, RPh

Research/Scholarship Experience

January 2011– Present	Johnson KL, Bookstaver PB, **Brown ML**, Bailey SS, Perry JK, Rogers KL, Peters SB. Role of raltegravir in HIV-1 management. Ann Pharm (Accepted in Press, December 2011).
April 2011– Present	**Brown ML**, Bookstaver PB, Johnson KL, Peters SB. Update on raltegravir and the development of new integrase strand transfer inhibitors. South Med J. (Decision pending/submitted December 2011).

Abstracts

December 2011	**Brown ML**, Rudisill CN, Bookstaver PB. Adverse events secondary to sulfamethoxazole/trimethoprim in hospitalized HIV-infected patients. Presented at the 46th ASHP Midyear Clinical Meeting & Exhibition; December 4-8, 2011, New Orleans, LA. (Abstract # I-243)
March 2011	**Brown ML**, Rudisill CN, Bookstaver PB, Johnson RR. Adverse drug events with sulfamethoxazole/trimethoprim in hospitalized patients. Presented at South Carolina Society of Health-System Pharmacists 2011 Annual Meeting; March 13-15, 2011, Hilton Head, SC. (Abstract # 10)

Published Abstracts

October 2011	**Brown ML**, Rudisill CN, Bookstaver PB. Adverse drug events secondary to sulfamethoxazole/trimethoprim in HIV-infected hospitalized patients. Pharmacotherapy 2011;31:429e [Presented at the American College of Clinical Pharmacy 2011 Annual Meeting; Pittsburgh, PA, October 16-19, 2011; #431]

Grant Submissions

October 2010	**Undergraduate Scholar Award** Lower South University, Office of Undergraduate Research. Adverse drug events with sulfamethoxazole/trimethoprim in hospitalized patients. Amount: $3,000 (Non-Funded)

Figure 7-2: *(continued)*

Selected Professional Presentations

March 2012	Vancomycin Dosing in an Obese Population Senior Grand Rounds Presentation To be presented to colleagues and faculty at the Lower South University College of Pharmacy Columbia, SC
July 2011	Polydipsia and Intermittent Hyponatremia in the Psychiatric Patient Presented to staff, residents and students Eastern South V.A Medical Center Columbia, SC
July 2011	Kratom (*Mitragyna speciosa korth*) Provided for the mental health and pharmacy departments Eastern South V.A. Medical Center Columbia, SC
July 2011	Migraine Headache Presenting as Bipolar Disorder Presented to mental health staff, residents and students Eastern South V.A Medical Center Columbia, SC
November 2009	Gardisil Informational Presentation Immunization Committee- APhA-ASP Presented to members of the Alpha Psi Omega Sorority Columbia, SC

Honors and Awards

Fall 2006, Fall 2007, 2008–present	**Lower South University Dean's Honor Roll**
Fall 2011	**John J. James Scholarship** St. Peter's Foundation, Greenville, SC
Spring 2010	**Top Ten Finalist** Academy of Student Pharmacists Local Patient Counseling Competition
August 2009–May 2012	**Pharmacy Alumni Scholarship**
Spring 2007	**Lower South University President's Honor Roll**
Fall 2006–Spring 2010	**South Carolina LIFE (Legislative Initiative for Future Excellence) Scholarship**

Professional Organizations/Leadership Experience

American Academy of HIV Medicine
    Student Member, 2011–present

American College of Clinical Pharmacy
    Student Member, 2011–present

American Pharmacists Association- Academy of Student Pharmacists
    Member, 2008–2011
    Heartburn Awareness committee Co-Chair, 2010-2011
    Patient Counseling Competition Participant 2010, 2011

Figure 7-2: (*continued*)

Phi Lambda Sigma Leadership Society
    Member, 2011–present
    Taking Charge of Your Life: The Ultimate Leadership Skills for Success
    Charleston, SC, January 2011

Kappa Psi Little Sisters
    Member, 2008–present
    Treasurer, 2009

Student Society of Health-Systems Pharmacists
    Member 2010–2011

Volunteer/Community Service Activities

December 2011   **Christmas Food Baskets**
                     Knight of Columbus Council, Southeastern, SC
                     Pack and delivery volunteer

July 2011   **Effects of Therapeutic Ultrasound in Delayed Onset
                     Muscle Soreness and Force Production Recovery
                     After Muscle Damage**
                     Lower South University
                     Study Subject

April 2011   **Dining with Friends Dessert Finale**
                     AIDS Benefit Foundation of South Carolina
                     Event Volunteer

April 2009, 2010   **Relay for Life**
                     Volunteer, Columbia, SC

October 2008,   **Walk For Life/Race for the Cure**
2009, 2010   Hospital Health Foundation, Columbia, SC

Other Activities and Interests

Lower South University Intramurals
    Coed Softball, 2008
    Coed Basketball, 2011

Certification, Training, and Licensure

2010–Present   **Pharmaceutical Care for Patients with Diabetes**
                     American Pharmacist Association

2010–Present   **Pharmacy Based Immunization Delivery**
                     American Pharmacists Association
                     Certified Immunizer

2010–Present   **Basic Life Support for Healthcare Providers**
                     American Heart Association

2009–Present   **Collaborative Institutional Training Initiative**
                     Biomedical Research Investigators: Basic Course

2008–Present   **Pharmacy Intern License No. 7893**
                     South Carolina Board of Pharmacy

References

Available upon request

Figure 7-2: (*continued*)

ANNA R. COX, PharmD

807-555-7905 (Mobile)   535 Sycamore Lane, Unit 654   arcox@webmail.edu
                          Charleston, SC 29407

Education

August 2007–May 2011   *Doctor of Pharmacy*
                         Royal West College of Pharmacy, Royal West University
                         Sacramento, California

August 2005–May 2007   *Pre-Pharmacy Coursework*
                         Royal West University
                         Sacramento, California

Post Doctorate Training

July 2011–Present   *Pharmacy Practice Residency (Post-Graduate
                            Year One)*
                         Medical University of California
                         Los Angeles, California
                         Residency Program Director: Brenda Ward, PharmD,
                            MSCR, BCPS

Licensure and Certification

Licensure

June 2011–Present   *Registered Pharmacist*
                         California; License #134365

June 2011–Present   *Registered Pharmacist*
                         Nevada; License #23237

Certification

July 2011–Present   *American Heart Association*
                         Advanced Cardiovascular Life Support

November 2010–Present   *American Pharmacists Association*
                         Pharmacy-Based Immunization Delivery Certification

April 2010–Present   *American Heart Association*
                         Basic Life Support for Healthcare Professionals
                            Certification

Rotation Experience

PGY1 Pharmacy Practice Experiences
Medical University of California; Los Angeles, California

June 2012   *Neurosurgical Intensive Care Unit*
                         Preceptor: Christopher Murphy, PharmD

May 2012   *Cardiothoracic Intensive Care Unit*
                         Preceptor: William Peterson, BS, PharmD

April 2012   *Pulmonary*
                         Preceptor: Nia Perez, PharmD, BCPS

March 2012   *Psychiatry*
                         Preceptor: Amy London, PharmD, BCPS

Figure 7-3:
An Example CV for a PGY-1 Resident Candidate.

February 2012	*Drug Information* Preceptor: Jorge Ramirez, PharmD
January 2012	*Transplant Surgery* Preceptor: Nancy Jones, PharmD, MSCR, BCPS
December 2011	*Transplant Clinic* Preceptor: Darrin Torres, PharmD, BCPS
November 2011	*Practice Management* Preceptor: Peter Sanders, PharmD, MBA
October 2011	*Transplant Nephrology* Preceptor: Sarah Stevens, PharmD, MSCR, BCPS
September 2011	*Pediatric Hematology/Oncology* Preceptor: Treater Phillips, PharmD, BCPS
August 2011	*General Pediatrics* Preceptor: Treater Phillips, PharmD, BCPS

Advanced Pharmacy Practice Experiences
South Carolina College of Pharmacy

April 2011	*Cardiology* Special Heart Hospital; Los Angeles, California Preceptor: Jon Robertson, PharmD
March 2011	*Advanced Institutional* Tops Health Children's Hospital; Sacramento, California Preceptor: Riley Jones, PharmD, BCPS
January 2011	*Infectious Diseases* California Special VA Medical Center; Sacramento, California Preceptor: J. Bradley Watson, PharmD, BCPS (AQ-ID)
November 2010	*Ambulatory Care* California Special VA Medical Center; Sacramento, California Preceptor: Jason Wong, PharmD, CDE
October 2010	*Pediatric Critical Care* Tops Health Children's Hospital; Sacramento, California Preceptor: Priya Patel, PharmD, BCPS
September 2010	*Oncology* Cancer Specialists; San Francisco, California Preceptor: Saurabh Gaya, PharmD
August 2010	*Academic* Royal West University College of Pharmacy; Sacramento, California Preceptor: Brandon Bookstaver, PharmD, BCPS (AQ-ID), AAHIVE
July 2010	*Advanced Community (Retail Independent)* Special Care Pharmacy; Van Nuys, California Preceptor: John Graham, RPh
May 2010	*Solid Organ Transplantation* Medical University of California; Los Angeles, California Preceptor: Brooks Griffin, PharmD, BCPS

Figure 7-3: *(continued)*

Professional Experience

July 2011–Present

Clinical Staff Pharmacist (Resident)
Medical University of California; Los Angeles, California
Supervisor: Donna Hayes, PharmD, BCPS

June 2010–May 2011

Pharmacy Intern
Special Drugs Pharmacy; Buena Vista, California
Supervisor: Jack Woods, PharmD

September 2008–
June 2010

Pharmacy Intern
Chain Pharmacy #2277; Los Angeles, California
Supervisor: Juanita Morales, PharmD

May 2007–August
2008

Pharmacy Intern
Chain Pharmacy #11663; Los Angeles, South Carolina
Supervisor: Sabrina Gomez, RPh

Scholarship

Publications

Cox AR, Johnson SS, Morales NM, Patel JM, Jones TD, Miller AD, Bookstaver PB. Use of alternative pharmacologic treatment strategies in the prevention and treatment of Clostridium difficile infection. International Journal of Infectious Diseases. 2011 Jul;15(7):e138–48.

Cox AR, Havita J. Secondary prophylaxis of pediatric stroke. Tops Health Children's Hospital PharmSTAT Jr. Newsletter. 2011;11(2):1–4.

Abstracts

Blackwell JP, **Cox AR**, Smith JR. Analysis of the use of paralytics in the intensive care unit setting. To be presented at the UHC Pharmacy Council Pharmacy Resident Poster Session; December 3, 2011; New Orleans, Louisiana

Cox AR, Bookstaver PB, Rudisill CN, Fong P. Impact of an infectious diseases pharmacist-driven stewardship initiative on medication errors in hospitalized human immunodeficiency virus (HIV)-infected patients.
Presented at the Southern California 2011 Annual Meeting; March 15, 2011; San Diego, California; Poster #17

Cox AR, Bookstaver PB, Rudisill CN, Fong P. Pharmacist-driven stewardship to reduce medication errors in HIV-infected patients
Presented at Royal West University Scholarship Day 2011; April 23, 2011; Sacramento, SC

Cox AR, Bookstaver PB, Rudisill CN, Fong P. Impact of an infectious diseases pharmacist-driven stewardship initiative on medication errors in hospitalized human immunodeficiency virus (HIV)-infected patients.
Presented at the 45th ASHP Midyear Clinical Meeting & Exhibition; December 11, 2010; Anaheim, California; Poster #4-210

Current Research

"Evaluation of pharmacist involvement in the transplant discharge process"
Preceptors: Juanita Morales, PharmD, MSCR, BCPS; RonFord, PharmD, BCPS; Carl Russell, PharmD, BCPS

"Analysis of the use of paralytics in the intensive care unit setting"
Co-investigators: Rickey Diaz, PharmD; James Griffin, PharmD
Preceptors: Ron Ford, PharmD, BCPS; Melissa Owens, PharmD, BCPS; William Cole, PharmD, BCPS

Figure 7-3: *(continued)*

"Use of antimicrobial lock solutions in pediatric patients: a review of the literature"
Preceptors: Brandon Bookstaver, PharmD, BCPS (AQ-ID), AAHIVE; Christina Piro, PharmD

Grants

"Impact of an infectious diseases pharmacist-driven stewardship initiative on medication errors in hospitalized human immunodeficiency virus (HIV)-infected patients."
Grant: Undergraduate Scholar Program
Total amount awarded: $1500
Funding agency: Royal West University Undergraduate Research Department
Mentors: Brandon Bookstaver, PharmD, BCPS (AQ-ID), AAHIVE; Celeste Rudisill, PharmD, BCPS

Journal Referees

Manuscript peer review for *Infection and Drug Resistance*
Preceptor: Brandon Bookstaver, PharmD, BCPS (AQ-ID), AAHIVE

Selected Presentations

"Maintenance Immunosuppression in Solid Organ Transplant Recipients"
Team teaching presentation; Presented to pharmacy students and residents; Medical University of California; Los Angeles, California; October 2011

"Overview of Common Pediatric Chemotherapeutic Agents"
Inservice; Presented to medical residents and students; Medical University of California; Los Angeles, California; September 2011

"Alemtuzumab as Induction Immunosuppression in Kidney Transplantation"
Seminar; Presented to pharmacists and pharmacy students; Royal West University; Sacramento, California; March 2010

"Have a Heart! The Pharmacist's Basic Guide to Heart Transplantation"
Topic presentation; Presented to clinical pharmacists, pharmacy residents, and pharmacy students; Best Health Hospital; Van Nuys, California; April 2011

"Infectious Diseases in Sports: An Important Player"
Topic presentation; Presented to pharmacists and pharmacy students; Best Health Hospital; Columbia, Van Nuys, California; January 2010

"Sickle Cell Disease"
Patient case and disease state presentation; Presented to clinical pharmacists, pharmacy residents, and pharmacy students; Best Health Hospital; Van Nuys, California; October 2010

"Ixempra® (Ixabepilone)"
Nursing inservice; Presented to oncology nurses, clinical pharmacists, and pharmacy students; California Cancer Center at Best Health Hospital; Van Nuys, California; September 2010

"Acute Promyelocytic Leukemia"
Patient case and disease state presentation; Presented to clinical pharmacists and pharmacy students; Royal West University College of Pharmacy Sacramento, California; September 2010

Figure 7-3: *(continued)*

Awards and Honors

May 2011	*Summa Cum Laude graduate;* Royal West University College of Pharmacy
May 2011	*Teva Pharmaceuticals USA Students Award;* Royal West University College of Pharmacy
April 2011	*Undergraduate Research Day Poster Presentation Award;* Health & Medical Science division; Royal West University College of Pharmacy
Fall 2005–May 2011	*President's List,* Royal West University College of Pharmacy
2009–2010	*Jorge Reynolds Pharmacy Scholarship, Royal West University* College of Pharmacy
Spring 2009	*The Rho Chi Award, Royal West University College of Pharmacy* (Highest GPA after three semesters of professional coursework)
2008–2009	*Robert Fisher Pharmacy Scholarship, Royal West University* College of Pharmacy
2005–2009	*National Merit Scholar,* Royal West University
2005–2009	*Woods Scholar,* Royal West University
2005–2009	*California Fellows Scholar,* Royal West University

Professional Affiliations

September 2010–Present	*American College of Clinical Pharmacy* Clinical Pharmacy Challenge, Campus-Level Participant, Fall 2010
August 2009–Present	*American Society of Health-System Pharmacists,* Member Clinical Skills Competition, Campus-Level Participant, Fall 2010
March 2010–May 2011	*The American Academy of HIV Medicine,* Student Member
April 2009–April 2011	*Royal West University Student Government Association* Student Senator for the College of Pharmacy; Academics Committee member
May 2009–May 2011	*The Rho Chi Society,* Member
May 2008–May 2011	*Phi Beta Kappa,* Member
August 2007–May 2011	*American Pharmacists Association – Academy of Student Pharmacists,* Member
Fall 2007	*Kappa Epsilon Professional Fraternity,* Member

References

upon request

Figure 7-3: (*continued*)

one more thing. RPDs, while looking for strengths in considering you as an applicant, will also be looking for things they wish to explore further. They will function like an offensive coordinator looking for gaps in a defense to attack. Look at your CV. Have others look at your CV. Answer the question, where are my "gaps." What can be questioned or explored further in an interview? For example, you have a bunch of great service activities during your undergraduate years, however, there is very little listed during pharmacy school. A RPD may look at that and wonder why the gap. Was school too difficult to be able to do this service or does the applicant really not like service anymore? At this point, can you think of a valid answer to their concern or do you hope they never ask the question in the first place? If the latter is true, you may wish to delete some activities from your CV. Otherwise, get your defense in good working order and get ready to play!

Developing your CV and submitting it for a residency position is only the first step. By this time, we hope you have developed something that, in the context of your experiences, does the job to get you in the door for a residency interview. In this next step, it is important not to forget about your CV, but to use it with intention when discussing your qualifications, experiences, and fit for the residency. The interview is no time to be modest and talking about yourself can be difficult for some people. In these times, it is important to lean back on your CV as the framework for addressing questions and making statements. After you've exposed yourself to or thought about the questions you'll be asked, think about your experiences on those CV pages. Make connections to these documented and easily referenced items. Show directors that you can reflect on the meaning and implications of what you've done as it relates to your continuous professional development. Be prepared to talk about how that ambulatory care rotation you did that sparked your interest in the content and patient interactions you wish to further pursue in an ambulatory setting. Use the CV to ask questions of your own. For example, if you helped out at a free clinic and wish to do that again, be prepared to talk about what you did and what the experience meant to you to frame the question of if you can do that sort of activity as a part of or complementary to your residency program. The depth of thinking and evidence of progressing development will be likely to impress!

ADDITIONAL RESOURCES

It is important to use resources when developing your CV. The most important of these is a set of close confidants that know you well who can proofread and help you ensure completeness. In addition, a career mentor may provide some valuable insights to help you develop and use your CV. A plethora of other resources exist, but given the many different formats and opinions on what could be in a CV, it is important to solicit input from those that know you well. Below is an outline of resources you may use, request at your school or explore further.

Professional Meetings

Student organizations or national and state professional societies will often hold career development workshops where they will discuss CV development. Watch for these events at meetings of these groups to gain perspectives from workshop facilitators and participants.

Web Sites

The content on the Internet for CVs is pretty general. Given the more specific nature of pharmacists' activities, it may be advisable to use templates and samples on the Web to get an idea for how people format their CVs.

University Resources

Sometimes our best resources are closer than we think. Many universities have career centers that may provide counseling and tools to help in your CV development. Additionally, writing centers on campus may provide assistance with proofreading and general writing skills.

Chapter Takeaways

- ▶ A CV is document used extensively in health professions to describe your career history of education, employment, accomplishments, and involvement.

- ▶ There are no "right" answers when deciding what to include on your CV. The content may vary for different job or residency applications.

- ▶ The content of your CV will evolve and change over time. Updating your CV on a regular basis is imperative and helps prevent the task from becoming too daunting.

- ▶ There is not a "right" way to create a CV, but you must always proofread a CV carefully, be consistent with the little details throughout the document, and make your CV easily readable by others.

- ▶ Look for gaps in your CV and be prepared to answer questions about them.

- ▶ Mentors can be valuable resources in reviewing the content of your CV, proofreading the document, and highlighting important areas of emphasis.

- ▶ Be prepared to discuss anything on your CV in detail.

ROLE OF THE MENTOR

Proofing—Asking your mentor to be one of the many people you should ask to review your CV is a possibility. Make sure they aren't the only ones though, because your mentor's knowledge of activities may lead them to easily skip over errors because they know you did them and expect to see them on your CV.

Content review—Depending on when you draft your CV and how often you update it, you may miss some things. Having a mentor that knows what you've done may result in identifying some things you may have forgotten in a draft.

Talking off your CV—Ask your mentor what they would "play up" or highlight from your CV if they were in your shoes. In addition, your mentor can play the role of prospective RPD and ask you questions or clarify discrepancies.

Reassurance—Having a mentor provide a thorough review of and discuss your CV may be most helpful to your self-esteem and belief in yourself as an attractive residency candidate.

FREQUENTLY ASKED QUESTIONS

Q: Should I list my grade point average?

A: One of the most common questions we hear when students are starting their CV is whether they are required to include their grade point average (GPA) somewhere in the document. If you have a very good GPA from pharmacy school, it is certainly appropriate to include this information. However, if you would prefer that an interviewer or potential employer focus on your leadership skills and involvement in professional organizations, it may be prudent to leave this information off. If you do choose to include your GPA, it is a good idea to also include the scale that your GPA is measured on (e.g., 3.86/4.00). Not all pharmacy schools use 4.0 scales and including this information up front prevents the reader from interpreting the value incorrectly. Consistency is also key. Don't list your undergraduate GPA and exclude your pharmacy school GPA.

Q: Should I include a career objective statement?

A: While a career objective statement may provide additional input in to why you're doing what you're doing and provide a framework for the history of you that is reported in your CV, career objectives can look boring if safely stated or potentially be misinterpreted if boldly stated. In addition, most programs ask you to include a cover letter that provides the opportunity to detail your intent and rationale for applying to this program. With the space confines and the need to be concise in a CV, the cover letter may be the more optimal location to discuss your career objective.

Q: What presentations should I list?

A: Since you are now at the point of applying for postgraduate training or employment, it is probably time to pare down that list to only include significant presentations. You should always include invited presentations and presentations given outside of your required pharmacy school or residency curriculum. Presentations delivered during APPEs are also relevant to your residency application.

Q: **Should I list my references on the CV?**

A: It is generally not necessary to include contact information for your references in your CV. Most frequently, this section of a CV contains a statement suggesting that the information is available upon request. If you choose to streamline the process and include your references up front, be sure that the people you have listed know that you are listing them and know what kind of position you're applying for. As their contact information can change, ensure that this is current.

Q: **Should I include languages that I speak in my CV?**

A: Your CV is not the place to include personal information, and this can include items such as languages that you speak. Depending on the position or residency that you are applying for, this information may be very relevant to your application. A cover letter is the ideal place to describe languages (other than English) that you are fluent in. You should never include languages that you only know minimally or cannot speak fluently.

Q: **Should I include the date my CV was last updated?**

A: Typically, employers expect that the CV you are submitting was just updated before it was submitted. You could include this because potential employers may hang on to CVs and review them again when positions open up. When they do, it may be nice to have something there to remind them when it was last updated. Should you include this piece of information, make sure it is in a location that you won't forget to update. If you wish to know when your CV was last updated, use a file name that indicates the date updated.

Q: **Should my special computer skills be included in my CV?**

A: The profession of pharmacy is highly dependent on technology. Many pharmacy school graduates have significant experience with statistical software, electronic medical records, or other relevant computer hardware and software. This information may be important for your individual residency application (especially if you are applying for a PGY-2 specialty residency in pharmacy informatics), but it is better housed in your cover letter. This strategy also allows you to describe these skills in more detail during an interview.

Q: **How do I represent my APPE rotations since they will only be partially completed by the time I need to apply for residency?**

A: As you apply for residency, it's important to include your APPE rotation information. RPDs will look to this section of your CV to gauge the depth and breadth of your experiential education and determine your areas of interest. Even though you will not have completed your APPE year when you apply for residencies, it's important to include as much information as you know about the upcoming rotations. This is the perfect time to use subheadings. For example, you could title this section of your CV "Experiential

Education" and then have subheadings of "Planned Advanced Pharmacy Practice Experiences" and "Completed Advanced Pharmacy Practice Experiences." Just be sure to maintain your reverse chronological format and review the planned rotations frequently in case your rotations change unexpectedly.

Q: The residency program I am applying to wants me to email my CV to them. What is the best way to do this?

A: Undoubtedly you will create your CV electronically using a version of Microsoft Word or some other word processing software. However, there are almost as many versions of Microsoft Word as there are ways to write a CV. In addition, firewalls and other computer security measures within health systems may prevent suspicious documents from successfully being emailed. An ideal way to electronically send your CV is as a pdf document. These documents can be viewed almost universally on any computer. This file type also helps to ensure that the formatting you've worked so hard on is maintained in the final copy that your prospective employer views. There are many Web sites available to convert a Microsoft Word document into a pdf file...just type "free pdf converter" into your favorite search engine and pick your favorite site. Recent versions of Microsoft software now have the option to save documents as a pdf.

Q: Should I put my match number on my CV?

A: While making sure a potential RPD is aware of your match number is a good thing, this is not something we would suggest putting on your CV. Since your CV represents more of a lifetime of work and accomplishments, the listing of something you only use for the purpose of identification in the match system isn't consistent. In addition, it may be one of those things you forget to take off your CV. The letter of intent is a place where information specific to your application, such as your match number, may be included.

References

1. Cole MS, Rubin RS, Field HS, Giles WF. Recruiters' perceptions and use of applicant resume information: Screening the recent graduate. App Psych. 2007;56(2):319–343.

2. Roach CF, Behling O. *Functionalism: Basis for Alternate Approach to the Study of Leadership*. Elmsford, NY: Pergamon; 1984:36.

Recruitment Activities at Professional Meetings 8

Heather M. Draper

MEETINGS OF PROFESSIONAL PHARMACY ORGANIZATIONS

Your decision is as good as final—you are going to pursue postgraduate pharmacy training. You've been asking around a bit, and word on the street is that the American Society of Health-System Pharmacists Midyear Clinical Meeting (ASHP MCM) is *the* place to be if you're planning to do a pharmacy residency or fellowship. And now that you've made your decision to pursue residency training, you may feel like you are right back at the beginning again, trying to figure out if there's a professional pharmacy organization meeting you should attend. There are numerous opportunities and benefits associated with attending a meeting, particularly as you begin your search for a postgraduate training.

First, a few notes about what to expect at a meeting. When you attend a meeting, you can expect to be able to attend presentations, networking opportunities, exposition halls, student competitions, and advocacy and policy sessions. Meetings offer numerous programming opportunities designed to assist you in preparing for and pursuing postgraduate training programs, such as guidance for preparing your curriculum vitae (CV), preparing for residency interviews, and participating in the Residency Match. Networking is perhaps one of the most important aspects of professional pharmacy meetings, as it allows you to begin developing relationships with colleagues, learn about pharmacy practice trends, and discuss critical issues facing pharmacy practice. Most meetings offer numerous opportunities, formal and informal, for pharmacy students and pharmacy residents to network with each other and with practitioners in various fields of pharmacy practice.

THE ROLE OF PROFESSIONAL PHARMACY ORGANIZATION MEETINGS IN THE RESIDENCY RECRUITMENT AND SELECTION PROCESS

Professional pharmacy organization meetings are a critical step in the residency selection and recruitment process, both for the candidate and the program. Meetings offer you the opportunity to meet and speak with numerous training programs in a single location over a specified period of time. Meetings allow you to cast a wide net and explore the potential programs you may consider, and then to narrow your search to those programs to submit a formal application.

> "Networking is absolutely vital to your pursuit of a residency. Joining organizations and attending professional conferences are two of the best ways to build your network early on and help your chances of obtaining a residency in the future."
>
> *Amin E. – Pharmacy Student, Texas*

This is particularly beneficial if you are considering applying to postgraduate training programs located outside of your immediate geographic location. To put it simply, consider that you live in Knoxville, Tennessee. You are interested in pursuing residency training programs in North Carolina, Florida, Illinois, Michigan, Texas, and Colorado. You have identified programs within each of these states as a result of completing research and after speaking with a mentor about each of the programs. On the most simplistic level, the next step in your pursuit of residency training is to continue to investigate the opportunities available within each program in light of your training and career goals, to ask any questions that you have for each program, and to express your interest in a program. To accomplish these tasks, you must efficiently manage your time, schedule, and money. How is this possible? Of course, the answer is to attend a meeting with a residency showcase, where you can meet with each of the programs that you are interested in, all in one location and within just a few days. Likewise, programs utilize meetings in a similar way. They help maximize their efficiency in meeting with potential candidates, provide information and answer questions for a large audience, and identify those candidates to consider inviting for an on-site interview.

INDIVIDUAL MEETINGS OF PROFESSIONAL PHARMACY ORGANIZATIONS

Now that you have determined that you are going to complete a postgraduate training, it is critical to decide which meeting(s) to attend. Professional pharmacy organizations hold meetings at the local, state, regional, and national levels. The focus of this chapter is to investigate the role of meetings held at the national level, including meetings of the ASHP, the APhA (American Pharmacists Association), the ACCP (American College of Clinical Pharmacy), the

AMCP (Academy of Managed Care Pharmacy), and the NCPA (National Community Pharmacists Association), and to highlight the unique aspects of each meeting to guide you in determining which meetings best compliment your individual needs in pursuing postgraduate pharmacy training opportunities. The ASHP MCM offers you access to the greatest selection of postgraduate training programs, including Postgraduate Year One (PGY-1), Postgraduate Year Two (PGY-2), and fellowship programs, and should be considered a key meeting to attend as you begin your search.

AMERICAN SOCIETY OF HEALTH-SYSTEM PHARMACISTS

ASHP offers two national meetings per year: the MCM, held in December, and the Summer Meeting, held in June. Of all of the professional pharmacy organization meetings, the ASHP MCM is perhaps the most significant, as it represents the greatest opportunity to gain knowledge and information, to network, and to begin your official search and exploration of individual postgraduate training opportunities. The ASHP MCM offers programming designed specifically for pharmacy students, including presentations on how to prepare your CV, how to set yourself apart from other candidates on residency applications, and what to expect in postgraduate pharmacy training. The ASHP MCM also offers the Clinical Skills Competition, providing pharmacy students the opportunity to showcase their clinical thinking and problem solving skills in a patient case-based competition. There are several leadership opportunities available to you through ASHP, with formal leadership activities and events held at the MCM. There are numerous networking opportunities at the ASHP MCM, both formal and informal, allowing you to meet and speak with fellow pharmacy students and pharmacy residents, as well as practicing practitioners representing a broad range of practice specialties throughout the United States and from countries around the world. Two of the most notable opportunities for you to consider and attend at the ASHP MCM include the Residency Showcase and Personal Placement Service (PPS).

The ASHP MCM Residency Showcase

In general, the ASHP MCM Residency Showcase is a 2-day event consisting of several sessions in which ASHP-accredited or ASHP-accreditation pending programs offer you the opportunity to gather information and speak with program directors, preceptors, and current pharmacy residents. The Residency Showcase is by far the largest gathering of postgraduate training programs of all meetings, representing hundreds

"I found it really valuable to attend ASHP MCM as a third year student because the residency showcase can be overwhelming and seeing it the year before allows you to feel more prepared for what will happen the following year when it is most important."

Brittany S. – Pharmacy Student, Ohio

of PGY-1 and nearly all PGY-2 residency and fellowship training programs available.

This allows you to speak with a large number of programs in a single location over a short period of time, which is particularly helpful if you are interested in programs from a large geographic distribution. The general setup for the Residency Showcase consists of a large exhibit hall where each program is located in a predesignated space that contains either a booth or table with information. Program directors, preceptors, and current pharmacy residents are available at the booth to meet with you. You can then walk throughout the Residency Showcase and speak directly with the programs that you are interested in. The Residency Showcase is considered a general information session, and formal interviews do not occur.

> "Take initiative to review basic information about a program before talking with them at a residency showcase or in an interview."
>
> *Danielle Y. – Pharmacy Resident, Tennessee*

There are several things to consider when planning to attend the Residency Showcase. First, each residency program is allotted time and space in one of several sessions lasting 3 hours. You will want to complete research of the Residency Showcase to determine which day and time the programs that you are interested in will be available.

A map of the Residency Showcase, indicating the day, time, and location of each program, is made available on the ASHP MCM Web site well in advance of the meeting. If you arrive at the Residency Showcase without a plan, it is likely that you are to spend a majority of time searching for the program location and wasting time that might otherwise be spent speaking and researching various programs. Plotting out a plan for each session of the Residency Showcase will ensure that you have ample time to interact with each program that you are interested in. Your time is the only limit to the number of programs that you can speak with at the Residency Showcase. In general, plan to spend approximately 10 minutes speaking and asking questions of a program. Based on this guidance, you should be able to navigate the Residency Showcase and speak to 10 programs during each 3-hour session.

> "At the showcase, take notes after meeting with each site. (The backs of business cards are a great place for these notes). If you don't take notes, you will likely have difficulty keeping the details of the sites straight when you walk out of the showcase."
>
> *Brittany S. – Pharmacy Student, Ohio*

The ASHP MCM Personal Placement Service

PPS is another opportunity for you to interact with postgraduate training programs, but on a more personal level. PPS offers a more formal setting than the Residency Showcase, and is intended to serve as a more traditional interview between a single candidate and a single program or institution. The format for these interviews depends somewhat on the position, but in general, last 30 minutes, and can be described as a cross between an informative meeting and an interview. PPS is most frequently used for PGY-2, fellowship, and employment opportunities, but its use for PGY-1 programs is increasing. For example, residency programs may participate in PPS with the goal of assisting in determining which candidates to extend an invitation for an on-site interview, particularly when there are likely more applicants than on-site interview slots. It is important to note that not all postgraduate pharmacy training programs participate in PPS and the only opportunity to interact with some programs, particularly PGY-1 residency programs, may be at the Residency Showcase.

PPS is located within the same location as the ASHP MCM, although participation in PPS requires a separate registration and fee in addition to that required for the ASHP MCM meeting. You can register in advance for PPS, or do so once arriving at the meeting. Note that you'll save money and have some advantages if you register in advance. When you register for PPS, you will be asked to create a profile. Your profile should contain key information related to you and your search, including your CV, the type of opportunity you are seeking, and your professional interests. Your information is then entered into a database that can be accessed by residency program directors and potential employers who are also registered in PPS. Likewise each program registered with PPS will provide a profile, which generally consists of a job description and contact information. After establishing a profile, PPS serves as a search engine for you and programs or employers to seek one another for matching interests and to determine if an interview can be scheduled at the ASHP MCM. Generally speaking, employers attempt to schedule as many interviews as possible prior to arriving at the meeting, although some will offer opportunities to schedule interviews on-site. Therefore, it is beneficial for you to register early and schedule as many interviews in advance of the meeting as possible.

AMERICAN PHARMACISTS ASSOCIATION

The APhA Annual Meeting & Exposition, typically held in March, offers programming for preparing for postgraduate training, leadership development, and formal and informal networking opportunities. The APhA Annual Meeting & Exposition hosts the National Patient Counseling Competition, which offers you an opportunity to showcase your skills in providing patient counseling. Two highly desirable workshops offered at the APhA Annual Meeting & Exposition include the Student Leadership Development Workshop and the Preparing for the Pharmacist Licensure Examination Workshop, which require additional registration. If you are active in the APhA-Academy of Student Pharmacists (APhA-ASP), there are several events offered at the APhA Annual Meeting & Exposition related to hosting, developing, and coordinating ASP events at your college. You can also attend the Student Information

Showcase, which is similar in format to the ASHP MCM Residency Showcase, but much smaller in scope, that primarily represents community pharmacy residency programs. The Student Information Showcase is followed by the Student Information Showcase Roundtables, which provides opportunities to network with experienced practitioners and gain insight into community pharmacy residency programs.

AMERICAN COLLEGE OF CLINICAL PHARMACY

ACCP offers two major national meetings per year, the Annual Meeting, held typically in October, and the Updates in Therapeutics Meeting, held each spring in April. The Annual Meeting hosts the Career Development Symposium, which offers you the opportunity to gain insights into developing your CV, navigating the Residency Match process, and other helpful tips for transitioning into the role of a pharmacy resident. You may also participate in the Career Development Roundtable, which offers the opportunity to network with practicing pharmacists in a variety of specialty practice areas. You can also participate in the ACCP Residency and Fellowship Forum, which is similar in format to the ASHP MCM Residency Showcase, consisting of both PGY-1 and PGY-2 residency programs. However, there are not nearly as many programs as the ASHP MCM. The ACCP Annual Meeting hosts a Mock Interview Session, where you can gain valuable insight and tips on preparing for professional interviews, along with the opportunity to participate in a mock interview with experienced pharmacists. Finally, you can participate in the Clinical Pharmacy Challenge, which allows you to showcase your skills as a clinical pharmacist. Of note, there is a competitive process for applying for funds for travel expenses and/or free meeting registration for both pharmacy students and pharmacy residents to attend the ACCP Annual Meeting, which requires submission of a completed application, a CV or resume, letters of reference, and an essay. These opportunities could not only save your money but would also be well-respected honors.

In addition to the Annual Meeting, ACCP now offers a separate 2-day meeting in the spring specifically designed for pharmacy students pursuing postgraduate training opportunities. This 2-day course offers a broad array of informative presentations designed to provide you with key insight and advice in preparing yourself to be a competitive candidate for postgraduate training, including aspects related to leadership, professional experience, networking, and research and scholarly activity. This 2-day program is beneficial for pharmacy students at all levels, from the first to the fourth year of training.

ACADEMY OF MANAGED CARE PHARMACY

AMCP offers two national meetings per year: the AMCP Educational Conference, held in October, and the AMCP Annual Meeting & Showcase, held in April. While both meetings offer educational programming, networking, and leadership opportunities for students, you may be particularly interested in attending the Annual Educational Conference, which offers a residency show-case. The format of the AMCP Residency Showcase is similar to the ASHP MCM, although it offers access specifically (and only) to managed care train-ing opportunities (see Chapter 16 for more details on available managed care residencies). The AMCP National Meeting & Showcase also hosts the student Pharmacy and Therapeutics Committee Competition, which allows you to competitively showcase your critical thinking skills related to medication for-mulary decision making.

NATIONAL COMMUNITY PHARMACISTS ASSOCIATION

NCPA hosts two national meetings per year, the Annual Convention and Trade Exposition, held in the October, and the Annual Conference on National Legis-lation and Government Affairs. The Annual Convention and Trade Exposition offers educational programming, networking, and leadership opportunities specifically designed for pharmacy students with an interest in community pharmacy practice. Educational programming is targeted to key consider ations and concepts in community pharmacy, including developing business plans, political advocacy, and innovative practice models At the Annual Con-vention and Trade Exposition, a Community Pharmacy Residency Showcase is held. It is similar in format to the ASHP MCM. In addition, you can participate in the Good Neighbor Pharmacy NCPA Pruitt-Schutte Student Business Plan Competition, which allows you to showcase your skills in creating a business plan for ownership of a community pharmacy.

PREPARATION FOR PROFESSIONAL PHARMACY ORGANIZATION MEETINGS

At a glance, the number of activities available to you at a meeting seems over-whelming. In order to ensure success and capitalize upon the opportunities available, you must prepare yourself in advance. Doing so will maximize your experience and ensure that you are successful at the meeting. So, how should you prepare for a meeting?

Registration and Accommodations for the Meeting

Registration for meetings typically begins several months in advance. You can register to attend a meeting on each individual organization's Web site. It is in your best interest to complete your registration as far in advance of the meet-ing as possible. Early registration is typically at a reduced rate, and it will offer you the greatest price and selection for travel accommodations (e.g., airfare and lodging). Early registration also ensures that you maximize the amount of time that you have to prepare and research for the meeting, and will provide you with useful meeting information and updates. When completing meeting registration, be sure to investigate whether you just need to register for the meeting, or if separate registration is required for other events that you plan to participate in. For example, PPS requires separate registration in addition to the ASHP MCM general meeting registration. Finally, most professional pharmacy organizations negotiate a reduced rate for lodging accommodations (e.g., hotels) within close proximity to the meeting location. You can find specific information related to registration, lodging, and transportation for each meeting on individual professional pharmacy organization Web sites.

Preparation for the Meeting

What is the bottom line to ensure that you get the most of out of a professional pharmacy organization meeting? Preparation and research.

It is absolutely critical and cannot be stressed enough. Your plan for the meeting should be established well in advance of traveling to the meeting. For this very purpose, professional pharmacy organizations provide a wealth of information about the meeting on their Web site months in advance, including information specifically designed for students.

> "Careful planning is the key to successfully navigating the ASHP Residency Showcase. Printing out schedules and floor plans beforehand, identifying where your programs of interest are located, and having good questions to ask each program will ensure that you get the most out the Showcase."
>
> *Amin E. – Pharmacy Student, Texas*

Specifically, you will want to review the meeting itinerary, taking note of events of interest. You should consider developing your own meeting itinerary, specific to the days that you plan to be at the meeting. Most meetings now offer several options to assist you in creating your meeting itinerary, including online scheduling tools that you can print out to bring with you to the meeting and smartphone applications that allow you to download your meeting itinerary to your phone. Your meeting itinerary should include some flexibility in scheduling, as you may be invited to other activities, such as networking events after meeting with a program during a session.

Prior to networking with residency programs that interest you at the meeting, research each program and develop an understanding of the basic components. You can conduct a search of the program's Web site or by using the ASHP online residency directory. Specific aspects to research include

> "Be prepared for MCM! Prioritize your time to get a good sense of the programs that are important to you and demonstrate that you are interested and are well informed about what they have to offer."
>
> *Kathryn E. – Pharmacy Student, Arizona*

the type of institution, the general patient population served and areas of patient care provided, the number and type of postgraduate training

TABLE 8-1 • Using Geography to Guide Your Program Priority List for a Professional Pharmacy Organization Meeting

One way that you may want to prioritize your list of programs is to consider the geographic location of the programs relative to your current location. For example, you may not want to visit and get information on those residency programs in your hometown to the same extent as those that are 500 miles away. For programs close to you that you have already spoken with in the past, you may quickly stop by and verbalize your interest in the program and say that you look forward to speak with them in the future. In general, most residency program directors, preceptors, and current pharmacy residents at the meeting have the understanding that you have not come to the meeting to speak solely with local residency programs, and a general "quick stop" is all that is necessary. Take your time at the meeting to maximize your exposure to those programs with geographic locations further away, that you are less familiar with, and that you are most interested in.

programs offered, and required and elective rotations. Based on your interest areas, training and career goals and objectives, the information that you obtain through your research of each program and the geographic location of each program, you should develop a list of the programs that you want to speak with at the meeting (Table 8-1). It will also be helpful to prioritize your list based on your interest in each program. This will ensure that you maximize opportunities to speak with key programs on your list and will prevent haphazard decision making on the day of meeting events, which could result in a significant loss of time. Finally, you should prepare a list of questions for each individual program. For example, questions to ask the current pharmacy residents in a program are to describe a typical day, to ask about their research projects, or to ask about the pharmacy resident's involvement in various teaching and learning experiences. Potential questions to ask program directors and/or preceptors include asking about the career paths of former pharmacy residents or fellows, or opportunities to be involved in teaching. Ensure that your questions are professional and appropriate—at this point in the postgraduate training research process, questions regarding staffing requirements, salary, benefits, or vacation time are not appropriate. You will have a limited amount of time to speak with each individual program; likewise, each program has a limited amount of time to speak with each individual candidate. You don't want to waste this time by asking questions that can easily be answered on the program's Web site, as this makes you appear unprepared and prevents you from asking other vital questions.

What to Bring to the Meeting

There are several items that you will want to bring with you to the meeting, which are summarized in Table 8-2.

TABLE 8-2 • Packing Checklist for Professional Pharmacy Organization Meetings

Professional business attire
Travel reservations: airfare, lodging, transportation (when applicable)
Personal Identification (e.g., driver's license)
Meeting registration confirmation
Personalized meeting itinerary
Contact information for scheduled interviews
Copies of curriculum vitae
Electronic copy of curriculum vitae
Business cards
Notes/research applicable to meeting events and/or appointments
List of prepared questions, separated by individual institution
Blank notepad to record notes/questions
Professional portfolio to store documents for meeting events

Current copies of your CV should be brought for all formal networking events, such as a residency showcase and interview activities. Generally speaking, provide a copy of your CV only when requested. Conservatively, you should plan to bring one copy of your CV for every three programs that you plan to interact with at a residency showcase, and one copy for each program that you formally interview with, such as at PPS. Programs may not ask for your CVduring the showcase, but it's better to be prepared. During PPS, there is a very high likelihood that an interviewer will ask for a copy of your CV. You should consider having professional business cards made to bring with you to the meeting. Business cards serve as a simple yet professional means to share your contact information when a full CV is not needed, such as at social networking events. There are many options available for having personalized professional business cards printed inexpensively, either through your local college or university, professional printing shops, or online merchandisers. Information printed on your business card should be brief and limited to key contact information. Ensure that all contact information listed on your business card is professional, especially your email address. Likewise, do not include contact information related to social media (e.g., Twitter© and Facebook©), unless used specifically and solely for professional purposes. Any symbols or decorations, if included, should be kept to a minimum and should be professional; your college or university logo is appropriate, if allowed by copyright. A sample professional pharmacy student business card is provided for your reference in Figure 8-1. Plan to bring your business cards with you to all formal and informal meeting activities to ensure that you are always prepared to provide your contact information when requested.

Finally, you may want to bring along a bottle of water and mints with you. You may be surprised at the resulting effect of a dry mouth on your speech,

ALLISON HORNE, B.S., PHARM.D. CANDIDATE

Doctor of Pharmacy Candidate, Class of 2013
Class President, Class of 2013
Chair, APhA-ASP Project Heart
The University Health Science Center
College of Pharmacy
Telephone: (865) 555-2013
E-Mail: ahorne@email.edu

Figure 8-1:
Sample Pharmacy Student Business Card.

which can come from a combination of speaking for long periods of time during a residency showcase or interview and the adverse effect of increased sympathetic outflow that you are likely to experience from interviewing with potential future program directors, preceptors, and/or employers! Gum may seem like a good idea for this purpose, but is not the most professional. You will also want to have a watch with you, as a clock may not be readily available in all meeting locations. This will ensure that you remain on time with your schedule.

GENERAL GUIDANCE WHEN ATTENDING A PROFESSIONAL PHARMACY ORGANIZATION MEETING

Networking, Discussions, and Informal Interviews

Networking opportunities including receptions and social business functions allow you to introduce yourself, meet others, gain valuable insight into current issues in the profession of pharmacy, and ask questions related to pursuing postgraduate training opportunities and professional/career development. Prior to attending networking activities, ensure that you have adequately prepared in advance and are familiar with the format, the location, and the length of the networking session. Depending on the activity, you do not have to stay for the entire session, but you should stay for important announcements or keynote speakers. As a general rule, wear professional attire to all networking sessions. After speaking with individuals or programs of interest, it will be valuable for you to quickly jot down notes on the key discussion points from your interaction—for example, the names and titles of those who you spoke with (which can easily be obtained through an exchange of business cards), specific aspects of the program that you discussed, and responses to the questions that you asked. This information is important in assisting you in determining which programs to further pursue and when writing personalized thank you cards. With this level of importance in your career decision making on the line, combined with the massive number of potential opportunities presented to you, you should not solely rely on your memory to track each interaction you had at the meeting, as it can be easy to either forget or confuse the details of one program with another. Again, keeping a basic notepad in your business portfolio, along with your CV and business cards, is an easy, organized way to record your interactions at the meeting.

Formal Interviews

Formal interviews at professional pharmacy organization meetings follow the same general rules as other professional, formal interviews, though they may be shorter in length. When participating in a formal interview opportunity at a professional pharmacy organization meeting, it is important to recognize that your performance during this interview may dictate whether or not you are invited on-site for an interview! Therefore, you will want to follow all of the rules and guidance for interviewing (see Chapter 10). For interviews occurring at professional pharmacy organization meetings, plan to arrive approximately 15 minutes prior to your scheduled appointment time, if possible, to ensure that you have ample time to locate the assigned location for the interview and are on time. Whenever possible, coordinate as many interviews as possible prior to the meeting. As the date of the meeting approaches, interview time slots for each program will be filled; therefore, it is to your advantage to try to schedule interviews as soon as the information on schedules is available. Again, keep in mind that interviews at meetings are generally reserved for PGY-2, fellowship, and employment opportunities, and interviews for PGY-1 residency training programs may not be available.

Be sure to thoroughly review the guidelines associated with interview sessions at the meeting. For example, determine the length of the interview, which are usually brief, lasting 30 minutes. When scheduling interviews, it is advisable not to schedule more than one interview per hour time slot; that is, try to avoid scheduling interviews back-to-back (e.g., one interview at 1:00 PM and a second interview at 1:30 PM). There are several reasons for this recommendation, but perhaps the most powerful reason is that if you are having a positive interaction with a program, you don't want be forced to stop the conversation to leave to go on to your next interview. In addition, if your first scheduled interview ends on time, you will want to have a buffer of time in between interviews to be able to locate your next interview location, to record your thoughts about the interview that you just completed, take a break, gather your thoughts, and review your research notes for the next interview. Not only will you personally feel less rushed and more prepared by allowing this buffer of time in between interviews, but you will appear less rushed and more prepared to the interviewer, as well. Depending on availability and meeting schedules, the ideal situation of scheduling one interview per hour may not be feasible. In that case, ensure that you have adequately prepared yourself for those interviews that occur back-to-back and have researched and located the physical location for each interview prior to going to the first interview.

Maintaining Professional Demeanor

What do you consider the three most important attributes of determining whether or not candidates are asked on-site for an interview, ranked preferably in the Match, and offered a position in a program? Among these, do you include professionalism? Professionalism is a key attribute sought in candidates by postgraduate training programs. Perhaps the most critical consideration that differentiates your professional image from being a student on rotation to being a resident, even in the same institution, is that as a resident, you *represent* the institution. When residency or fellowship programs consider you as a potential candidate, they are considering you from the perspective of being a representative of their program and institution. Certainly, at this point in your training, you have heard about professionalism on numerous occasions. It may not come as a surprise, but it is worth pointing out that a professional demeanor is critical in all communication and interactions as you pursue the residency training—this applies to residency recruitment events at any professional meeting, whether at the local, state, or national level. So, what exactly is professional behavior, what are programs looking for, and how can you portray a professional demeanor when interacting with programs at a meeting?

While you may have some internal objections to this thought, a meeting is neither the time nor environment to test out the latest trend or to push the boundary of fashion—this is an insignificant sacrifice to make relative to your future career. In terms of outward appearance, a general guideline is to wear business casual attire when attending educational programming sessions, and to wear professional business attire during networking sessions, residency showcase events, and for all interviews. If it is unclear to you whether business causal or professional business attire is appropriate for a particular meeting event, you should err on the side of more formal attire, wearing professional business attire. If you are still unclear about what constitutes professional business attire, it would be in your best interest to conduct some basic research (you can even look online) or check with a mentor or advisor. Wear comfortable, yet professional, shoes, as you are likely going to be doing a fair amount of walking and standing. To complete your look, place all documents in a nicely organized portfolio. A portfolio with your college or university emblem or seal, if available, serves well for this purpose. Avoid using a binder with drug advertising, or one covered with bumper stickers from every garage band you've seen over the last 7 years. You may bring a nice looking, small backpack or briefcase if you feel it is absolutely necessary, but keep the size to a minimum, as large briefcases and bags are a major inconvenience. Illustrative examples of "do's" and "don'ts" of attire for a meeting are provided in Figures 8-2 and 8-3. Unfortunately, as the saying goes, the "names are made up but the problems are real" when it comes to the examples provided in this textbook—and you don't want to end up being an example in the next edition of this book!

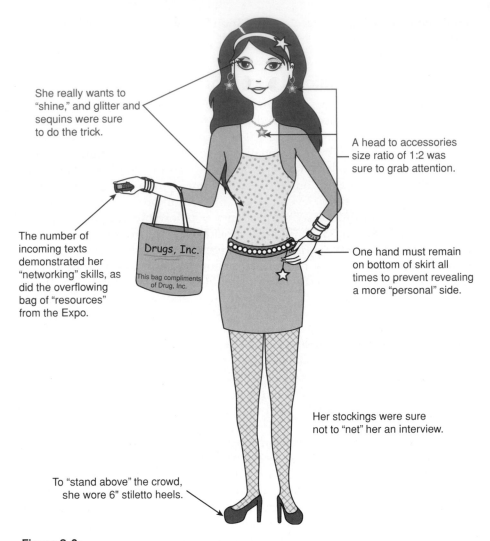

She really wants to "shine," and glitter and sequins were sure to do the trick.

A head to accessories size ratio of 1:2 was sure to grab attention.

The number of incoming texts demonstrated her "networking" skills, as did the overflowing bag of "resources" from the Expo.

Drugs, Inc.

This bag compliments of Drug, Inc.

One hand must remain on bottom of skirt all times to prevent revealing a more "personal" side.

Her stockings were sure not to "net" her an interview.

To "stand above" the crowd, she wore 6" stiletto heels.

Figure 8-2:
The "Star" Candidate–In Case Programs Did Not Figure Out She Was a "Star" Based on Her CV, She Wanted to Send the Message. If Only She Knew the Message She Would Send.

Professionalism applies to both the inside and the outside—what you wear, how you wear it, what you say, how you say it. A summary of key points to consider when portraying a professional demeanor are summarized in Table 8-3. If you are unsure about your communication skills and how you may come across in a professional setting, practice your response to key interview questions in a mirror, speaking out loud to yourself, and conduct a practice interview session with trustworthy friends, colleagues, or a mentor or advisor.

And one final note about professionalism—when meeting events are over for the day, you may want to spend some time enjoying yourself and all of

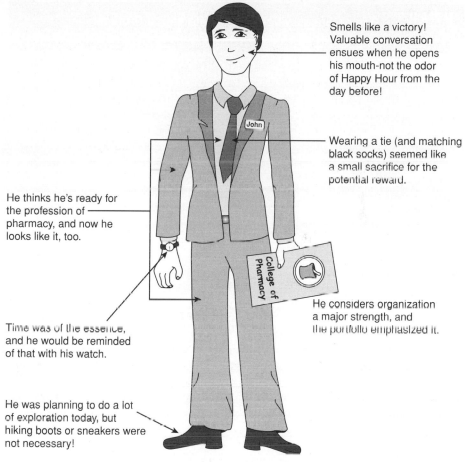

Figure 8-3:
A Real Star Candidate. True Star Candidates Speak for Themselves—Accessories Are Not Needed to Prove It. Head-to-Toe, He Is Ready to Go—Leaving No Doubt of the Message He Would Send from Beginning of the Meeting to the Very End.

the attractions that the meeting location has to offer. While you are certainly encouraged to have a good time and enjoy yourself at the meeting, you should do so in a way that you will not regret in the morning. Consider it this way—the ASHP MCM is the largest formal meeting of pharmacists *in the world*—more than 20,000 pharmacists attend the ASHP MCM each year.[3] Chances are, wherever you go, you are going to be in the company of pharmacists, and potentially in the company of future program directors, preceptors, or current pharmacy residents and fellows. Be aware of how your behavior may potentially be perceived, while at the same time, enjoy yourself—it is possible to do both! And finally, a reminder about the basic kinetics of ethanol—ethanol is excreted by exhalation (which is why law enforcement can use "breathalyzers" during vehicle road stops). Keep this in mind when enjoying yourself the night before and the day of major meeting events—

TABLE 8-3 • Basic Considerations for Maintaining a Professional Demeanor at a Professional Pharmacy Organization Meeting

DO's	DON'Ts
Wear professional business attire	Wear blue jeans and a T-shirt
Wear comfortable, but professional, shoes	Wear tennis shoes/sneakers
Bring a professional business portfolio or folder	Bring an extra-large bag from the pharmaceutical industry exposition hall
Maintain good posture	Slouch because you are tired
Offer a firm handshake and smile as you introduce yourself	Fumble with your backpack and forget the handshake
Maintain eye contact when speaking and being spoken to	Look around the room to see what you might be missing
Wait for your time to speak with a program	Interrupt an ongoing conversation
Listen carefully and completely to each statement and question	Interrupt and state, "Yeah, I already know that"
Prepare for potential questions	Read question responses from a script
Turn off cellular telephone	Answer every incoming text message
Briefly greet potential colleagues in passing	Ignore a potential colleague or invite yourself into their conversation at dinner
Attend networking events or receptions when invited	Show up at a networking event that you were not invited to

while you might not be aware of the odor that exude, those around will be, and will take note of it! It is in your best interest to avoid indulging prior to meeting events.

CONSIDERATIONS AFTER RETURNING FROM PROFESSIONAL PHARMACY ORGANIZATION MEETINGS

Thank You Cards

After you return from a meeting, the hard work can begin. Your first step after returning from a meeting should be to send a follow-up message, or thank you card, to the individuals that you interacted with at a residency showcase or in a formal interview (see Chapter 10 for further guidance on writing thank you cards). In general, a thank you card should be written to those individuals from a program that you spent a significant amount of time speaking with, including program directors, preceptors, and residents. A thank you card is not necessarily needed for all of the people that you were introduced to, but rather should be focused, intentional, and personalized to those people that answered your questions, spent time speaking about the program with you, or that you spent time networking with formally and informally. Keeping a business card from each program and person that you interacted with will provide the necessary contact information needed for sending a follow-up message. You do not need to include your CV in a thank you card, as the thank you card is not an official application and should not be treated as one. Do not make any assumptions in the thank you card. When you return from a meeting, you likely will not have submitted your application materials yet, nor will you know if you will be invited on-site for an interview. Don't make an assumption in the thank you card that you are automatically invited on-site for an interview based on your interaction at a meeting alone.

CONCLUSION

Professional pharmacy organization meetings are key in the search for postgraduate training opportunities. Meetings offer you an opportunity to seek out information and interact with representatives from numerous programs all in one location and within a short period of time, which in turn allows you to focus your efforts on the programs to submit an application to. In general, the ASHP MCM offers you the greatest opportunity to speak with PGY-1, PGY-2, and fellowship training programs of all meetings available. Once you have made a decision to attend a meeting, take the time and effort to prepare yourself for the opportunities available. Your time will be well-spent!

Chapter Takeaways

▶ Meetings of professional pharmacy organizations play a key role in the pursuit of postgraduate residency training, particularly through the breadth of knowledge afforded and the numerous networking opportunities available.

▶ Participating in a professional pharmacy organization meeting at the national level is particularly useful for pursuing postgraduate training opportunities that span a large geographic distribution.

▶ Pharmacy students and pharmacy residents pursuing postgraduate residency training opportunities should strongly consider participating in the ASHP MCM Residency Showcase and Personal Placement Service.

▶ Research and preparation of activities to participate in during a professional pharmacy organization meeting is *essential*. Be sure to research meeting activities on the organization's Web site well in advance of the meeting, taking note of meeting activity tools designed specifically for pharmacy students. Use this information to create your own individualized itinerary of activities for the meeting.

▶ When seeking information and networking opportunities related to postgraduate training at a professional pharmacy organization meeting, conduct thorough research of each individual program prior to the meeting, and develop a list of questions individualized for each program.

ROLE FOR THE MENTOR

Assist the pharmacy student or pharmacy resident in determining which professional pharmacy organization meeting to attend that will best meet their individual needs in the pursuit of postgraduate training.

Review the pharmacy student's or pharmacy resident's curriculum vitae (CV) prior to attending a professional pharmacy organization meeting, ensuring that formatting and organization are appropriate and consistent.

Assist the pharmacy student or pharmacy resident in developing a list of appropriate questions to ask postgraduate training programs that are appropriate, professional, and are designed to explore relevant program information.

FREQUENTLY ASKED QUESTIONS

Q: Should I write thank you cards for interactions that occurred at a professional pharmacy organization meeting? Whom should I write a thank you card for, and what is the preferred method for writing a thank you card?

A: Yes. It is considered professional etiquette and courtesy to thank a program and the representatives of the program that you met with at the meeting for their time and information provided. A thank you card should be written to those individuals that spoke with you directly, spent a significant amount of time with you, and/or answered your questions. Preferably, thank you cards should be handwritten, should be personalized and individualized to each person or program, and should contain an expression of your interest and appreciation for the program. In general, thank you cards should be prepared and sent immediately after returning from the meeting.

Q: What is an appropriate number of residencies to meet with at the ASHP MCM Residency Showcase given the limitations in time?

A: For each individual 3-hour session of the Residency Showcase, you should generally consider meeting with up to 10 programs. This will allow you ample time to record notes after speaking with one program, coordinate your notes/questions and locate the next program, and account for time spent speaking with each program. Since there are 3 Residency Showcase sessions at the ASHP MCM, you could potentially meet with up to 30 programs at the meeting through the Residency Showcase alone.

References

1. Mancuso CE, Paloucek FP. Understanding and preparing for pharmacy practice residency interviews. Am J Health Syst Pharm. 2004;61:1686–1689.

2. Huang L, Galinsky AD, Gruenfeld DH, Guillory LE. Powerful postures versus powerful roles: Which is the proximate correlate of thought and behavior? Psychol Sci. 2011;22:95–102.

3. American Society of Health-System Pharmacists. Meetings and Conferences. American Society of Health-System Pharmacists Web site. http://www.ashp.org/menu/Meetings/Conferences.aspx. Accessed February 3, 2012.

Application Process— The Holiday Rush 9

Jacob P. Gettig

At this point, it is probably clear to you that competition for pharmacy residencies is at an all time high. Although there is no way of calculating the exact number of residency program applications submitted to programs last year, the National Match Service reported that almost 12,000 rankings of Postgraduate Year One (PGY-1) Pharmacy Residencies were submitted to the 2011 Match.[1] By extrapolation, we know that there were *at the very least* 12,000 applications submitted to the 880 PGY-1 Pharmacy Residency programs that participated in the 2011 Match. A recent survey of deans of colleges of pharmacy in the United States projects a 58% increase in the number of residents/fellows by 2015.[2] It appears that an already competitive market for residency programs will only get more competitive in the near future. This competition is all the more reason for your application to be your "best foot forward" attempt at securing an on-site interview and eventually a position with your preferred residency program.

> "There is not much time in between Midyear, application submissions, and interviews. Everything will happen fast, so stay organized, motivated, and keep your eye on the prize!"
>
> *Vi D. – Pharmacy Student, Texas*

The temptation to relax after coming back from a busy American Society of Health-System Pharmacists Midyear Clinical Meeting (ASHP MCM) or other meeting will be strong. Instead, fight the temptation and transition immediately into residency application mode!

If you haven't already, now is the time to seriously reflect on the pros and cons of potential residency program options (see Chapter 5) and make any final additions or adjustment to your curriculum vitae (CV) since it will be an integral part of any residency application (see Chapter 7). Now, before you begin your residency applications with writing your letters of intent and requesting letters of recommendation and college transcripts, you will need to get organized and make a final decision about the residency programs to which you will apply.

PLANNING AND ORGANIZING

Organization is *imperative* to be successful in the residency application process.

> "The residency application process is daunting, but when you feel overwhelmed, remember to focus on your personal and professional goals and the characteristics that are most important to you in a residency."
>
> *Christina T. – Pharmacy Student Texas*

Common questions you should answer for yourself when starting the application process are as follows:

- To which programs will I be submitting an application packet?
  - Do I have any questions about any programs that I need to have answered before making a final decision? If so, who do I contact for these answers?
- What does each program require in their application packet? Typical components of an application packet are described below; however, some programs may require additional forms, essays, examples of projects, etc.
- What are the deadlines for submitting application materials? Are these deadlines for receipt of materials or are they postmark deadlines?
- Do I need to submit all of my application materials together or can they be submitted as they are completed (e.g., letters of recommendation and college transcripts)?
- Does the program require I submit hard copies of application materials or electronic copies? Do they require both or is either format acceptable? If electronic, is a certain file format required (e.g., .doc vs. .pdf)?
- Who is the contact person at each program to which my letters and application materials should be addressed?
- Who has agreed to write me positive letters of recommendation and have I given my letter writers all of the relevant deadlines and other information they need?
- How do I request transcripts from my college of pharmacy/undergraduate college(s)? How much time does it take to process these requests? Are there fees for this? Does the residency program require that my fall quarter/semester grades are included? If so, when will the Registrar post these to my transcript?

Once you have these basic questions answered, create a filing system that works for you. While most residency candidates probably use and prefer electronic means of filing, if you prefer a hard copy filing system, use it! Create a secure set of e-folders or file folders in which you can store important documents, communications, etc. related to residency applications. If you are using an e-filing system, create a folder for each residency program to which you are applying. Within each program folder, create a subfolder entitled "Application

Materials" or something similar. Only save application materials that belong in the final application packet in this folder. If you use a hard copy filing system, usually separate manila folders for each program work nicely. Now is the time to break out that fancy label-maker you've had sitting around since you finished your classroom coursework!

Table 9-1 is an example of a tracking tool that you may find useful during the residency application process. This checklist includes the name of the residency program and the appropriate contact person. The rest of the checklist consists mostly of important dates such as the date on which your application materials are due and the dates on which these application materials were requested, sent, and received by all involved institutions or individuals. There is also a place to record which individuals agreed to write letters of recommendation for you and a space for additional notes specific to each application. There are many variations in this checklist that you could devise depending on your preference for details, but at the very least, you should include the name of the residency program, the contact person at the program, the due date for application materials, and the dates on which you requested materials and confirmed that the program received all of the necessary materials.

HOW MANY APPLICATIONS?

Applying to only a couple of residency programs in the past may have been sufficient, but given that 38% of candidates did not match to a PGY-1 Pharmacy Residency in the 2011 Match, applying to more residency programs may now be advisable.[1] However, there are considerations you need to make when applying to numerous residency programs. The first consideration is the concept of "fit" (see Chapter 5). Also, consider the time it will take to prepare each application packet . . . and prepare each application packet well. Each application will probably require a letter of intent (described below in more detail). While you may want to write a generic letter of intent for all programs to save you some time, a truly personalized and targeted letter of intent for each program will make you a more successful candidate. Another thing to consider is whether you have the time and money to afford going to every on-site interview that is offered to you. Each interview usually lasts 1 to 2 days, and most residency programs expect candidates to pay for their own lodging and travel expenses associated with the interview. Since most residency programs interview candidates during the week, unless you are not scheduled for an Advanced Pharmacy Practice Experience (APPE) rotation during January/February, you may have to miss days on your APPEs. Rotation preceptors and the Offices of Experiential Education at colleges of pharmacy usually understand this and are supportive of students' residency pursuits, but do not be surprised if they ask you to make up the time away from the rotation.

A final consideration is the probability of your success in securing a residency based on your level of preparation throughout pharmacy school. If you have been preparing for applying to residency programs since your first professional year by getting involved in student organizations or committees, doing research, taking challenging electives, excelling on rotations, and networking

TABLE 9-1 • Detailed Checklist of Residency Application Materials

Program	Contact at Program (Name/Email Address)	Deadline (Postmark or Date to Receive Materials?)	Transcripts Req[a]	Sent[b]	Conf[c]	Letter of Recommendation No. 1 Name: John Doe, PharmD			Letter of Recommendation No. 2 Name: Sally Johnson, PharmD			Letter of Recommendation No. 3 Name: Greg Brown, RPh			Letter of Intent/CV Sent	Conf	Notes
PGY-1 General Health System	Jane Smith (jsmith@general.org)	1/5/12 (postmark date)	12/15/11	12/28/11	12/3/12	Req	Sent	Conf	Req	Sent	Conf	Req	Sent	Conf	12/28/11	1/5/12	Met with Dr. Johnson 12/11/11 per her request to discuss career goals LORs nos. 1 and 3 were received on 1/9/12 but postmarked by 1/5/12
						11/25/11	1/3/12	1/9/12	11/25/11	12/18/11	1/5/12	12/7/11	1/2/12	1/9/12			
						Name:			Name:			Name:					
						Req	Sent	Conf	Req	Sent	Conf	Req	Sent	Conf			

[a]Date that applicants request transcript/letter.

[b]Date that college or letter writer sends (mails or emails, depending on what the program prefers) transcript or letter to residency program.

[c]Date that applicant confirms receipt of materials with residency program contact.

appropriately, the strength of your application may speak for itself. You may only need to apply to a few programs that are high on your list because of your accomplishments, experiences, and positive reputation as a candidate. If you are not necessarily a highly competitive candidate as compared to your peers, you may wish to apply for more programs to increase your chances of securing an on-site interview. A strategy you could consider is to apply to a variety of highly competitive, moderately competitive, and less competitive programs to increase your odds of securing an on-site interview, but you may want to consult with your mentor(s) to help guide you through this approach. Chapter 6, which describes aspects of the ideal residency candidate, may help you determine whether you are a highly competitive candidate. As a point of clarification, if after some reflection you determine you fall into a less competitive category, that's ok! There are no guarantees in the residency application and matching process, so if you know that residency training is the right path for you, pursue it fervently. Just recognize you need to be honest with yourself and aware of the fierce competition for pharmacy residencies.

THE APPLICATION PACKET

By now you probably just completed some serious self-examination and soul-searching. You have a plan and all the information about the residency programs you need. Now is the time to stop thinking and talking about applying and actually apply. Most programs are going to require the same types of application materials: your CV, a letter of intent, letters of recommendation, college transcripts, and often additional miscellaneous items. These types of application materials can further be divided into two categories: materials you create and materials that others create.

Curriculum Vitae

A full CV is almost always a necessary component of a residency application packet. Details of writing CVs are covered in Chapter 7. Remember to always print the CV you will submit with your application packet with a laser printer on high-quality paper that matches your other application materials. There is no universally agreed upon acceptable color of paper, and while off white may be a little easier on the eyes than traditional white paper, both are acceptable choices. Avoid using obnoxiously bright colors or colors on which black print is barely visible. Remember your application can stand out for aesthetic reasons in a good or a bad way. Although programs are unlikely to dismiss your application based on the color of paper you choose for your CV, it's best not to take that chance. Let your CV shine with your accomplishments and not with the chartreuse paper on which you printed it.

Letters of Intent

Most programs will simply ask for a letter of intent with no qualifications. Some programs, however, may ask for a letter of intent that addresses certain items. Pay close attention to the instructions and make sure you cover these items in your letter. In general, a good letter of intent does the following:

- Includes a personal touch—You can add a personal touch to your letter of intent by including a specific description of how you first learned about the residency program or how you learned more about the program. For example, if you and the residency program director (RPD) discussed the program at ASHP MCM, consider mentioning the specific part of the discussion that resonated with you. If you had discussions with other preceptors and residents at the Residency Showcase, you may also mention that.

- Explains specific aspects of the program that make it a good fit for you— This is one of the true tests of a targeted letter of intent, and those involved in the decision process will use this information to determine if you truly did your homework about their program. For example, instead of writing that you are interested in a program because it offers an ambulatory care rotation, be more specific. What is it about that ambulatory care rotation that interests you? Are you passionate about diabetes management and impressed with the level of care that clinicians provide patients with diabetes in the clinic? You obviously have limited space in a letter of intent, and there may be many examples of specific aspects about the program you could include. Just focus on a few specific examples and do your best to allow sincerity and passion to come through in your writing.

- Explains specific skills or accomplishments that demonstrate how you are the ideal candidate for the program—This should be tied directly to the previous bullet. Instead of describing yourself with trite adjectives, pick out something you are passionate about and highlight an experience you had during pharmacy school, in your job or even in your personal life that demonstrates this. For example, if you had an APPE rotation in which you worked with diabetic patients or were involved in an extracurricular activity such as the American Pharmacists Association's Operation Diabetes, use these experiences to describe how you would excel at diabetes management during the PGY-1 ambulatory care rotation. You might consider highlighting specific experiences that the residency could provide that will allow you to expand your knowledge and skills about diabetes management. For example, this could include more experience with dosing insulin regimens in treatment-resistant patients or more experience honing your motivational interviewing skills with diabetic patients. This level of introspection tells residency application reviewers that although you know you have strength in a particular area and may quickly adapt and learn their program, you recognize that the additional training their program would provide would help you grow even more.

- Is concise—A good letter of intent usually should be about one single-spaced typewritten page in a reasonable, professional font and should never exceed two typewritten pages. Remember that RPDs and other individuals involved in reviewing applications may receive more than 100 applications in any given year. You do not want to be the person who submits the unnecessarily long letter of intent that attracts the RPD's attention, but in a bad way.

Conversely, some things to avoid when writing a letter of intent include the following:

- Long tales of personal hardship—Letters of intent can be used to briefly explain lapses in the CV (e.g., if a CV shows a candidate was not enrolled in college or was unemployed for a period of time), but it should not recount irrelevant tales of woe from your personal life. If you are pursuing a Postgraduate Year Two (PGY-2) residency program in pain management partially because you have known family members who suffered with chronic pain, it is acceptable to mention this in your letter of intent since it may speak to certain members of the decision-making committee. However, the details of their trials and tribulations regarding pain management are unnecessary. The sample letter in Figure 9-3 provides an example of how to appropriately address hardships or gaps within your CV.

- An overabundance of buzzwords—Buzzwords are commonplace in any profession, and they certainly abound in pharmacy. Besides being annoying when overused, buzzwords are not an effective way of informing your application reviewers that you truly understand a concept. Any applicant can dish out a buzzword, but the applicants with outstanding letters of intent will replace buzzwords with specifics and context that ensure reviewers that the applicants clearly comprehend the concept behind the buzzword. For example, a common buzz phrase in a letter of intent is "optimizing patient care outcomes." While the idea of "optimizing patient care outcomes" is something that pharmacists embrace and strive for, what does it mean to you? Revisiting the passion for diabetes management described in previous examples, do you feel you need residency training to be able to better promote medication adherence in diabetic patients and thereby get patients to their therapeutic goals? By being specific, this is not implying your need to mention the hemoglobin A1c goal and reference the latest American Diabetes Association's treatment guidelines, but including something specific about your area of interest tells those reviewing your program what "optimizing patient care outcomes" means to you.

- A regurgitation of your CV—The letter of intent can be used effectively to highlight certain important aspects of your CV, but you should provide more detail about an activity or an accolade than what is provided on the CV. If your CV format includes bulleted descriptions of activities you did while on an APPE rotation, do not reiterate these bullets on your letter of intent without including another layer of depth. Always make sure you are linking this activity or accolade to why the program is a good fit for you or why you are a good fit for the program.

- A generic description of the program or of you—Avoid explaining what the residency program entails since the residency application review committee already knows what the residency entails. Especially avoid using the exact verbiage in the program's description on the ASHP Online Residency Directory or on the residency program's Web site to describe the program in your letter.[3] Use your own words and focus on the aspects of the program that truly speak to you. Avoid generic descriptions of yourself as well. Anyone pursuing residency training is likely "motivated" and "goal-oriented." What does that mean? Specificity will go much farther than catch-all descriptions or phrases.

One PGY-1 RPD recommended "the letter contain an overview of what, how, and why their [residency candidates'] pharmacy training experience occurred."[4] They called for a "letter of life" rather than a letter of intent. Such a letter would clearly explain experiences on CVs and transcripts and provide application reviewers more insight into the quantity and quality of learning opportunities you have had to date. As you can probably tell, there is not one absolute right way to write a letter of intent. Overall, it should be specific, concise, and sincere and set you apart from your peers. See Figures 9-1 through 9-3 for example letters of intent.

Other Materials

Some postgraduate training programs may require you to submit forms, additional essays, or examples of projects or presentations you have completed as part of your application packet. If forms are required, make sure you have the most up-to-date copy of the form, either from the program's Web site or from the appropriate contact person at the program. If you are asked to write an additional essay, make sure you explicitly follow directions and similar to the letter of intent, be specific, concise, and sincere. If you are required to submit examples of projects or presentations you have done, make sure they are examples of your best work that clearly demonstrate a skill set in which you have confidence. It is important to make sure you are intimately familiar with whatever example project/presentation you choose to submit because you may receive questions from application reviewers and/or from interviewers on an on-site interview. For example, if you feel you have particularly strong primary literature evaluation skills that you would like to showcase and you recently gave a well-received journal club presentation, a copy of the journal club handout might be an appropriate choice. If you end up getting an on-site interview, it will be important to revisit the journal club handout in case you get any questions during the interview. The "other" category is another clear reason why you will need to be very organized in your application approach. If the program is taking the time to collect and review other materials, then these materials are important contributions to their decision-making process. If you miss submitting an "other" something due to lack of organization or going through the motions, it will probably cost you the on-site interview you have already worked so hard to get!

Letters of Recommendation

Remember the first time in pharmacy school you heard someone tell you "networking is important," "Pharmacy is a small world," or "get to know your professors and preceptors"? Well, residency application season is the

Sample Letter of Intent #1 with Comments

[Jane Smith
123 Main Street
Anytown, USA
800-555-8888
Jane_smith@myemail.com]

December 20, 2011

[April Miller, Pharm.D., BCPS
PGY1 Residency Program Director]
University Hospital
5 Hospital Lane
Residency Town, USA

Dear Dr. Miller,

It is with much enthusiasm I share with you my reasons for pursuing the PGY-1 pharmacy practice residency at University Hospital. I was initially drawn to the program [after meeting John Carter] at the Midyear Clinical Meeting. The genuine enthusiasm he expressed made a huge impression on me. As I learned more about pharmacy at University Hospital, I knew I wanted to be a part of it. From the inter-disciplinary practice model to the focus on exceptional patient-centered care, it is a program I feel reflects my passion for what pharmacy has to offer now and in the future.

My short-term professional goal is to become a confident and effective general clinical practitioner through the completion of PGY-1 training. Therefore, my ideal residency is one that fosters the transition from student to practitioner by offering the right balance of support and independence. I believe PGY-1 training at University Hospital will help me accomplish this goal by enhancing my abilities to solve complex medication problems and make drug therapy recommendations in a variety of patient care settings.

My long-term professional goals include PGY-2 training and obtaining a clinical practice position. I intend to pursue a PGY2 residency, but have not yet been able to narrow down my interests to one area. Thus the multitude of rotational experiences, as well as the offering of two PGY-2 residencies is appealing to me. [I would be interested in completing a second year at University Hospital if the opportunity were to be available to me.]

I believe I am an excellent fit for University Hospital and am prepared to handle the challenges of residency training. Through my introductory and advanced pharmacy practice experiences, I have developed a great foundation. I am committed to working hard and am dedicated to expanding my clinical skills. [I have conducted and presented several research projects, which have not only prepared me for future residency projects but have also strengthened my time management abilities.] I also enjoy interacting with patients, students, and healthcare professionals alike and look forward to many future teaching and precepting opportunities.

Thank you for considering my candidacy for the PGY-1 pharmacy practice residency at University Hospital. I would be honored to be a part of such a dedicated and team-oriented program. [Please find my curriculum vitae enclosed for your review.]

Sincerely,
[Jane Smith]
Jane Smith, PharmD Candidate
University of USA

Comments:

Many word processing programs have letterhead templates. You may consider using one of these or create your own to make your letter of intent look more visually appealing.

Under the contact person's name, it is customary to include an additional line with his/her official job title.

This is a nice personal touch. Besides mentioning his enthusiasm, you may want to mention you and he specifically discussed that really resonated with you.

While it may be appropriate to share the fact that having PGY-2 programs at the same institution for which you are applying to a PGY-1 program is appealing to you, remember to keep your letter focused on the current program you are seeking. Don't get too ahead of yourself.

This is good. It highlights a specific accomplishment or set of accomplishments that, in turn, the candidate uses to demonstrate improvement in a specific skill set, time management.

Although there is nothing explicitly wrong with mentioning your CV is enclosed, stopping with the previous sentence ends the letter on more of a high note.

An actual signature should be included here. If letters are provided electronically, you can print and sign, then scan into a PDF for electronic transmission. Alternatively, you can create your own 'electronic signature' to be able to cut and paste into each letter.

Figure 9-1:
Sample Letter of Intent.

Sample Letter of Intent #2 with Comments

[December] 23, 2011

April Miller, PharmD, BCPS
Residency Program Director, PGY-1 Residency Program
Community Hospital
456 Oak Street
Department of Pharmacy
Columbia, MO 24924

Dear Dr. Miller,

[My name is Sally Student, and I am a Doctor of Pharmacy candidate currently attending the University of East College of Pharmacy]. I am writing to express my interest in the PGY1 residency program with Community Hospital. I have researched your program and also spoken with Dr. Joseph Jones and current residents in order to become familiar with what the program has to offer. I believe your residency program would be an ideal learning experience for me to enhance my abilities and grow as a pharmacist.

[During my four years of school], my goal has been to pursue a pharmacy residency after graduation in order to become a [well-rounded pharmacist] and a valuable member of the medical team. I think a post-graduate residency program can help me to develop skills and abilities that will shape me into a better pharmacist. My ultimate career goal, which has been based on my practice rotations so far, is to pursue a position as a [pediatric clinical pharmacist.]

Community Hospital has an outstanding reputation as a respectable institution and the pharmacy residency program seems to offer unique learning experiences. The residency program offers a broad range of opportunities for rotations that I am eager to gain experience in, [especially pediatrics, critical care and cardiology]. The fact that the required core rotations include oncology, pediatrics and cardiology assures me that I will be able to spend a substantial amount of time immersed in the areas that I am most interested in. Another goal that I would like to achieve during a residency program is the completion of a teaching certificate. I think lecturing and serving as a preceptor to pharmacy students would be a rewarding experience, and it would allow me to share my knowledge to help foster the growth of the pharmacy profession. [Finally, I am enthusiastic to complete a research project and publishable manuscript on a topic relating to my interests that has important applications in pharmacy.]

The advanced practice pharmacy rotations I have completed to date, along with my rigorous pharmacy school education, have prepared me for pursuing a residency position. I have gained experience in a wide range of areas, including pain management, [neonatal pharmacy practice and adult critical care]. I have presented on numerous occasions to pharmacy staff, nursing staff and medical residents. I have maintained a strong active role in multiple pharmacy organizations and for my college of pharmacy. [Each year, I have competed in the local ASHP Clinical Skills Competition and represented the University of East at the national ASHP competition during my third professional year]. I have also worked as a pharmacy intern for five years at Walgreens pharmacy, while maintaining excellent academic standing. All of these experiences have helped me prepare for a position as a pharmacy resident at your institution.

[I look forward to interviewing for a PGY-1 residency position at Community Hospital.] Thank you for your time and for considering my candidacy for this excellent program.

Sincerely,
Sally Student
PharmD Candidate 2012
University of East
[ASHP Match #: 13432]
(800) 555-6300
Sally.student@internetmail.edu

Consider putting your return address information or letterhead above the date. If you do this, the signature line at the bottom does not need to contain as much information.

These types of overly simplistic introductory statements are usually not necessary since the reader can garner this information from your return address/ letterhead or your signature.

This is good. It lets the readers know that you've been considering residency training for a long time.

One might argue that a pharmacy school curriculum can make you a well-rounded pharmacist. Is there something more specific to residency training that this could be replaced with?

Specifics like this are good and show readers that you have given a lot of thought to your career path.

Mentioning the specific rotations that appeal to you help set you apart from a generic candidate that's interested in everything. The fact that pediatrics is included here makes since given the candidate's career goal.

I have not seen a lot of letters intent that specifically list the required research project as an interest. This is good and could set you apart from peers.

The candidate does a nice job of mentioning specific APPE rotations she did that prepare her for similar residency rotations.

This is an accomplishment definitely worthy of high-lighting in a letter of intent.

This sounds a little overconfident and assumes you will get an interview. While confidence is appreciated, a more humble approach is advised.

It never hurts to include your match number in multiple places so reviewers have easy access to it!

Figure 9-2:
Sample Letter of Intent.

Sample Letter #3 with Comments

James Jones
PharmD Candidate
University of Atlantic College of Pharmacy
Columbia, MO 65201

[12/14/2011]

April Miller, Pharm.D., BCPS
University of North USA
7 College Way
Department of Pharmacy
North, GA 40572

Dear Dr. Miller,

Thank you for speaking with me to discuss your residency program. I am currently a fourth year pharmacy student at University of Atlantic College of Pharmacy. I am writing this letter to declare my interest in the pharmacy practice residency at University of North. [After completing two rotations at your institution, researching your program, and meeting with you at the ASHP midyear residency showcase, I have been very impressed with the opportunities that would be afforded to me within your program.]

There is undoubtedly much to be said for how well a student has performed academically. Maintaining balance between work, school, and extracurricular activities is also needed to excel. Throughout both undergraduate and pharmacy schools, I consistently held two to three jobs at any given time, and was also involved in playing or working with various athletic teams. [While I have always been a hard worker, it was not until my fourth year of pharmacy school, upon beginning clinical rotations, that I truly found my niche.] After two rotations, I knew that I would not be satisfied settling into community pharmacy practice. After being exposed to both ambulatory and acute care rotations, I feel that an acute care setting would be the area where I could contribute the most to patient care. Thankfully, it is also in these settings I will find the most career satisfaction.

Pursuing a residency will help facilitate my short and long-term career aspirations. This [job] provides me the opportunity to interact with patients and strengthen my pharmacotherapeutic knowledge of specific disease states. My short-term career goals are to obtain a [pharmacy practice residency, followed by either a specialty residency] or fellowship. During this time, I hope to continue to refine my clinical expertise, as well as expand my skills in research and teaching. After completing my post-doctorate training, I plan to obtain a position as a clinical pharmacist in a [specialized patient population. I realize that being exposed to different areas of pharmacy practice will undoubtedly shape my direction. At this point I am very interested in pediatric pharmacy practice.] In this role, I would hope to teach or precept students, conduct research, and maintain a clinical practice site.

The program at University of North has everything that I am looking for in a pharmacy practice residency. [I want a program that offers a diverse selection of elective rotations, primarily in pediatrics.] Also, I want to complete a residency in a teaching hospital setting, where interprofessional collaboration is most in tune. I have no doubts that after the completion of this residency, I would be a competent and successful clinical pharmacist.

Thank you again for your time and consideration, and I look forward to hearing from you.

Sincerely,
James Jones,
PharmD Candidate 2012

Comments (right margin):

Spell out December 14, 2011 in a formal letter of intent

This is a good example of personalizing a letter of intent with multiple ways the candidate learned about the program/institution.

This is the case with many students who may not consider residency training until they do their APPE rotations in their fourth professional year. The letter of intent is a good place to share with application reviewers how you came to the decision about pursuing residency training, especially if you did not get involved with extracurricular or research opportunities early on in pharmacy school.

This is a minor point, but avoid referring to a residency as a job. "Program", "educational opportunity" or "training opportunity" are better choices.

Although these terms are still used in conversation, avoid using them in a formal letter to a program. PGY-1 Pharmacy residency and PGY-2 [insert specialty, if known] Pharmacy residency is the terminology used by ASHP.

The candidate does a nice job of elaborating on his current interest in pediatric pharmacy while recognizing that a PGY1 program has the capacity to change his interests based on his residency rotations.

The candidate ties in his interest in pediatrics again, which is good. He should consider tying the "diverse selection of elective rotations" and "teaching hospital setting" points more explicitly back to the program at University of North. This will give the application reviewers a clearer understanding of how his interests fit their institution/program.

Figure 9-3:
Sample Letter No. 3.

perfect time to find out how well you listened. The two biggest broad questions that residency applicants have about letters of recommendation are as follows:

- Who should I ask to write me a letter of recommendation?
- To the best of my ability, how do I ensure that I will get a positive letter of recommendation?

Who Should I Ask to Write Me a Letter of Recommendation? Most programs will require at least three letters of recommendation as part of your application packet, but they won't give you any more guidance than that. Therefore, you will need to choose your letter writers carefully and thoughtfully. Your letter writers should be very familiar with your knowledge, skills, and abilities. Common choices include faculty at your college of pharmacy, rotation preceptors, advisors of student organizations with whom you worked closely, research mentors, or supervisors at your place of employment. You may consider asking individuals who can comment on *different* skills/abilities you have because of the capacity in which they worked with you. For example, a faculty member who worked closely with you as part of a student organization may be able to comment on your excellent leadership and time management skills, whereas a research mentor may be able to comment on your attention to detail technical skills and written communication abilities. The choice of letter writers should also make sense to the program decision makers. If you are applying to a PGY-1 Pharmacy Residency at General Health-System, and you completed an APPE rotation there, it makes sense to ask the preceptor of that APPE rotation to write you a letter. If you are applying to a PGY-2 Infectious Diseases Residency, it makes sense to ask your PGY-1 Infectious Diseases rotation preceptor to write a letter of recommendation for you.

You may be tempted to ask individuals who do not know you that well but who you perceive as having significant clout (e.g., the dean of your college) to write you a letter. Although titles hold significance with some program decision makers, most who review residency applications would rather read letters that add richer perspective to your application as a whole. Application reviewers have had a lot of experience reading between the lines of letters of recommendation. It is abundantly apparent when a letter is written by someone who barely knows the candidate. Do yourself a favor and enlist letter writers who can provide specific details about all of your many wonderful attributes! In addition, if a program asks you for three letters of recommendation, they mean three. Although there may be numerous individuals who could write positive letters of recommendation for you, application instructions exist for a reason. The application review process is systematic for most programs, and the programs may not have a way to process or score the fourth or fifth letter of recommendation. What you thought was going to make your application stronger may just be a point of confusion or frustration for the program decision makers, who are probably reviewing many other pages of many other applications. *Always* follow instructions!

How Will I Know They Will Write Me a Positive Letter of Recommendation?
Chances are you will not. Unless the letter writer chooses to share their letter
with you, it is unlikely you will ever see your letters of recommendation. In fact,
some programs ask that applicants waive the right to see their letters of recommendation. ASHP has an example of a letter of recommendation form with a
waiver on their Web site.[5] But besides having done everything in your power to
build professional connections with your letter writers, here are some other comments and courtesies you can employ to make sure the process goes smoothly:

- Ask your letter writers whether they are willing to write a *positive* letter of
  recommendation for you—It may seem obvious, but simply adding "positive" or "good" to qualify the type of letter they will write could save you a
  mediocre or at worst a bad letter of recommendation. Although most letter
  writers are not out to demolish your professional aspirations, they may not
  have as high of an opinion of you as you think they do. Asking whether one
  will write you a positive letter takes more courage on your part because
  it opens you to a potentially uncomfortable situation, but by adding one
  qualifier to your question you will be doing due diligence to secure letter
  writers who undoubtedly have your best interests in mind and will be root-
  ing for you with every word they write.

- Give your letter writers as much notice as possible—Many of these individuals will have already been asked to write letters for other applicants,
  so the more time you can give them to write you a letter, the better. As soon
  as you know you will be applying to a program and you have your letter
  writers selected, let them know. Although there is no universally agreed
  upon time line, you should contact and confirm your letter writers the week
  after you get back from ASHP MCM at the very latest. Confirming them by
  November is preferred.

- Give your letter writers all the necessary information about the programs,
  preferably all at once. Different individuals will have different needs about
  the information they need or want from you, but in general, your letter
  writers will need to know the following:
  - The names of the programs, the appropriate contact person, and the mail-
    ing address and/or email address depending on the delivery method the
    program prefers.
  - The deadlines for submitting the letters and whether the letters need to
    be received or postmarked by the deadline.
  - Whether they need to mail and/or email their letters directly to the con-
    tact person or whether they are to seal their letters in an envelope for
    you to retrieve and include in your application packet. If there is nothing
    on the ASHP Online Residency Directory or the program's Web site that
    explains how they want letters of recommendation delivered, the con-
    servative option would be for the letter writer to mail a hard copy of the
    letter directly to the program contact.[3]
  - Whether there are forms they need to complete and whether these forms
    are intended to accompany or replace traditional letters of recommenda-
    tion. If the program does not mention a letter of recommendation form

in its application requirements, then do not include one! However, if a program is using the form on the ASHP Web site, for example, you will need to complete the top portion by indicating whether you waive the right to review the letter and provide this to your letter writers to complete the rest of the form.[5] You will also need to be very clear whether the program needs the completed form *only* or whether the program needs the completed form *in addition to* a traditional letter of recommendation. If there are no explicit instructions about the form, the conservative option would be to instruct your letter writers to complete the form and write a traditional letter of recommendation.

o Letter writers may require additional information from you in order to complete their task well. You might consider proactively providing a copy of your CV, a copy of your letter of intent, a link to the program's Web site, or a hard copy of information about program specifics. Some letter writers may ask you to email them a brief explanation of why you are pursuing a particular residency, especially if you have not provided them your letter of intent. If you do not know your letter writers as well as you would like, do not be surprised if they ask to meet with you to discuss your application prior to agreeing to write a letter for you. You can also be proactive with this. If you feel unsure about how well your letter writers know your intentions and desire for residency training, consider setting up a brief meeting or at least arranging a time to drop off all necessary materials to them face-to-face, so they have an opportunity to gauge your commitment to the residency application process. The key with the "other" category of information that may be requested is to be courteous and as accommodating as possible. Chances are they are not asking for these materials because they are trying to make things difficult or test you, rather they need this information to write a letter of recommendation with additional depth.

• Give your letter writers any other ancillary materials they might need—Some letter writers may value this differently than others, but it is better to be overly courteous and accommodating than the opposite! Providing your letter writers with envelopes complete with the contact person, program addresses and paid postage are appreciated. If your letter writers would prefer to use their own business envelopes, you may offer to take some envelopes in advance and prepare them with program information and the appropriate postage. Most individuals you ask to write you letters will be happy to manage the envelope/postage on their own, but if you proactively provide these materials, it will not go unnoticed. Table 9-2 provides a sample of the types of information you should provide to individuals providing letters of recommendation for you.

> "It is very helpful to develop organized packets of program information (program contact, addressed envelopes, due dates, etc.) for your preceptors writing recommendation letters."
>
> *Danielle Y. – Pharmacy Resident, Tennessee*

The process of selecting individuals to write you positive letters of recommendation and making sure they have everything they need in order to

TABLE 9-2 • Sample of Information to Provide for Individuals Providing Letters of Recommendation

Residency Program	Residency Program Director	Due Date	Mailing or Email Address	Special Forms or Instructions	My Interest in the Program
Baptist Medical Center, South City, Oregon	Mark Griffin, PharmD, BCPS Email: mgriffin@baptist.org	1/15/2012	Mail to: Mark Griffin, PharmD, BCPS Residency Program Director, Baptist Medical Center, Department of Pharmacy, 1523 S. Rural Highway South City, OR 70121	Written letter of recommendation. No additional form required. Mail directly to Dr. Griffin.	Wide variety of rotations, including internal medicine requirement and three outpatient clinic electives to choose from. Cardiology elective. Focus on patient interaction—medication reconciliation, counseling, etc. Many chances to precept students.
Special Veterans Affairs Medical Center, Anytown, TX	Dan Johnson, PharmD, BCPS Email: dan.johnson@specialva.gov	1/6/2012	Mail or email to: Dan Johnson, PharmD, BCPS Director, Pharmacy Practice Residency Program, Special VA Medical Center, 1032 VA, Way, Anytown, TX 23212 danjohnson@specialva.gov	Require both a written letter of recommendation and a completed recommendation using the ASHP Residency Applicant Recommendation Request form. Email (preferred) directly to Dr. Johnson.	Cardiology, geriatrics, home-based primary care rotations. Emergency medicine longitudinal rotation. I will likely apply for job at new VA in Texas post residency training.

accomplish this important task can be a nerve-wracking part of the application process, mostly because so much of it is outside your realm of control. Letters of recommendation, however, are a very important part of the application packet because they offer residency programs vital external perspectives on the candidate. By being courteous, respectful, and organized with your approach to asking for letters of recommendation and by being responsive and accommodating to those who agree to write them, you will be doing everything within your control to ensure three glowing letters of recommendation!

College Transcripts

Most pharmacy residencies require college transcripts, but programs may differ on whether they require transcripts from pharmacy school only or *all* college transcripts including prepharmacy coursework. As with the other parts of your application packet, check instructions carefully to make sure you are requesting the correct transcripts. In addition, check to see whether the residency programs you are applying to require grades from the fall quarter or semester of your fourth professional year to be on the transcript. Because of the timing of the residency application process, you may need to wait for your institution's Registrar's office to include these grades on the transcript that will be submitted with your application packet. Once you have verified which transcripts are required for your application, contact the Registrar's office at each institution to get the process started.

Allow as much times as possible for processing. Policies vary per institution, but at least 2 weeks should be sufficient. You may be charged fees for requesting transcripts, and some institutions offer expedited processing and mailing for additional fees. A word of caution: The Registrar's office may not fulfill a transcript request if you have unpaid charges against your account. Now is the time to make sure all of those pesky campus parking tickets and library fines are paid off!

Residency programs may want transcripts mailed directly to them, but some may prefer that they are included with the rest of your application packet. Most programs require official transcripts, but some may accept unofficial transcripts, which typically do not have a university seal, stamp, or signature. If you are not collecting the transcripts to submit with the rest of your application packet, make sure you follow up with your Registrar's office(s) to confirm that they have processed and mailed your transcripts by the appropriate deadlines. You can always email or call the residency program contact to double-check that they have received all of your transcripts as an additional safety check.

REVIEWING AND SUBMITTING YOUR APPLICATION MATERIALS

Proofread, Proofread, Proofread!

The importance of thoroughly proofreading all of your application materials cannot be stressed enough. While a basic spelling and grammar check in your favorite word processing program can prevent most flubs, it is worth

> "Ask a trusted friend or family member to review *each* part of your application, particularly essays. This allows you to catch mistakes, such as misspellings of names, and provide an external perspective on your applications."
>
> *Kathryn F. – Pharmacy Student, Arizona*

reviewing your application materials multiple times and asking trusted peers or mentors to read your materials provided they are willing and have the time.

Some common proofreading mistakes and suggestions for preventing or correcting these mistakes include

- Mistake no. 1—Misspelling the name of the contact person or institution to which you are applying.
  - Solution—Always double-check the names of contact persons and institutions against a trusted resource. The ASHP Online Residency Directory can be used as a reference source, but if the spellings are different on the institution's Web site, go with the institution's Web site.[3]
- Mistake no. 2—Addressing your letter to the wrong contact person/institution. This may occur if you go into a copy and paste frenzy and are managing multiple letters of intent simultaneously.
  - Solution—Focus on one application at a time. Be systematic, consistent, and descriptive with the file name you give your letters (e.g., John Doe Hospital LOI_Gettig JP.doc and Jane Smith Clinic LOI_Gettig JP.doc). Finally, *always* double-check that the contact person's name and institution are consistent with the address label of your envelope before sealing the envelope.
- Mistake no. 3—Using the wrong homonyms. Forget what a homonym is? Examples include their, they're, and there; or two, too, and to. Since these may be spelled correctly and are real words recognized by spell check, they are unlikely to get flagged in a word processing program.
  - Solution—After finishing what you think is your final draft of any of your application materials, set it aside and find something to distract yourself. Take a quick walk, get a snack, etc. Come back to the draft and reread carefully, sentence by sentence. This is also a good opportunity to enlist the eyes of a friend or mentor whose proofreading skills you trust.
- Mistake no. 4—Misspelling words, especially high-stakes words. Because of the wonders of modern technology, this doesn't happen as often as the previously mentioned mistakes, but it is certain to raise some eyebrows if it does happen. For example, if you are applying for a residency, and you misspell it "residensy" or perhaps you meant to mention pharmacy practice, but instead you wrote "pharmcay" practice because you were tpying too fast and not proofraeding. See how this works? A candidate can quickly lose credibility with a program for such careless mistakes, similar to how I may have lost credibility with you for lecturing you on the importance of proofreading while not thoroughly proofreading myself. Fortunately for me, I have section and copy editors to catch my mistakes. You will not.

○ Solution—Fortunately most spell-checking programs will catch these rather blatant mistakes. Otherwise, there is no simple solution other than repeatedly reviewing your application materials and having other individuals review them before submission if possible.

This is by no means an exhaustive list of proofreading mistakes. The possibilities are, unfortunately, endless. In addition, if you find written communication challenging or if English is your second language, you will need to give yourself even more time to review, rewrite, and revise until your application materials are grammatically superb. Your own keen attention to detail and openness to constructive feedback from peers and mentors during the final review of your application materials are critical to deliver the neatly wrapped package that will be your residency application packet.

Special Delivery!

When you send something as important as a residency application, you want to be sure it gets to the intended person by the intended time. It is not advised to fold everything in thirds, stuff it into a regular letter-sized envelope, and drop it in a mailbox. Application reviewers prefer handling documents that do not have creases in critical places. What if that crease fell right over the most prized accolade on your CV? At minimum, ship your application materials in a 12 ½" × 9 ½" cardboard envelope and splurge on a confirmation service of some kind. The United States Postal Service offers its Priority Mail® Flat Rate service, which ensures delivery within 2 to 3 business days for about $5.00. Delivery Confirmation™ costs less than a dollar more and allows you to track when your application was delivered or if delivery was attempted, but failed. For an additional $3.00 or so, you can purchase a Certified Mail® service, which tracks when you mailed your application out in addition to when it was delivered or if there were failed delivery attempts.[6] Shipping companies like FedEx®, United Parcel Service (UPS), and DHL are other options, and they will offer similar services. Keep in mind that if you wait until the last minute, you may need to use an overnight shipping option, which can cost up to $20.00 per application package. Working ahead of schedule can help save a small fortune on delivery fees.

If the program requires you submit your materials electronically, first make sure you send them from your *professional* email address. If you are a fourth year pharmacy student, an obvious choice would be your college of pharmacy email address; however, another professional sounding address from a commercial email service would also be acceptable. Although most people love a good play on words, especially when it incorporates pharmacy, now is not the time. Avoid sending materials from your hotpharmgurl@yahoo.com or iknowmydrugz@hotmail.com email addresses.

The actual text of your email does not need to be long because the focus is on the attached application materials. You may open with "Dear Dr. X" and close with a professional closing and your name. Similar to snail mail, electronic mail programs will usually have a delivery receipt/confirmation option. Another approach is to save your sent email, so that you have evidence of this important communication later. All things considered, electronic submissions are easier to track than hard copy submissions.

This advice is not meant to scare you. Provided you give yourself enough lead time, submitting your application materials will probably go off without a hitch. Still, it is just as important to be as organized and systematic about the delivery of your application as you were when preparing it.

E-PROFESSIONALISM

Email Etiquette

Besides using a professional email address for correspondence with residency program contacts, here are a few other tips for presenting yourself professionally through this commonly used communication medium:

- Open and close your emails professionally. Use "Dear Dr. X" or "Hello Dr. X" (if the contact person, does in fact have a doctorate degree) to open and close with such words as "sincerely" or "regards" and your name. There are other options for appropriate opening and closings of emails, but refrain from jumping directly into the body of an email, especially if this is the first email you are sending to someone.

- Avoid informal abbreviations and emoticons. Emailing residency programs is not the time to LOL, and it certainly is not the time to LMAO. Avoid using numbers to represent syllables (e.g., b4 for before and 2 for to). For example: "Plz find attached my letter of intent. Sorry it was 18. ☺" is probably not going to be met with the compassion you are looking for—even if you use a teary-eyed frowny emoticon.

- Always make sure you have all of the appropriate files attached. Before hitting send, open each attachment and make sure it's the correct version and is addressed to the correct program. Do not get overzealous and hit send before making sure everything that's supposed to be attached is attached.

- Always double-check to whom you are sending or carbon copying your emails. Do not inadvertently send application materials intended for one program to the wrong program.

- Don't forget to include a subject line. While it can sometimes be difficult to think of one, with residency materials including your name is best. For example, "Application Materials for Jacob Gettig."

- Respect the time of the individuals you email. Make sure you have your thoughts organized, and that your emails are comprehensive and clear. Avoid emailing residency program contacts repeatedly for minor clarifications when possible.

This is not a comprehensive list of email etiquette pointers, so you will need to use your best judgment when communicating with residency programs. Remember that any emails you send can be forwarded, printed, and shared among those who will review your residency applications. Residency programs may use professionalism and/or writing skills to guide their decision to invite you for an interview. U don't want ur bad email skillz to ruin ur chances of getting an interview.

Your Online Image

Remember that Facebook or Twitter account on which you shared your deepest, darkest secrets and posted *hilarious* pictures at parties, bars, or other venues in which seemingly unprofessional behavior may occur? If you haven't already checked 10 times today, now is the time to check it. The appropriateness of using one's image on social media to make a judgment call on whether they are fit for a residency program is debatable. But, the fact is, it's happening. In a 2010 survey of RPDs, 20% of the 454 respondents admitted to reviewing social media for residency applicant information.[7] The majority (52%) of respondents who did this found professionalism concerns, and almost 90% of respondents felt that it is fair to assess a candidate's character from the types of information they voluntarily share online. A detailed how-to-list for managing your online image is outside the scope of this chapter, but some basic advice includes

- Check the privacy settings on any platform you have an online profile. Each platform will treat privacy a little differently, but make sure you know what is visible to whom and tighten up privacy settings when appropriate.

- Make sure your profile picture is appropriate if it's visible to everyone who searches for you. There is no definition of what constitutes appropriate, but a simple shot of your face is probably appropriate. The list of what could be considered inappropriate is outside the scope of this chapter since values vary and perceptions vary widely among individuals involved in the residency application review process.

- Check if any comments you have made in a public forum in which you can be identified are not disparaging, lewd, or unprofessional in any other sense of the word. If you find some and can still delete them, do it.

The residency application process is a time when the old saying that "an ounce of prevention is worth a pound of cure" is most certainly true. By this time in your professional career, you have probably heard repeatedly how important your professional image is. You probably have even attended presentations in which e-professionalism was specifically discussed. Hopefully, you have heeded advice to refrain from posting things that could be construed as unprofessional somewhere down the line. However, if you didn't and if your image is in need of a serious spring cleaning, now is most certainly the time to do so—even if you technically complete your applications in winter.

THE FUTURE OF THE RESIDENCY APPLICATION PROCESS

Although some residency programs have established fully electronic means for submitting residency application materials, there is currently no centralized electronic application system for pharmacy residencies.[8] However, at the December 2011 ASHP MCM, Janet Teeters, Director of Accreditation Services at ASHP, announced that a new online application management system for residency applications is on the horizon for fall/winter 2012. Pharmacy Online Residency Centralized Application System (PhORCAS) will work similarly to

Pharmacy College Application Service (PharmCAS) and is managed by the same company, Liaison International.[9] Since most pharmacy students will have applied to pharmacy school using PharmCAS, the process may be at least partially familiar. Exact details of the PhORCAS are forthcoming, but similar to PharmCAS it will act as a repository for all application materials and serve as a means to efficiently collect letters of recommendation and transcripts. Also similar to PharmCAS, residency applicants will be able to more efficiently apply to many programs quickly. Chapter 27 contains additional information about PhORCAS.

Chapter Takeaways

▶ Securing a pharmacy residency position is getting increasingly competitive. You will need to be organized and systematic if you want to be a successful candidate.

▶ Your letter of intent should include a personal touch and should concisely describe why you and the residency program are a good fit for each other by using specific examples.

▶ Choose authors for your letters of recommendation that know you well and will write you positive letters. Be respectful, courteous, and organized with your request and be responsive and accommodating with their needs throughout the letter writing process.

▶ Proofread all application materials multiple times and ask trusted peers and/or mentors to review your materials before you submit them.

▶ If you have not already done so, review your online image and modify it if necessary. Tighten privacy settings and remove anything that could be perceived as unprofessional by residency application reviewers.

ROLE FOR THE MENTOR

Mentors can help you decide which programs you should move forward with applying to by recognizing which appear to be a good fit for you and conversely which programs you would be a good fit for. By helping you through this process, they can also help decide on an appropriate number of programs to which you should apply.

Mentors may have additional insight for the types of things they like to see in a letter of intent. This insight may be even more valuable if they have experience on committees that review residency candidate applications.

Your mentor might be an appropriate person to ask for a letter of recommendation. They may also be able to guide you in your selection of other letter of recommendation authors.

Mentors may be willing to review your application materials prior to submission. Be respectful of their time, however, since they may be receiving similar requests from multiple students.

FREQUENTLY ASKED QUESTIONS

Q: How many residency programs should I apply to? Is there a certain number to aim for?

A: Given that the competition for pharmacy residencies is at an all time high right now, you may increase your odds of successfully getting an interview and ultimately matching with the program if you cast a broad net and apply to 8 to 10 residency programs. However, you should seriously reflect on your career plans and interests to make sure each program you apply to is an appropriate fit for you. You should also consider the time it will take to complete application, the time away from APPE rotations you may need if you are offered on-site interviews, and the possible travel and lodging expenses you may incur with each on-site interview you complete. Your mentors can help assess the strength of your application as a whole and may be able to suggest how many programs to which you should apply to remain competitive.

Q: Who should I ask to write my letters of recommendation?

A: This may vary depending on the programs you are applying to, but the best letters of recommendation will come from individuals who have a deep understanding of your knowledge, skills, and abilities. Instead of asking individuals to write you a letter because you perceive they have important titles or high ranking positions, consider asking faculty, preceptors, mentors, or work supervisors who can provide specific examples of the great characteristics about you that set you apart from your peers.

Q: Should I ask the same individuals to write letters of recommendations for all of my residency program applications?

A: Not necessarily. For example, assume your standard three letter writers are a faculty mentor, a preceptor, and a work supervisor, but you completed two of your APPE rotations at the institution where you are applying to a PGY-1 residency. You could consider asking both of the preceptors of these rotations (instead of the faculty mentor or work supervisor) to write you a letter of recommendation because they might have better rapport with the residency application reviewers at that institution. Using a checklist like the one suggested in Table 9-1 can help you keep track of which individuals you asked to write letters for you for each residency program application.

Q: What type of information do I need to give to the individuals who agree to write me good letters of recommendation?

A: Simply put—anything they ask for within reason. The typical information they will need includes your CV, information about the residency program(s) to which you're applying including deadlines, contact persons, and elements of the programs that particularly interest you. Being very organized and responsive to your letter writers' needs will go a long way and possibly even positively influence the content of their letters of recommendation.

References

1. National Matching Service. ASHP Resident Matching Service. http://www.natmatch.com/ashprmp. Accessed February 1, 2012.

2. Knapp KK, Manolakis M, Webster AA, Olsen KM. Projected Growth in Pharmacy Education and Research, 2010 to 2015. Am J Pharm Educ. 2011;75(6):108.

3. American Society of Health-System Pharmacists. Online Residency Directory. http://accred.ashp.org/aps/pages/directory/residencyProgramSearch.aspx. Accessed February 1, 2012.

4. Paloucek FP. Better letter of intent for pharmacy residency applications [letter]. Am J Health Syst Pharm. 2011;61:2218.

5. American Society of Health-System Pharmacists. Residency Applicant Recommendation Request Form. http://www.ashp.org/DocLibrary/Residents/Recommendation-Form.aspx. Accessed February 4, 2012.

6. United States Postal Service. Compare Services and Prices. https://www.usps.com/ship/service-chart.htm. Accessed February 4, 2012.

7. Cain J, Scott DR, Smith K. Use of social media by residency program directors for residency selection. Am J Health Syst Pharm. 2010;67:1635-1639.

8. Clark JS, et al. Using a novel approach to collect, disseminate, and assess residency application materials. Am J Health Syst Pharm. 2010;67:741–745.

9. Liaison International. Home Page. http://www.liaison-intl.com/clients/. Accessed February 7, 2012.

Interview Process 10

Ann M. Philbrick and Todd D. Sorensen

By now you've come a long way in your journey to securing your desired residency. You've researched programs, scrutinized them at the Residency Showcase, polished cover letters and curriculum vitae (CVs), and anxiously awaited responses from the residency program director (RPD). Now a very important part of the process is on the horizon—*the interview!*

In this chapter, we will share insights on a number of issues related to residency interviews. First, it's important to note that the style and tone of residency interviews can vary widely. Some programs plan long itineraries (full day); some are short (a couple of hours). Programs may have a very structured interview process or take a more laid-back approach. Some take on a very serious tone when hosting candidates; others seek to make it more light and fun. It may be difficult to predict which personality style the program will display during the interview, so you have to be ready for any of these. This chapter will discuss several universal elements important to interviews so that you can feel confident and prepared during the day.

SCHEDULING YOUR INTERVIEW

You should expect to be contacted by a residency program approximately 2 to 4 weeks after the application deadline.

> "Programs may contact you by phone. Be sure to update your voicemail greeting so that it sounds professional!"
>
> *Mandey M. – Pharmacy Resident, South Carolina*

Should a program decline to interview you, they will most likely email or send you a letter with this information. Invitations to interview will either come via email or personal phone call. Be prepared for this type of call during the month of January so you aren't caught off guard when you answer. Also, it is important to ensure that you have a voice mail message that sounds professional. Regardless of how the program contacts you, you should reply as soon as possible, preferably within 24 hours. The number of candidates that a program chooses to interview can vary widely, but most will likely interview somewhere between 5 and 10 candidates for each position they offer. Occasionally programs will require a preliminary phone interview to narrow down their applicant pool.

When considering a date to interview, it is important to remember that you are a student first, so you should keep your preceptor informed of your other commitments. If you will be scheduled for an Advanced Pharmacy Practice Experience (APPE) during the interview period, you should contact your preceptor in January to let them know that you have applied to residency programs and anticipate needing to take time to attend interviews during the experience. Then, as you receive invitations to interview, keep your preceptor informed and confirm available dates with them prior to scheduling interviews. They may have suggestions regarding which days during the rotation would be better for interviews (e.g., preceptor vacations or days without activities planned). You should also be prepared to offer to schedule time at the site to "make up" for time that you'll be away for interviews. This could be accomplished by being at the site nights or weekends or it could include taking on additional projects that can be done away from the site.

Some residency programs organize "interview days" on which they host several candidates, usually on Mondays and Fridays. Programs that manage interviews in this way may only offer 2 to 3 dates for interviews, and you will need to be flexible with your availability in order to make arrangements to visit on one of these dates. It is unlikely that these programs will make accommodations for individual candidates who cannot interview on one of the designated dates. If these dates conflict with available interview times with other programs, this may be the point where you will need to begin prioritizing the programs to which you applied, choosing to interview with one over another.

TRAVEL

If you are going to need to travel for your interview, you may wish to consider scheduling your interview on a Monday so that you have the weekend to travel. This can also minimize your time away from an APPE. If a Monday interview is not possible, consider traveling in the afternoon or evening to lessen time away from an APPE. When air transportation is required to travel to your interview, try to travel the day before to lessen the chance that unexpected delays will prevent you from arriving to your interview on time. If your arrival is delayed, keep the program updated on your situation. Most programs will understand these situations. Occasionally, you may have an opportunity to have dinner or take a tour of the town outside the specific interview time, so try to confirm the interview itinerary prior to scheduling your flight. Additionally, it is a good idea to only use a carry-on if possible as luggage can get lost. If a checked bag is required, place all items you will need for the interview in your carry-on.

> "Keep everything you might need for an interview in your carry-on luggage – you never know when checked bags may get lost!"
>
> *Mandey M. – Pharmacy Resident, South Carolina*

Programs may offer you transportation to/from the airport. If they do not, remember to allow plenty of time for a shuttle or taxi to get you to your location.

HOTEL ARRANGEMENTS

Some exceptions may exist, but generally speaking, residency programs will not provide funds for your travel or lodging expenses during interviews. The cost of traveling to multiple interviews will need to be considered when applying to programs and then again when receiving interview invitations from programs. While they may not provide financial support for lodging, most programs will have recommendations for affordable accommodations. If not, you should feel comfortable asking for suggestions. Programs may have an arrangement with a local hotel to provide discounts to candidates. Additionally receiving recommendations from the program will likely ensure that you will find lodging close to the interview site and in a safe location. Provided you aren't staying an extra night, you can go ahead and check out of the hotel in the morning prior to your interview. Most programs are fine with storing your luggage in a closet on site for the day. Otherwise, most hotels have the capability of storing luggage after you check out.

ATTIRE

Just like with professional meeting attendance, what you wear to an interview matters. Like it or not, it will influence the perception that RPDs and preceptors have of you, and you should dress professionally. This means a business suit in black, charcoal, navy, or brown with a coordinated shirt and for men, a tie. For women, skirts are acceptable but they should be an appropriate length—just above the knee. As uncomfortable as they are, if you (women) chose to wear a skirt, panty hose are required. For men, shoes should be clean and polished. Women should wear dress shoes, preferably a short, comfortable heel (see illustrations and suggestions in Chapter 8 for more details). Keep in mind that there will likely be a tour as part of the interview, so you will want a shoe in which you can walk long distances. You should make a point to cover tattoos that may be visible. Table 10-1 gives a summary of appropriate interview attire.

TABLE 10-1 • Appropriate Interview Attire	
Men	**Women**
• Suit of black, charcoal, navy, or brown	• Suit of black, charcoal, navy, or brown
• Coordinating shirt and tie	• Coordinated shirt
• Matching socks	• Short, comfortable heels
• Polished shoes	• Conservative makeup
• Minimal, or no cologne/aftershave	• Minimal, or no perfume
• Neat, professional hairstyle	• Minimal jewelry and accessories
• Short, trimmed/manicured fingernails	• Neat, professional hairstyle
	• Short, trimmed/manicured nails

It is a good idea to carry a small portfolio with you. Here you can place extra copies of your CV and business cards, keep a list of questions you'd like to ask during the interview, and have paper and pen available to take notes during your time with the program. Briefcases or laptop bags are appropriate, but remember you will have to carry it with you during the day, which may be a hassle. For women, it is acceptable to carry a small coordinating purse during the day. Also, keep in mind many programs will offer to store these items if needed during the day.

THE INTERVIEW

It is finally time for the big day.

Remember that from the moment you arrive at your destination, you are being interviewed. The way you interact with the program's administrative assistant could get back to the RPD. Make sure to make positive impressions wherever you go. Be polite and use formalities (Dr., Mr. Mrs., etc.) unless told otherwise.

> "Nothing eases your mind during residency interviews like proper preparation."
>
> Matthew W. – Pharmacy Student, Michigan

> "Refer to interviewers by their conferred degree and not by their first names unless permitted to."
>
> Lola A. – Pharmacy Student, Tennessee

You may be the only candidate to interview that day or there may be other candidates present as well. If other candidates are present, your actual interview time with the RPD and preceptors will likely be individualized. Listening to a program overview, tours, and meals are the activities likely completed as a group. Some places may also offer some group interviews.

Prior to your interview, you should receive an itinerary for the day, which will show you all scheduled activities. While you should be willing to be flexible if plans change, there should be no surprises about the day's activities! Sample itineraries can be found as Figures 10-1 through 10-3 in this chapter. Do your homework—make sure you know who each person you'll be meeting is within the residency program. It is a good idea to try and research information about the individuals you'll meet if possible. Check out the program Web site and see if you can identify their clinical or research interests. Search a database such as PubMed® or OVID® to see if they have had recent publications. If you have a mutual interest, make sure that you bring that up in the interview so that they are more likely to remember you after the interview.

You should expect to spend 30 to 60 minutes of the interview with the RPD. This is one of the most important parts of your visit as the RPD will likely have the most influence with respect to ranking candidates. Make sure that

PGY-1 PHARMACY PRACTICE RESIDENCY

University Hospital
Interview Schedule for

Aidan Jones

Jim Jones, PharmD, BCPS Assistant Director Clinical Services PGY-1 Residency Director	9:00–10:00 am Ground Floor Pharmacy Administration
Celeste Rudisill, PharmD Pharmacy Clinical Manager Residency Coordinator	10:00–10:30 am Ground Floor Pharmacy Administration
Mark Williams, PharmD, BCOP Clinical Specialist Hematology and Oncology	10:30–11:00 am Ground Floor Pharmacy Administration
Brandon Bookstaver, PharmD, BCPS, AAHIVE Clinical Specialist Infectious Diseases	11:00–11:30 am Ground Floor Pharmacy Administration
Lunch and Tour Current PGY-1 Residents	11:30 am–1:00 pm
April Miller, PharmD, BCPS Clinical Specialist Surgery	1:00–1:30 pm Ground Floor–Ardmore Tower Pharmacy Administration
Jim Jones (Wrap up)	1:30–1:45 pm

Figure 10-1:
Sample PGY-1 Interview Schedule with Individual Interviews.

you have prepared questions for the RPD as this is also the time to have your most pressing questions answered. You should also expect to spend time with program preceptors as well as current residents. You may be tempted to relax a bit with the current residents; however, it's important to note that current residents often have significant input with the program's ranking selection process, so consider that part of your interview as important as any other. Interviews may be conducted in a variety of ways. You may have one-on-one interviews throughout the day, as seen in Figure 10-1 or you could have a situation where you are being interviewed by several people at once, as outlined in Figure 10-2. In the situation where you have multiple interviewers in one room, answer questions directly back to the person who asked it, while making eye contact with other individuals. Figure 10-3 provides a sample Postgraduate Year Two (PGY-2) interview schedule.

Also included in a typical interview is a tour of the facilities, which may include travel to several buildings or sites. The tour will be helpful as it will familiarize you with the layout of the facility and give you an idea of how the day-to-day operations work. You may also be asked to attend patient care

ACADEMIC COMMUNITY HOSPITAL: RESIDENCY APPLICANT INTERVIEW SCHEDULE

Time	Jose Martinez	Ricky Jones	TJ Smith
8:00–9:00 am	Overview of Residency	Overview of Residency	Overview of Residency
9:00–9:30 pm	Clinical Application Assessment	Clinical Application Assessment	Clinical Application Assessment
9:45–10:15 am	Clinical Experience Site–Heart Hospital		Clinical Experience Site–ICU
10:30–11:00 am	Clinical Experience Site–ICU		Clinical Experience Site–Cardiology
11:00 am–12:00 pm	Hospital/ Department Tour	Hospital/ Department Tour	Hospital/ Department Tour
12:00–1:00 pm	Lunch with residents	Lunch with residents	Lunch with residents
1:00–1:30 pm	Clinical Preceptors Interview (Pharmacy Conference Room)	Pharmacy Operations Experience	Manager's Interview (Director's office)
1:30–2:00 pm	Manager's Interview (Director's office)	Clinical Preceptor Interview (Pharmacy Conference Room)	Pharmacy Operations Experience
2:00–2:30 pm	Pharmacy Operations Experience	Manager's Interview (Director's office)	Clinical Preceptor Interview (Pharmacy Conference Room)
2:30–3:30 pm	Wrap-Up and Questions	Wrap-Up and Questions	Wrap-Up and Questions

Figure 10-2:
Academic Community Hospital: Residency Applicant Interview Schedule.

rounds. This can be helpful as it gives you an idea of how the healthcare team incorporates clinical pharmacists into its activities. You may consider having a question or two for the clinical pharmacist, attending physician, or other members of the healthcare team to ask in this situation.

ANSWERING INTERVIEW QUESTIONS

While there are many activities in the interview day, candidates often find the actual "interviews" to be most stressful. Rather than being nervous, consider these sessions as your opportunity to share all the wonderful things about

INTERVIEW SCHEDULE

PGY-2 Oncology Residency
April Miller, PharmD

9:30–10:30 am	Sally Martin, PharmD, BCOP Clinical Specialist, Hematology and Oncology Director, Hematology and Oncology Residency
10:30–11:00 am	Tour Sarah Smith, PharmD PGY-2 Oncology Resident
11:00–11:45 am	Jose Johnson, PharmD, BCOP Clinical Pharmacist, Cancer Center
11:45 am–1:00 pm	Lunch with PGY-2 and PGY-1 Residents
1:00–1:30 pm	Interview Presentation
1:30–2:00 pm	Cathy Jons, PharmD, BCPS Clinical Specialist, Drug Information
2:00–2:45 pm	Decentralized Oncology Pharmacists
2:45–3:30 pm	Wrap-Up and Final Questions Sally Martin

Figure 10-3:
Sample PGY-2 Interview Schedule.

yourself that make you a great residency candidate. Examples of common interview questions are listed in Table 10-2.[1] You will find this list (and possibly others) as a good way to help prepare for interviews. Read over it and think through an answer to each of these questions. Unlike a formal presentation, you should have general ideas of your feelings on the questions, NOT exact, completely formulated, typed out responses. You want to come across genuine—not rehearsed. That way interviewers can see your unique personality and get an idea of who you are. It is also a good idea to have a solid idea of what goals you have for your pharmacy career, what you are looking for in a residency and your preferred learning style. These questions will almost always come up, so be prepared to answer them.

> "Be familiar with everything on your CV. If it's written down, it's fair game for questioning."
>
> *John M. – Pharmacy Resident, Wisconsin*

Two common questions asked during interviews have to do with your greatest strengths and weaknesses. *What is your greatest strength?* is one of the easier questions that you will have to answer. When answering, it is important that you tie your strengths to the position that you are seeking. Even more important is that you have examples and stories that you can share that provide evidence that your answer is valid. For example, you

TABLE 10-2 • Sample Interview Questions

- Why do you want to do a residency? Why are you interested specifically in this residency program?
- Where do you see yourself after residency? Are you considering a specialty residency or fellowship?
- What makes you a better candidate than the other candidates we have/will interview?
- What areas of pharmacy interest you most?
- What is your definition of pharmaceutical care? What is your definition of a clinical pharmacist?
- Describe your ideal preceptor.
- What is the most important issue facing the profession of pharmacy today? In what ways do you believe you can help address this issue?
- How do you handle stress?
- Describe a situation of conflict with another person. How did you handle it?
- Provide an example of how you've provided leadership during your time as a student pharmacist.
- Provide an example of how you've worked within a team during your time as a student pharmacist.
- Describe the most significant contribution you made to a patient's care this past year.
- Describe your most memorable experiences from your rotations.
- If I were to ask a preceptor to describe you, what would he/she say? Using three adjectives, how would a friend describe you?
- (For PGY-2 candidates) Describe your PGY-1 residency. What were your most valuable experiences?
- Look ahead to your retirement party—who do you hope attends this party to recognize your career in pharmacy? What will be said when people offer toasts to your career?
- Describe the most interesting journal article you have read recently.
- What do you do for fun?

might say that time management is a strength and it enables you to be organized, efficient, and meet deadlines, all important characteristics in a future resident. But the interview will be deemed much more positively if you then can go on to tell about a specific time where your time management skills were tested and you were able to succeed by relying on them. Consider using the STAR method: S Situation, T Task, A Action, and R Result. For example, you could say that you were doing a group project in pharmacotherapy (situation) and had to make a presentation for the class (task). I delegated responsibilities to my group members and gave them deadlines to meet (action). We gave an excellent presentation and received top marks (results).

What is your greatest weakness? can be a little more difficult to answer. Common sense may suggest that you do not want to expose your faults during an interview and it's often been said that you should try to "turn a negative into a positive attribute" when asked this question. However, that can backfire as your answer may seem insincere and that you are trying to avoid the question. For most interviewers, this question isn't about trying to uncover a weakness that will hurt your chances of being highly ranked. Rather, this question can provide insight into the candidate's honesty, knowledge of their personal limits, and highlight their ability to be self reflective. It is best to address this question with an honest answer about an area in which you may be challenged, but then link it to reasons why you want to pursue postgraduate training and how you are looking forward to achieving growth over the residency experience.

There are certain questions that should never be asked of you during an interview. These include questions regarding marital status, children, religious preferences, nationality, age, or health-related questions. This can be tricky because shouting, "you're not allowed to ask me that!" will certainly not win any points. Should you get asked these questions, answering in vague terms or politely stating "I would rather not answer that question" are appropriate. For example, if asked your age, you could say, "I look a lot younger than I am" or similar.

QUESTIONS TO ASK

Every residency program expects you to ask questions.

> "Don't run out of questions to ask during residency interviews! Coming prepared with questions goes a long way in demonstrating initiative and interest."
>
> *Christina T. – Pharmacy Student Texas*

When asked if you have any questions, you should try your best to always have one ready. Be prepared, you'll have many opportunities to ask questions throughout your interview day. Asking questions shows that you are interested in the program and have thought through things that you might want to know about it. Some sample questions to ask of a program are listed in Table 10-3; however, you should also think creatively and develop questions unique to you and the program you are interviewing at. The quality of questions asked during an interview is frequently one of the elements that can leave interviewers with a positive impression about a candidate. Do not ask questions that could be answered by looking on the program, or facility Web site. This may make you look unprepared. Also, don't be afraid to ask the same question of multiple people. For example, it might be helpful to ask the RPD, a preceptor, and a resident what the program's overall philosophy of training is. You might be surprised if those answers vary greatly. Keep in mind that the answers to your questions will be key in helping you decide how to rank a particular program.

TABLE 10-3 • Sample Questions to Ask at an Interview

- What do you believe are the greatest strengths of your residency program?
- Do you anticipate any significant changes to the residency program design in the next year?
- Why has this organization invested the time and financial resources into residency training? What are the benefits to the organization?
- What types of pharmacists are most successful in this organization?
- Do the staff and residents socialize outside of work?
- What is the average length of tenure of the staff?
- What unique knowledge and skills will I gain from this program compared to other programs?
- What do your residents like the most about this program and this organization? What do they like the least?
- How frequently are residents hired by the organization following their residency?
- What types of relationships do pharmacists have with physicians and nurses at this institution?
- What is your idea of the perfect resident?

INTERVIEW PRESENTATION

Some interviews will require a presentation. Presentations are more common in specialized residencies (PGY-2) but may also occur for Postgraduate Year One (PGY-1) residencies.

> "Remember to e-mail Powerpoint® presentations to yourself. It's a good backup if your jump drive doesn't work."
>
> *Mandey M. – Pharmacy Resident, South Carolina*

The purpose of the presentation is not simply to gauge your level of knowledge on a topic, but more often intended to evaluate your confidence, sense of presence in front of a group, and your ability to "think on your feet" fielding questions. It is okay to use the same presentation for multiple interviews, but be sure to customize it for each interview. Some programs will ask for a copy of the presentation in advance.

The length of the presentation may range from 15 to 60 minutes, and you should ask whether or not you need to provide handouts. Most programs will let the candidate choose the topic of their presentation. With that said, it is important that you choose your topic and develop your presentation so that it will be of interest to the attendees—you may want to inquire about who is expected to attend the presentation. When choosing a topic, you should consider topics with which you are comfortable, but also try to develop the presentation that shows something unique about you or your experience. Remember that there will be several other candidates giving presentations— consider how you can use this opportunity to make a positive impression not only based on your presentation skills, but by allowing the attendees to learn more about who you are, your interests, and the unique experience you can bring to the program.

CLINICAL ASSESSMENTS OR EXAMS

Some programs present candidates with a clinical assessment or exam during the interview. This may range from a straightforward multiple choice type test to a more complex clinical case where you must develop a SOAP note that outlines your evaluation. These assessments are designed to evaluate your knowledge of basic disease states (hypertension, diabetes, pneumonia, etc.) and will not address rare clinical issues. Inclusion of a clinical assessment during an interview is usually done to assess basic clinical competence and critical thinking skills. In preparing for the clinical assessment portion of the interview, ensure that you are familiar with treatment guidelines for disease states or clinical situations common to the program's practice setting. For example, in an institution with a large cardiac population, be familiar with how to treat myocardial infarction.

INTERVIEW DINNER

Occasionally, there may be a meal associated with the interview. While most interviewees may think of this as a simple necessity, it is actually an opportunity for your potential employer to gauge how you handle extra pressure—eating food and making a good impression is no easy task! First of all, do not worry about paying for your meal. If the program invites you to lunch or dinner, they are planning to cover the expense of the meal. With that said, be judicious in your menu choices. If it is a fine dining situation, do not order the most expensive item on the menu. Avoid items that can be messy (food with sauces, food eaten with your hands, etc.). Alcohol may be available and you should take a cue from your host regarding ordering a drink. If the host offers an alcoholic beverage, you can feel comfortable accepting it. On the other hand, if you do not drink alcohol or are not comfortable drinking in an interview setting, you also should feel confident choosing nonalcoholic beverages. For more basic dining etiquette recommendations, we refer readers to the following Web sites:

http://www.findalink.net/diningetiquette.php

http://www.etiquettescholar.com/etiquette_scholar/dining_etiquette.html

AFTER THE INTERVIEW

After you have finished the interview, conduct a debriefing session on your own. Write down things that you liked and disliked about the program. Recall the answers to the questions that you felt were important for you to get answers. It is also okay to evaluate how well your personality will mesh with that of the RPD, the preceptors, and the program itself. This will make it much easier to evaluate the programs in an objective manner, once you have finished all of your interviews. You may want to revisit the chart provided in Chapter 5 to see how each program stacks up after the interview.

THANK YOU NOTES

Expressing gratitude to the program for hosting you following an interview is always a good idea.

> "Thank you cards are so important – the first day I arrived to my residency, I noticed a preceptor had my hand-written card hanging in her cube. Don't underestimate how far a thoughtful note goes!"
>
> *Anokhi S. – Pharmacy Resident, Pennsylvania*

It is not necessary to send a note to every person that you interviewed with—one note addressed to the RPD is sufficient. Handwritten notes remain a nice gesture, but with the reliance on email, that mode of communication is also appropriate. It's not as much how you follow up, but what you say. This is one last chance to leave a positive impression with the program and thus your note shouldn't sound like it's the same one sent to all of the programs with which you interviewed. Make it personal. Highlight unique elements from the interview day. Express genuine enthusiasm for the opportunity to join the program.

LAST MINUTE TIPS

- Forget about your cell phone. Checking your phone for text messages, missed phone calls, or emails sends the signal that you are not interested. If you can, leave your cell phone in your car. Otherwise, it should be off, or on silent and tucked away.
- Everyone loves a firm handshake. It displays confidence.
- Do not speak negatively about past/current jobs or rotations. This can suggest that you may be likely to complain about the job for which you are interviewing.
- Control nervous behaviors. The tapping of a foot or a pen can be very distracting to an interviewer. It may be a good idea to ask a close friend if you have any annoying behaviors as you may not be aware of them.

Remember that interviews are about you finding a good fit just as much as they are finding a good candidate.

With good preparation, pharmacy residency interviews can be a great experience. Think about them as a series of "first dates." Think about who you are and what you want from a residency program and your future career, then just be yourself. Just like a first date, use your interview day to get to know the program, just as much as the program gets to know you. And as a plus, no awkward "good night kiss" at the end of the day (well, you hope so at least!)

Chapter Takeaways

▶ Interviews will be scheduled within 2 to 4 weeks after you submit your application. Be prepared to respond to interview requests within 24 hours.

▶ Dress professionally—half of a person's first impression is how you look.

▶ You will meet with several people throughout the day. Know who they are and their professional interests.

▶ Your time with the residency director is most important. Come prepared with questions as it shows you are interested in their program.

▶ Know why you want to do a residency, and why the program you are interviewing at meets those needs.

▶ Be prepared for common questions—but do not sound rehearsed.

▶ Send a thank you note to the RPD within a week following the interview. Make sure to include why you think you are the best candidate for the residency.

ROLE FOR THE MENTOR

A mentor can help you by arranging for or conducting a mock interview.[2,3] This simulated experience can give you valuable feedback on nervous habits or way to improve your interview style.

If required, a mentor can review presentation content and provide helpful feedback on content and style.

FREQUENTLY ASKED QUESTIONS

Q: How long after I submit my application, when will I get an interview offer?
A: Anywhere from 2 to 4 weeks. Interview offers will come by phone or email, whereas denials will come via email or postal mail.

Q: How should I schedule an interview?
A: Most programs have set interview dates that you will have to choose from. If you have to travel long distances, consider scheduling on Monday so that you have the weekend to travel and decrease your time away from your current APPE. Make sure that your preceptor knows that you are expecting interviews prior to them being offered as they may have suggested days to be gone from the APPE. Be prepared to take on extra work for days missed.

Q: How should I dress for my interview?
A: Interview dress can be summed up in two words: professional and modest. A suit is required. Your tie or undershirt should be color coordinated and modest. Remember, less is more when it comes to accessories, makeup and perfume/cologne.

Q: How long do most interviews last?

A: This can vary anywhere from 2 to 8 hours.

Q: Who will I meet during my interview?

A: First and foremost, you will meet the RPD. You can also count on meeting with current preceptors and residents. Other people you could meet include department chairs, deans, pharmacy directors, and physicians.

Q: What questions should I be prepared for?

A: You should be prepared to talk about what you want out of a residency, what your career goals are, and how that program fits into these. You should also be able to answer questions regarding your biggest strengths and weakness.

Q: Do I need to send a thank you note to everyone I meet with?

A: No. One note to the RPD is sufficient. This can be handwritten or typed and sent through postal mail or email. Remember to include something personal about you, and why you would fit into their program.

References

1. Mancuso CE, Paloucek FP. Understanding and preparing for pharmacy practice residency interviews. Am J Health Syst Pharm 2004;61:1686–1689.

2. Prescott WA. Program to prepare pharmacy students for their postgraduate training search. Am J Pharm Educ 2010;74:1–8.

3. Koenigsfeld CF, et al. A faculty-led mock residency interview exercise for fourth-year doctor of pharmacy students. J Pharm Pract 2012;25(1):101–107.

The Match Process 11

Tibb F. Jacobs

You've finally finished your interviews and know exactly which residency programs you love and which you don't. Now it's time to start thinking about words guaranteed to strike fear into the heart of any self-respecting pharmacy student: the Match. Many students don't know how the Match works and are convinced its only purpose is to keep them from getting a residency! The Match is designed to help candidates completely assess all of their options before making final decisions. It allows candidates to interview at several programs and allows programs to interview all candidates before finalizing rank order lists. Since both programs and candidates find out Match results almost simultaneously, it provides a fair means of placing candidates and programs together. Without the Match, candidates may be pressured into making a decision before interviewing with all programs. Imagine if you interviewed at your third choice first and they offered you a residency position. You would not be able to interview with any other programs if you accepted their offer. The Match also prevents highly sought-after candidates from stockpiling multiple offers, while qualified but less sought-after candidates have none. And the Match protects both programs and candidates by creating a binding contract, so that neither party can change their mind and accept a more "preferred" candidate or offer at the last minute. Understanding the match process will help you use it to your full advantage.

The Match only helps place candidates with positions in residency programs, and you must still apply and interview directly with the residency program you are interested in. After all interviews are completed, candidates and program directors go online and submit a ranked list of their preferences. The Match then attempts to place candidates into open residency positions based entirely on their preferences listed on their rank order list. Match priority is given to candidate preference rather than program preference.[1]

> "The match works in the favor of the residency candidate. Rank the programs according to your interest and not how you think the programs will rank you."
>
> *Danielle Y. – Pharmacy Resident, Tennessee*

The process of matching could all be done by hand, but a computer is used due to the large volume of individuals involved. The Match works just like the social fraternity and sorority rush process. Programs and candidates submit their individual rank order lists, and the computer attempts to match the candidate with their first choice program. If the candidate can't be matched with their first choice, the computer moves to the second choice and so forth until the candidate is "tentatively" matched or their rank order list is completed. The match is only tentative because the candidate can be removed if a candidate more preferred by the program comes along. At this point, the computer again tries to match the first candidate with another program on their rank order list. This process is carried out for all candidates, and at the end of the match process, all tentative matches are finalized.[1]

For the 2011 residency cycle, 3982 students registered for the Match. A total of 705 students withdrew prior to submitting rankings, leaving 3277 students that submitted rankings for only 2173 Postgraduate Year One (PGY-1) positions. After the Match, there were only 146 open positions and 1250 unmatched candidates.[1] Those numbers may appear daunting at first; however, not all candidates are equal. Some are not able to move many miles away from home, and not all candidates are appropriately prepared for the application process. In other words, not all 3277 candidates are equally competitive. Since 2007, the number of applicants has increased from 1900 to 3277, while the number of positions available has only increased from 1605 to 2163. As more programs continue to develop and expand, these statistics should improve the candidate's likelihood of a successful match. It does appear that 2011 graduates were slightly more successful than pre-2011 candidates at obtaining a position through the Match (64% successfully matched compared to 42% of pre-2011 graduates). After seeing these data, you probably realize how important it is to fully understand The Match and make it work for you.

WHO PARTICIPATES IN THE MATCH?

Applicants

Any student or resident that is interested in obtaining an American Society of Health-System Pharmacists (ASHP)-accredited PGY-1 or Postgraduate Year Two (PGY-2) pharmacy residency position must register and participate in the Match.

In order to be eligible to register, you must be a graduate (or about to graduate) from an ACPE-accredited college of pharmacy. Candidates for PGY-2 residencies must have completed or be currently completing a PGY-1 residency. If you are a graduate of a foreign school of pharmacy and want to participate, you have to provide a copy of your state licensure or your Foreign Pharmacy Graduate Examination Committee (FPGEC) certificate.

Programs

Programs must offer all of their positions through the Match if they are ASHP accredited, have preliminary accreditation, or are in candidate or pre-candidate status. This means that nearly every program you will be interested in will be participating in the Match. The only possible exceptions would be a very new program (with no previous residents) or a program that has chosen not to be ASHP accredited.[1]

THE MATCH TIME LINE

Registration for the match usually begins in August prior to the program's start and continues through January (Figure 11-1). A list of programs participating in the Match will be available for you to review by November (prior to the ASHP MCM). Rank order lists can be submitted starting in February through early March (best to do this after your interviews have been completed). The final date for submission of your rank order lists is always due in early March, so please double-check the date very carefully. *No rank order lists can be submitted after this date.* Match results are released in mid- to late-March. You will get an email by noon EST on Match day letting you know which program you matched with, or whether you did not match. Residency programs find out if they matched candidates at the same time. Scramble for an open position begins immediately after Match results are released, so you will be able to view a list of available positions right away if you did not match.[1]

THE MATCH TIMELINE

August

Applicants can begin registering for ASHP Match online via www.natmatch.com website.

Pay nonrefundable registration fee

September

October

November

List of programs participating in Match are available for access by applicants

December

Attend ASHP MCM

Final date for Early Commitment positions (PGY-2 programs only)

Apply to residency programs of your choice

January

Recommended date to register for Match

February

Residency interviews

Submit rank order lists online at www.natmatch.com

March

DO NOT MISS RANK ORDER DEADLINE!!!

Match results revealed

Scramble process starts immediately after Match results available

Figure 11-1: The Match Time Line.

REGISTERING FOR THE MATCH

Prior to registering, you should read over the Applicant Agreement, Match Rules, and the Schedule of Dates provided on the Web site (http://www.natmatch.com/ashprmp/). The Applicant Agreement states that you must accept appointment to the program that you are matched with, unless both parties agree in writing to release each other from the Match result. *By registering, you are agreeing to honor this contract.* Violations of this Applicant Agreement will be reported to ASHP that has the right to penalize participants that violate Agreements or Match Rules.[1] Even if you escape without penalties, it could be very difficult to find a future residency and possibly a job if you do not honor your Applicant Agreement. Pharmacy is a very small world and breaking your contract could be detrimental to your future career. After reading through all the rules, you can register using the online registration system available on the matching services Web site. A fee is due upon registration, and ASHP recommends that you register prior to mid-January.[1] Remember that registering for the Match is not the same as applying to residency programs. You still have to apply individually to all programs that you are interested in. Each program may have a different application date may even be due as early as December and as late as February.[1]

After you register, you are assigned a five-digit applicant code number. Be aware that you may be asked to supply this code to programs that you apply to. All application requirements and interviews have to be completed prior to early March. This is to ensure that everyone (applicants and programs) can submit their rank order list by the March deadline.[1]

MAKING RANK ORDER LIST

Applicants

As you complete your interviews, you should begin to finalize your rank order list. There may be a program that you just didn't get a good feeling about when you interviewed. If you don't think you could be happy there for a year, don't rank that program. Remember, the Match is a binding contract.

Go through your list of programs and very carefully determine your favorites. It may be helpful to make a list of pros and cons for each program before determining your final ranking. It may also be beneficial to go through your pros and cons list with your mentor, but this decision should be yours though. You are the one that will spend a year there, and who has the most information to help make this decision!

Remember to make your rank order list in the order that you actually prefer each program and not how you think each program will rank you. There is no way to "beat the Match" and attempting to guess how programs will rank you is not of benefit. The Match is slanted toward your preferences over the residency programs, so be sure to be honest.

If you do not get invited for any interviews, you can either leave your name in the Match or withdraw from the Match. Regardless, you will still have access to the listing of post-match positions available on match day on the matching services Web site. Unfortunately, your fee is nonrefundable whether you are invited for interviews or not.[1]

TABLE 11-1 • Example Match Scenario: Applicants' Rank Order Lists

Jessica	Ryan	Ashley	Mike	Chris	Brandon	Heather	Daniel
1. Baptist	1. University	1. University	1. University	1. Baptist	1. Methodist	1. State	1. State
2. State	2. Methodist	2. Methodist		2. State	2. University	2. Baptist	2. Methodist
3. Methodist	3. Baptist	3. State		3. Methodist	3. Baptist	3. University	3. University
4. University					4. State	4. Methodist	

Programs

It's also not easy for programs to determine their rank order lists. While you may have interviewed at five or six places, an individual program may have interviewed 30+ candidates! Every interviewer and person you have contacted with during the interview process is likely to have some influence on the program's rank list. Keep this in mind when you are interviewing. Every single person that you come in contact during your interviews is evaluating you and will be asked at some point to provide feedback and possibly even rank you. Many programs have current residents fill out an evaluation as well.

At some point, the resident selection committee or some similar group is going to sit down in a room and fight it out in order to pull together that program's rank order list. At many programs, this is a fairly democratic process; however, sometimes the residency director or program director will make the final decision about the rank order list. Just like you may not rank all programs, programs may choose not to rank all candidates they interviewed.

EXAMPLE MATCH PROCESS

In order for you to fully understand the Match and how it works, here is a sample scenario with all the contingencies worked out. The example below takes you through the Match process for eight applicants and four programs. In order to mimic the real Match as closely as possible, these fictional programs have only six total positions available. So even in the best-case scenario, at least two students will end up unmatched. Table 11-1 includes the rank order list of candidates and Table 11-2 includes the rank order list of the various residency programs.

TABLE 11-2 • Example Match Scenario: Programs' Rank Order Lists

University (1 Position)	Methodist (1 Position)	Baptist (2 Positions)	State (2 Positions)
1. Mike	1. Mike	1. Daniel	1. Daniel
2. Daniel	2. Daniel	2. Chris	2. Chris
3. Ryan	3. Chris	3. Mike	3. Mike
	4. Ryan	4. Ryan	4. Jessica
	5. Ashley	5. Ashley	5. Ryan
	6. Jessica		6. Ashley
	7. Heather		7. Heather
	8. Brandon		

In this scenario, assume that all eight students interviewed with all four programs. What follows are the results of their match process (Table 11-3).

The process is now complete and all tentative matches are finalized. The final list is as follows:

- University (1 position): Mike
- Methodist (1 position): Ryan
- Baptist (2 positions): Chris, unmatched
- State (2 positions): Daniel, Jessica.

TABLE 11-3 • Example Match Process: Matching System Methods[2]

Applicant	Attempt to Match in Program	Current Program Status	Results
Jessica	1. Baptist	Baptist has two open positions; however, they did not rank Jessica.	The Match now moves to Jessica's second choice.
	2. State	State has two open positions. Jessica is no. 4 on their list.	Tentatively match Jessica with State
Ryan	1. University	University has one open position. Ryan is no. 3 on their list.	Tentatively match Ryan with University.
Ashley	1. University	University has one open position; however, they did not rank Ashley.	The Match now moves to Ashley's second choice.
	2. Methodist	Methodist is filled with higher ranked applicants.	The Match now moves to Ashley's third choice.
	3. State	State has one open position. Ashley is no. 6 on their list.	Tentatively match Ashley with State.
Mike	1. University	University's one position is filled, but they prefer Mike to their current tentative match (Ryan). Mike is no. 1 on their list and Ryan is no. 3.	Ryan is removed from University. Tentatively match University with Mike. Since Ryan was removed from University, another attempt is made to rematch Ryan.
Ryan	1. University	University is filled with higher ranked applicants.	The Match now moves to Ryan's second choice.
	2. Methodist	Methodist has one open position. Ryan is no. 4 on their list.	Tentatively match Ryan with Methodist.

TABLE 11-3 • Example Match Process: Matching System Methods[2] (continued)

Applicant	Attempt to Match in Program	Current Program Status	Results
Chris	1. Baptist	Baptist has two open positions. Chris is no. 2 on their list.	Tentatively match Chris with Baptist
Brandon	1. Methodist	Methodist is filled with higher ranked applicants.	The Match now moves to Brandon's second choice.
	2. University	University did not rank Brandon.	The Match now moves to Brandon's third choice.
	3. Baptist	Baptist did not rank Brandon.	The Match now moves to Brandon's fourth choice.
	4. State	State did not rank Brandon.	Brandon remains unmatched
Heather	1. State	State is filled with higher ranked applicants	The Match now moves to Heather's second choice.
	2. Baptist	Baptist did not rank Heather.	The Match now moves to Heather's third choice.
	3. University	University did not rank Heather.	The Match now moves to Heather's fourth choice.
	4. Methodist	Methodist is filled with higher ranked applicants.	Heather remains unmatched.
Daniel	1. State	Both of State's positions are filled, but they prefer Daniel to both of the other applicants (Jessica and Ashley). Daniel is no. 1, Jessica is no. 4, and Ashley is no. 6.	Ashley is removed (since she is ranked lower by State) and Daniel is tentatively matched with State. Since Ashley was removed, another attempt is made to rematch Ashley.
Ashley	1. University	University is filled with higher ranked applicants.	The Match moves to Ashley's second choice.
	2. Methodist	Methodist is filled with higher ranked applicants.	The Match moves to Ashley's third choice.
	3. State	State is filled with higher ranked applicants.	Ashley remains unmatched.

After the Match, there is only one open position at Baptist, but Ashley, Brandon, and Heather remain unmatched. So now in this particular post-Match scramble, there would be three students competing for one open position. However, in the real scramble, there could be many more students competing for each open position!

If you look at the results of this Match, a couple of things stand out. First of all, Mike got really lucky. He only ranked one program, and that program only had one position. This isn't really a smart way to make your rank order list. Even though the three other programs ranked Mike, he could have still ended up unmatched because he put all his eggs in one basket.

If Jessica would have only ranked one program, she would not have matched. Her first choice program filled up with candidates more highly ranked than she was. However, because she ranked additional programs, she got placed in her second choice position.

Ryan also got placed with his second choice (Methodist) even though they ranked him fourth on their list. Because the candidates that Methodist ranked higher than Ryan all chose other programs above Methodist, Ryan ended up with a position there. So, students' preferences are taken into consideration over the programs' preferences.

If Ashley would have ranked Baptist, she would have matched there. They ranked her, and they are left with an open position. If she wasn't willing to go there, then that was a good decision. If she was willing to go there, she should be kicking herself right now!

Brandon and Heather did not match because either the programs they were interested in didn't rank them or filled their positions with candidates who were more preferred. There is nothing in the match process they could have done differently to improve their odds of matching.

Since both Baptist and State selected Daniel as their first choice, the match process worked in Daniel's favor and he went to State (which was his first choice). And Chris placed with Baptist because he was one of their top two candidates.

TIPS FOR A SUCCESSFUL MATCH

- Rank only programs you are willing to go to. DO NOT rank a program if you aren't willing to go there. You can end up at ANY program that you put on your rank order List. If you don't want to go there, don't rank them. Ask yourself, "would I rather have this residency program or no residency program?" The Match is a binding contract, so you could end up stuck for a year with a program that you don't really care for.

- Do rank all programs that you are willing to go to. It's not going to increase your odds of going to your first choice if you only list one program in your rank order list. If you are willing to go to four different programs, then rank all four. The computer will keep going down your list until they find a tentative match for you. If you only list one program, but that program doesn't rank you or fills their positions with higher ranked applicants, you

> "Do not rank a program if you do not plan on accepting a residency position within that program."
>
> *Danielle Y. – Pharmacy Resident, Tennessee*

won't match. The computer has nowhere else to attempt to place you. The more programs you rank, the more likely you are to match somewhere. Occasionally, students feel like they have some kind of "understanding" with a particular program, and they will definitely get a spot there. Officially, no positions (outside of PGY-2 early commitment) can be offered before the Match, and doing so would a violation of the matching contract. So what you are hearing is probably not the definitive promise of a position that you think. Even if you feel very strongly that you have some type of "in" with a particular program, go ahead and rank all your other alternatives. That way you have the best chance of matching. If you really did have a real connection with your first choice program, no harm was done, but if you misinterpreted something, you won't be left looking for a position in the scramble.

- Rank programs honestly. Don't rank a particular program higher just because you think they will rank you high. This doesn't help you at all. The match process is designed to try to match YOUR choices first, not the residency programs'.[1] So, if you rank Program A high, the process will attempt to put you there first. The computer doesn't know that you really wanted to go to Program B or even Program C, but you thought you had a better chance with Program A! So you easily end up at Program A, even if Programs B and C ranked you also. The only reasons that you will not match with a particular program are if the program doesn't rank you or the program fills all their spots with higher ranked applicants. The bottom line is that you should rank programs according to your true preferences. Don't worry about where or even if a particular program will rank you. If you like them, then rank them in order of your preference. This gives you the best chance at matching with your first choices.

- Preference is given to you rather than residency programs. Remember that the match algorithm tries to match your preferences rather than the programs' preferences.[1]

- When in doubt contact National Matching Services Inc. If there is a scenario that comes up and you just aren't sure what to do and your mentor doesn't know the answer, contact NMS directly. They are very prompt at returning emails. All their contact info is listed on the www.natmatch.com Web site. Their email address is ashprmp@natmatch.com. There are also telephone numbers available.

PGY-2 MATCH

The good news is that the 2011 PGY-2 statistics are not quite as scary as the PGY-1 statistics. There were 370 PGY-2 positions offered with 294 of the positions filling during the Match. However, 397 people participated in the PGY-2

Match, which means 103 participants did not match for 76 unfilled positions.[1] This does not take into consideration that some PGY-2 specialties may be much more competitive than others.

In order to participate in the PGY-2 Match, you must have completed a PGY-1 or be in the process of completing a PGY-1. Naturally, your PGY-1 must end before your PGY-2 would begin! The PGY-2 Match works exactly the same way the PGY-1 Match does, with the exception of the Early Commitment Process. Current PGY-1 residents at an institution that offers a PGY-2 program in an area they are interested in have the option of using the Early Commitment Process, in which both the PGY-2 program and the resident forgo the Match and just select each other. The PGY-2 residency program must pay a nonrefundable fee to National Matching Services for each position that utilizes the Early Commitment Process.[1] If you are currently completing a PGY-1 residency and have chosen to go through with Early Commitment to a PGY-2 program at your current PGY-1 program, the fees and letters of agreement are due right after Midyear (in mid-December).[1]

COUPLES MATCH

What about if you are married or can't part with that special someone during your residency year, and don't want to leave being together up to chance? National Matching Services offers individuals the opportunity to match as a couple. Both you and your partner register individually for the Match, select the option to participate as a couple, and chose your partner. You and your partner make "pairs" of program choices, and both rank order lists have to be submitted individually (after working things out with each other of course)! You both have to submit the same number of ranks. These choices do not have to be the exact same programs; they may be in the same city or within driving distance. You can even choose for one of you to rank and the other to go unmatched.[1] ASHP provides a more detailed explanation and even an example on the Match Web site (www.natmatch.com). It works the same way as the regular Match process; it's just much more difficult to understand because of the logistics of attempting to match two people at once. A couple will match to their most preferred pair on their list where both partners can be matched.[1]

The major benefit of participating in the Match as a couple is that you can minimize the chances that you and your significant other will be separated for a year. It's almost impossible to predict where you will match, so if the two of you are both planning to pursue a residency, there is a very good chance that you will end up in different locations. However, participating in the Couples Match is not without risks. Since your final placement will depend on both of you (instead of just one individual), you may be less likely to get your first choices on your rank order lists because both your lists have to be taken into consideration. One important caveat, before you and your partner decide to go through the Match as a couple, you may want to make sure that you are both equally competitive. You could easily go unmatched if one person is far more competitive than their partner.

POST-MATCH POSITIONS (THE "SCRAMBLE")

Occasionally, programs don't fill all their open positions through the Match. Many students used to count on "scrambling" for these open positions after the Match. However, in recent years, there are very few spots left empty after the Match results are released. Remember in 2011, there were 1250 unmatched candidates and only 146 open positions![1] The bottom line: don't count on getting a residency post-match.

Keep in mind many very good candidates do not match. It is okay to be upset, but keeping a level head in the post-Match process will serve you well. When you find out you do not match, you will also get a list of programs that have unfilled or open positions. You have to IMMEDIATELY start contacting these programs. If you interview with a particular program during the scramble and you both like each other, they are free to offer you a position immediately and you can accept![3]

Before the match results are even revealed, you need to make a conscious decision as to whether or not you are willing to scramble and what your plans will be if you do not match. Are you going to be happy in another type of job? Are you geographically limited due to finances or family and you've already applied/interviewed with all places you can reasonably consider? Then you may not want to scramble for an open position. On the other hand, are you dead set that you WILL do a residency no matter where you have to move or even if you have to reapply next year? If yes, you are probably someone who will scramble for open positions. But the important thing is to decide that before emotions are running high and the clock is ticking. You will only have a limited amount of time to find a suitable residency, and in 2011 there were more than eight candidates available for each empty spot.

It wouldn't hurt to have an email drafted prior to the match results being revealed. If you match, awesome! You don't need your email draft. However, if you didn't match, you can immediately start contacting programs. A recent letter in AJHP mentioned how one residency program filled their two unmatched positions.[4] The program director started getting emails 2 MINUTES after the match results were released. They got a total of 86 applicants for their two open spots! Within 5 hours after the Match results, they made the decision about what four students they were going to interview![4] Interviews took place via phone and on-site (depending on the location of the applicant). Within 3 days, both positions were filled. So you don't have time to freak out or get depressed. You can cry, but you have to start emailing residency directors and preparing your applications while you cry (Figure 11-2).

It may also be a good idea to let your rotation preceptor know in advance that Match results are coming out on a certain day. Let them know that you are planning to scramble if you do not match. Then politely ask if it would be possible to send or respond to emails during regular rotation hours on Match Day. Since Match results are all available by noon EST, you may need a little time during business hours that day. Keep in mind that

TESTIMONY OF AN UNMATCHED CANDIDATE

Post-match scramble. I still can't help but shudder as I type those words. For some students, "match day" is a joyous occasion. It is the culmination of all their hard work and determination throughout pharmacy school and most likely the pinnacle of their young professional lives. But, for others, "match day" will forever be marred as the day where their world turned upside down. Where the plans they made for themself go out the window, taking their ego along with it.

I can still remember "match day" as if it were yesterday. I remember going to bed the night before without a care in the world. My CV was impressive, my grades were impeccable, and I had interviewed at 8 of the most prestigious programs. My pride was soaring, and I was somehow convinced that I was a shoe-in for any institution I desired.

The next morning during rotation my phone began to buzz with friends announcing that the match results were in. I pulled up my email and read the first line, "We regret to inform you…" What? They must have sent this to the wrong person? Those few sentences managed to turn my world upside down. According to my plan, I was supposed to go to the top ranked program and complete 2 years of residency and go on to a career in academia!

I felt numb. At that moment, I didn't know what I was going to do. I was in such shock that I didn't know how to proceed. I questioned whether the post-match scramble was even something I wanted to consider. I cried. And cried some more. And bled mascara all over my sweet preceptor's shirt.

The feelings that come in that moment may be different for every person. For me, it was a profound sense of embarrassment. How could I look at all my other friends who had matched and bear to say that I didn't? Would they think less of me? Would people think that I was a less capable, less intelligent person?

I did eventually pick myself up out of this hole. With some very wise counsel from trusted mentors, I realized that my career was not over. I moved past the feelings of inadequacy and realized that the results of the match are not a reflection of my abilities or talents. The residency application and match process is not only competitive, but also depends on some chance. I realized that I did in fact want to pursue a residency, even if it wasn't at one of my top 3 picks. I recognized that self-pity was getting me nowhere, and I needed to start focusing on the next steps.

I scoured the list of unmatched programs with the help of several mentors. I called every place that I would consider going. From South Carolina, I flew to Pennsylvania and drove to Kentucky and Louisiana within that week. On each of these interviews I took with me a new perspective on myself. The pride that once exuded from me was replaced with a healthy dose of humility. I approached each interview with an open mind and reinvigorated drive.

I consider the post-match scramble a great success for me. The program I accepted wasn't even a blip on my radar during my pre-match searching. But, come to find out they had everything I desired in a program. Sometimes when we get caught up in searching for the "best", we miss these hidden gems. My experiences were there were wonderful and prepared for the career plans I had had all along.

And now, 2 years later, I am an assistant professor and still practice in the same hospital where I completed my PGY-1 residency. Isn't it funny how life can take what feels like the worst of circumstances and turn it into a happy ending?

Figure 11-2:
Testimony from a Post-Match Scramble Candidate.

you may find out your results earlier, but everyone should know by noon EST.

One important thing to remember is that just because a program doesn't fill all its positions doesn't mean that it's a poor program. You're not going to be stuck in some awful residency for a year if you go through the scramble. Possibly, the program only interviewed and/or ranked their top candidates. Often newer programs are not on a lot of candidates' radar yet, so they just may not have had as many applicants as more established programs. And some programs are just not as geographically appealing as others. Programs in smaller towns or more rural areas may have fewer applicants and therefore be less likely to fill all positions.

So who should you contact first? How do you decide what programs to get in touch with? First, start with programs that you may have applied to but didn't get an interview with. They may have only interviewed a small percentage of their candidates. On the other hand, if you did interview with a program and YOU ranked them, and they still have an open spot, they obviously did NOT rank YOU. It's probably not worth your time to contact them.

Geography is also going to play a role. Look at the map, and decide how far from "home" you're willing to go for a year. Then look at all the states that includes and see who has an open spot. Maybe your friends have mentioned programs they were interested in that now sound appealing to you. Get as much information as you can from the ASHP directory or the program's Web site, or friends and other contacts and then start contacting residency directors. Right away! There's no time to waste!

Contact your mentor, and let them know you didn't match. Sit down and go through the list of available programs with them. They (or somebody they know) will probably have helpful information about several of the programs. They can certainly help you streamline your list. Consider the factors that went into your original decisions about programs and look through the list of available positions.

Once you've reduced your list of potential programs to a more manageable number, send an email stating that you see they have an open position. Make sure that you attach your CV to this initial email. Mention some things that you are hoping to get out of a residency, and let them know that you are interested in being considered for a position there. If there are specific questions that you have, you can inquire in this email. Most importantly, ask what other steps you need to do to "officially" apply for their residency. You see why it's a good idea to have that email already drafted and ready to go the morning of the match? You will probably have to send in a letter of intent and get your letters of recommendation and transcripts sent in as well. (Often directors will be willing to accept unofficial transcripts initially.) But before you make yourself completely crazy, ask what they require and what their time line is. Some programs may be planning to make a decision within 2 days while others may be planning on taking 2 to 3 weeks. Some may require on-site interviews, and some may only require phone interviews.

Just make sure you get them whatever information is required in order to meet all their deadlines.

Also, contact the individuals who wrote your letters of recommendation to let them know you did not match, but will be participating in the scramble. Ask them if they are still willing and able to write a letter for you. Things could have changed since they wrote your first set of letters.

Just remember many good candidates don't match. Obtaining a position with a PGY-1 program is super-competitive right now. If you don't match, it doesn't mean you shouldn't do a residency or you will be a terrible resident. It just means you didn't match. Stay focused and optimistic during the scramble, and keep in mind there are still "good" positions available.

TIPS FOR A SUCCESSFUL SCRAMBLE

Prior to Match

- Decide if you are willing to scramble for a position.
- Draft an email to potential programs stating your interest, and make sure you have an updated copy of your CV on hand.
- Recall the qualities you were looking for in programs in the first place.
- Inform your preceptor of the Match date and make sure that it will be acceptable to send and receive emails during regular rotation hours.

Post-Match

- Sort through potential program list with your list of nonnegotiable characteristics.
- Use your mentor to help narrow your list.
- Contact residency directors IMMEDIATELY after the match. Attach your CV and ask what you need to do to apply.
- Contact individuals who wrote your letters of recommendation and make sure they are still available for you.
- Start applying for open positions!

Chapter Takeaways

▶ Make sure that the rank order list that you submit is your "real" order and not in the order that you think you will match. The Match process is designed to take your preferences into account first. The only way you will NOT match with your first choice is if they do not rank you at all or all their positions are filled by more preferred candidates.

▶ Rank any program that you are willing to go to. Don't count on matching with only your first or second choice program. On the other hand, don't rank any program you aren't willing to go to. You could end up stuck with a program you hate!

▶ Long before the match results come out, make a decision about whether or not you are going to participate in the scramble if you don't match. The morning of the Match is not the time to be making this kind of decision.

▶ Be ready to hit the ground running if you are going through the scramble. Programs start getting inundated with emails and calls immediately after the Match results are released so you can't afford to wait around.

ROLE FOR THE MENTOR

Your mentor can help you review all the programs you interviewed with when it's time to make your rank order list. Your mentor may have helpful insight about some of the programs and may be able to offer pros and cons about different programs that you hadn't thought about before. Ultimately, the final rank order list will be your decision.

If for some reason, you do NOT match, your mentor can be an invaluable resource. Besides supporting you in a disappointing time, they can help you sort through the scramble list and help you decide which programs would be a good idea to contact. Time is short here, so you will want all the help you can get!

FREQUENTLY ASKED QUESTIONS

Q: What happens if I don't Match?

A: On the morning the Match results are released, you will get a list of programs with open positions. You will be able to contact these programs and "scramble" for any open positions. Only candidates who have registered for the Match will have access to this list of available positions. You will have to log on to the NatMatch Web site to view the list.

Q: Do I HAVE to go to whatever program that I match with?

A: Absolutely! By entering the Match, you are basically signing a contract and promising to go to whatever program you match with. That's why it's so important to only rank programs you are really interested in.

Q: How many programs should I rank?

A: You should rank the programs you are comfortable spending a year with. There is no right or wrong number to rank. Don't rank any place that you don't want to go to. If you are willing to go to all the programs you interviewed with, then rank them all!

Q: Should I rank a "fall back" program (a place you are fairly certain you can Match with)?

A: Only if you are willing to spend a year there. If you are, then knock yourself out. Otherwise, no.

Q: Should I rank a program high on my list even if I don't think I'm really competitive enough to go there?

A: Yes yes yes! The computer takes your preferences into consideration first. Rank programs in the order that you prefer them. You have a better chance of getting your first choice if you rank them first than if you rank them later on your list.

References

1. ASHP Resident Matching Program: for Positions Beginning in 2012. http://natmatch.com/ashprmp/. Accessed January 25, 2012.

2. National Resident Matching Program: How the Matching Algorithm Works. http://nrmp/res_match/about/res/algorithms.html. Accessed January 25, 2012.

3. Lifshin LS, Teeters JL, Bush CG. ASHP resident matching program: How does it work? Am J Health Syst Pharm. 2004;61:446.

4. Crannage AJ, Drew AM, Pritchard LM, Murphy JA. Managing the residency scramble. Am J Health Syst Pharm. 2011;68:110.

Post-Match Logistics 12

Nancy H. Goodbar

YOU MATCHED!

After months of anticipation, you find out that you matched! From the moment you find out the match results, your emotions go into overdrive and your mind becomes a whirlwind of questions. First, take a deep breath and think about the following: you have to finish pharmacy school, find a place to live, take your boards, get licensed in one or more states, and figure out your student loan situation. The key to taking care of all this business is to plan ahead. Even in the months before the match, you can create a timeline and begin the process of preparing for the upcoming changes. Before the match you can set a goal of when you would ideally like to take the boards, complete appropriate paperwork, and work with your loan provider to set up an alternative loan repayment program while you are a resident. The more organized and prepared you are for the changes that are about to ensue, the better you will be able to complete everything that needs to be done in the post-match days. You do not want to spend the last 2 months of pharmacy school running yourself ragged. You want to spend your time soaking up 2 more months of knowledge as a pharmacy student, celebrating graduation with your family and friends, and looking toward the next year of your life with excitement and anticipation.

RELOCATION

The match results are published in late March, and most residencies begin on July 1st. Do the math; that leaves you approximately 3 months to take care of some vital planning.

Just like a drug information question, the best thing to do here is utilize your resources. The current resident(s) at your future residency program probably experienced some of the same things last year as you are experiencing now. Before talking to them, you need to decide a few things: Do you want a roommate or do you want to live by yourself? Do

> "Prepare questions about relocation to ask current residents and/or preceptors during interviews."
>
> *Matthew W. – Pharmacy Student, Michigan*

you want to live in an apartment or a house? Do you want to live as close as possible to the hospital or do you mind a commute of some sort? What is your price range? Answering all of these questions lets you combine your questions into a single email or phone conversation with folks at your new program. Here are some things to consider that may help you decide on some of the nitty-gritty details. Having a roommate looks glamorous because you will be able to save money, but sometimes after working 80-hour weeks it may be nice to have a haven all to yourself in order to enjoy some peace and quiet. If you have the opportunity to live with someone that is going to be a coresident, consider the amount of time that you will be spending with them at work, as well as at home.

Also, with the busy life of a resident, an apartment may suit your lifestyle better because of the provided amenities including a gym, pool, business center, or laundry facility, as well as the access to maintenance staff that relieves you of the responsibility of even changing a light bulb! Living in an apartment may also provide you with the opportunity to expand your social life outside the walls of the hospital. A house, on the other hand, may suit your needs better if you have a family, yard work helps you unwind from a busy day, a walk around a neighborhood gives you a sense of peace, or you are just plain tired of apartment living and desire a place where you can't hear your upstairs neighbor's every footstep. The question of buying versus renting may come up. Obviously, a lot of personal factors go into a decision like that, but given the relatively short time of a residency, nearly all residents choose to rent.

Living close to the hospital is a consideration if you would like to be able to roll out of bed, take a shower, and be at work within 15 minutes, but what if all of your coresidents and friends live on the other side of town? If you are moving to a big city, especially one in which you may have to rely on public transportation, it would be worth your while to determine the most feasible living location based on travel time and/or public transportation schedules. The cost of living in bigger cities can also vary substantially from those of smaller ones; therefore, it is even more important for you to do your research and utilize your resources to determine the best living arrangement for you!

After determining exactly what you are looking for, seek the advice of the current residents. You probably met most, if not all of them, at your residency interview and have their contact information (or at least know where to find it). Residents will be able to give you firsthand advice on the best and worst places to live, where you can get the most "bang for your buck," what traffic is like around the city, and safety considerations of different neighborhoods and apartment complexes. Unless you want to end up with a train station as your next-door neighbor, a racetrack in your back yard, or a sewage treatment plant across the street, then make sure to use your resources to avoid any such inconvenience. The residents will also be able to prepare you for what parking is like around the hospital; either you will get VIP status in a parking garage or you will have to park in a lot that would take binoculars to see from the roof of the hospital. This information will be important to factor into your commute time.

The actual act of moving and taking care of all the logistics can be a burden, but there are many resources out there that can help guide you through the moving process. Searching the Internet for moving checklists can help ensure that you take care of changing your address, get your mail forwarded, find a good cable company, hook up electricity and water, and there may be other things that you would not even think about. This is where a moving guide or checklist can help to make your move as painless as possible.

At this point you may also consider contacting your soon-to-be coresidents (and hopefully new friends) to find out what their plans are. Starting an email chain with your coresidents will not only allow you to find out their living plans but also enable you to get to know each other before residency begins. Many soon-to-be coresidents start email chains prior to the start of residency, and it really helps to alleviate a lot of nervousness about such a big upcoming change. Discussions with coresidents can make relocating a lot easier because you feel like you are moving to a new place with a group of friends ready to take on the residency challenge together.

Another relocation tip is to find out what there is to do for fun in your destination city. Residency will certainly keep you busy, but the key to sanity is to allow yourself time to enjoy being in a new place, make new and long-lasting friendships, and have the chance to gain a new sense of independence and responsibility. Allow yourself the time to explore the local cuisine, historical sites, running trails, and dog parks. Relocating for residency training is a big step toward both your professional and personal growth so take this advice: work hard, learn a lot, work hard, and enjoy every single moment of the opportunity that has been given to you.

LICENSURE REQUIREMENTS

If prison stripes and heavy fines aren't your style, be sure to check with the board of pharmacy where you plan to do residency. Each state and their respective board of pharmacy holds the key to issuing your license to practice in that state. When applying to take the NAPLEX, you will be required to choose a state as your primary jurisdiction for licensure.[1] The state of primary jurisdiction will be the one that will make the decisions of your eligibility to take the boards. More information on choosing your jurisdiction state, examination eligibility, and licensure inquiries can be found on the National Association of Boards of Pharmacy (NABP) Web site at www.nabp.net or your college of pharmacy.[1] If during your career you foresee yourself potentially needing to practice in more than one state OR if you want to have a little more flexibility and less licensing "hoop jumping," post-residency you can choose the score transfer option, which allows your NAPLEX score to be transferred to an additional state(s). Keep in mind that right now you need a license in whatever state your residency program is in, but you should also consider whether there are state(s) that you plan on practicing in post-residency. As each state and their boards of pharmacy may have different eligibility requirements, it will be your responsibility to contact the state's board of pharmacy in ample time to ensure that you have completed all requirements to be eligible for licensure, whether it is for immediate or future licensure transfer. If you wait too long to discuss licensure requirements with the state's board of pharmacy, you could jeopardize the start date of your residency. Most residency contracts include a statement that your entrance into the residency program is contingent upon your successful licensure in the state by a given date. Therefore, you must play close attention to all of the contingencies, due dates, and licensure requirements. This is another area in which communication with current residents and future coresidents can be beneficial. Consider the following: Are there MPJE review courses available? Are there study materials and/or advice available from current residents regarding the MPJE? Would you and your coresidents like to form a study group and potentially share acquired study materials for the exam? Were there any hurdles you need to be aware of regarding licensure requirements, internship hours, etc. that you may not have had to deal with yet?

One of the biggest differences from state to state is the internship hour requirement. It is your responsibility to identify these differences and ensure that you have appropriately met the requirements. Wherever you went to pharmacy school, you most likely learned the specifics of the laws and intern hour requirements affiliated with the state of your pharmacy education. Most colleges do not teach you the specifics of other states licensure eligibility requirements because let's be honest, why would they want to let a phenomenal pharmacy student like yourself think about moving to another state? Another state may require more intern hours for licensure, and keep in mind that the board of pharmacy in the state in which you obtained your intern hours must send the verified hours to the board of pharmacy in the state that you plan on getting your license in. Unfortunately, this can be a rate-limiting step so the sooner you get the ball rolling, the better. Not only is it a busy time for you, but it is a busy time for the state pharmacy boards as well! Remember (almost) everyone graduates at the same time. If you know your residency starts July 1st, you need to have the goal of being a licensed pharmacist in the state of your residency training as close as possible to the residency start date.

What are the pros and cons of initially getting licensed in more than one state? First of all, getting licensed in more than one state on the front end is not necessarily a bad idea, even if you are certain about what state you are going to end up practicing in after the completion of your residency. While you are completing paperwork through the NABP and signing up to take the NAPLEX and MPJE, it may be less burdensome on you in the future to go ahead and fulfill all licensure requirements in more than one state if you foresee the real possibility of practicing in a specific state later in your career. You may have gone to pharmacy school in one state, have family in another state, and be beginning residency training in another state. All of these situations are very common and you must decide if you would rather take care of any and all NAPLEX score transfers, fees, and internship hour verification on the front end. By using NAPLEX score transfer and getting licensed in more than one state initially, you eliminate the need for reciprocity later. You can then avoid taking the MPJE post-residency and having to maintain licensure in more than one state over the course of your career. For example, I got my pharmacy degree in my home state but completed residency training in a different state. I got licensed in both states from the start, and it made my transition back to my home state hassle-free because I had already taken care of all the logistical licensing procedures. A few more things to keep on your radar regarding dual state licensure are the potential differences in license renewal (annually or bienni-ally), license renewal fees plus a possible professional tax, and whether or not your continuing education requirements are waived while you are a resident.

LIABILITY INSURANCE

Like going to the dentist, insurance is one of those things no one likes to think about. Buying insurance forces you to think about the "what ifs" of life and of your professional practice, but is necessary as you enter the profession of pharmacy. You don't need a book to tell you that you hold patients' lives and well-being in your hands, and mistakes (even unintentional ones) can be det-rimental to both patients and you. In addition, even if you did NOTHING wrong, you can be sued for your actions. You should strongly consider profes-sional liability coverage as you begin your practice as a pharmacist, even dur-ing residency. There are a number of policies available and you should shop around to compare coverage and costs. Also, be sure to check with your future residency program to see if they provide this coverage as a benefit to you.

HOW DO YOU HANDLE YOUR STUDENT LOAN DEBT?

So, you decide that you are in so much debt that you take a pay cut and pursue a residency. When the bill comes for your student loan this may not sound exciting, but in the long run you will be glad that you did! You have a few options on how to handle your student loan debt during your residency. Obvi-ously, you will not be making full pharmacist's salary during the year or two of your residency training; therefore, it will be crucial for you to come up with a student loan repayment plan that will give you peace of mind and allow you to focus on meeting your professional goals, while still putting food on the table, avoiding working by candlelight, and taking cold showers.

You must first decide one of two things: do you want to pay on your loans during residency or wait until you finish residency? This decision should be based on the amount of debt that you have accrued, your resident salary, deter-mined cost of living, and whether you can realistically afford to make student loan payments during your time of residency training, while also taking into account that there is a 6-month grace period for student loan repayment post-graduation. If you do decide that loan payments will cause you hardships, you must contact the servicer of your loan in order to discuss whether or not you would qualify for loan deferment, forbearance, or some other form of payment relief.

A deferment is a temporary suspension of loan payments for situations such as re-enrollment in school, unemployment, or economic hardship; how-ever, residents typically do not qualify for loan deferment but would qualify for loan forbearance. Forbearance is a temporary postponement, delay, or decrease in payments for a certain period of time because you are experienc-ing financial difficulty. As interest accumulates on loan forbearance, you are responsible for repaying it. You can be granted forbearance by the servicer of your loans anywhere from 1 to 3 years. In order to be considered for loan forbearance, you must apply to the supplier of your loan and continue to make payments until you receive notice that you met the qualifications and have been granted forbearance.

If you decide that you are ready to begin paying back your student loans while you are a resident, you can choose one of the following options: standard repayment, extended repayment, graduated repayment, or income-based repayment. Standard repayment is a 10-year, fixed monthly repayment plan. You can expect to have the highest monthly payments with this plan, but you will pay the least interest thus paying less in the long run. Extended repayment is a 25-year, fixed monthly repayment plan. This plan allows smaller monthly payments, but you will be paying more in interest thus paying more in the long run. Graduated repayment has a timeline of up to 10 years for repaying the loan. This plan has monthly payments that start at lower rate and gradually increase, which would be ideal for someone who expects their salary to gradually increase over time. Income-based repayment is a newer loan repayment plan that takes into account income and family size, and it basically caps monthly payments at an affordable amount based on the aforementioned criteria. Eligibility for income-based repayment is determined by your loan provider, and it can be determined based on the amount of student loan debt in combination with income and family criterion.

All of the loan repayment schedules and loan calculators to aid in your decision can be found on the Federal Student Aid Web site.[2] It will be vital for you to be in contact with your loan provider in order to stay on track with payments, ensure that you do not fall behind, and to make sure you are diligent in choosing a loan repayment plan that is right for you. Non-US citizens should consult appropriate personnel to alleviate any Visa issues associated with school, work, or loans.

Although post-match logistics seems relatively simple, it definitely entails some of the most crucial and important decisions that you make. Finding the perfect place to live, ensuring all appropriate state licensure requirements are taken care of, as well as coming up with a plan for paying off student loan debt are issues that hang over the heads of all graduating pharmacists, not just you. Take the advice provided in this chapter and run with it. It will surely help as you prepare to embark on a new and exciting journey for your future career.

Chapter Takeaways

▶ Remember that relocation should not be stressful as long as you plan ahead and utilize your resources.

▶ You have a responsibility to contact state-specific boards of pharmacy to ensure that you have met appropriate licensure requirements.

▶ Assess your financial status and work with your loan provider to choose a loan repayment plan that is right for you.

FREQUENTLY ASKED QUESTIONS

Q: Can my future residency program help with some of the issues related to my transition?

A: Yes! Current residents at your future program can provide advice on great places to live, restaurants, and general advice related to moving to the city.

Q: What should I do about my student loans during residency?

A: Everyone's situation is different in terms of the amount of payment, resident salary, and cost of living. But, you have options to help if your student loan payments are too large for you to handle. You may select forbearance where you can avoid payments during residency or reduced payment options to make payments more manageable.

Q: I'm doing residency in a different state than the one I went to pharmacy school in. What state(s) should I get licensed in?

A: It's an individual decision. Generally speaking, it's easier to get licensed up front in all the state(s) you plan to practice pharmacy in using NAPLEX score transfer. If you don't know this up front, you may opt to wait until you finish residency and reciprocate your license. More information on this is available through the NABP (www.nabp.net).

References

1. National Association of Boards of Pharmacy. NAPLEX/MPJE Registration Bulletin. www.nabp.net/programs/assets/NAPLEX-MPJE.pdf. Accessed February 1, 2012.

2. Student Aid on the Web, Federal Student Aid Web site. studentaid.ed.gov. Accessed February 1, 2012.

Mentorship Through the Postgraduate Training Process 13

Jeffrey J. Fong

Are you feeling overwhelmed after reading the previous chapters? By now, many of you are not sure where or how to start this next journey in your career path on the road to postgraduate training. However, you have probably already discussed your future goals with faculty and more experienced pharmacy practitioners. Over your time as a pharmacy student, many of you have interacted with individuals with advanced practice skills, professional qualities you admire, and who want to motivate and guide a younger professional trainee like yourself. Well, if you were wondering who a good mentor would be, it is someone that possesses these qualities. Especially in health care, mentorship is an important process in many professions. Appropriate mentorship is needed to develop younger colleagues and give students the guidance to perfect their knowledge base, skill set, and professional experience. A mentor is much more involved than an advisor in your professional growth and development, offer specific advice that impacts you on a personal level, and furthermore serves as an advocate for the mentee in their pharmacy network.

> "My mentor was the single most helpful tool for my journey in pursuing post-graduate training. Finding a great mentor is a must!"
>
> *Samantha P. – Pharmacy Student, Alabama*

In addition, one key difference is that advisors are typically individuals assigned by your college to help with specific issues such as signing up with classes. Mentors are individuals whom you identify and seek out to help you along the way.

Mentors become even more important during your residency search given the complexities and magnitude of the process. Mentors can guide you through this seemingly overwhelming experience by serving as a "sounding board" and providing invaluable feedback. The mentor(s) you ultimately choose will be heavily based how comfortable you feel with the individual, especially in a one-on-one situation. These individuals should be someone who you expect to be candid in offering feedback and guidance, challenge you on a personal and professional level, and provide you motivation to achieve your goals and objectives. Other factors to consider include (1) whether or not you admire and want to emulate this professional's career path and professional achievements, (2) if they are well respected by their peers and have established a professional network, (3) if you can work well with this individual, and (4) if this person has time to provide mentorship? Faculty members are a logical choice for a mentor, but anyone in practice who meets the previously mentioned criteria (alumni, recent graduates, current residents, fellows, clinical pharmacist, clinical coordinators, directors of pharmacy, or IPPE or APPE rotation preceptors), who has experienced the American Society of Health-System Pharmacists Midyear Clinical Meeting (ASHP MCM), or who has been involved in residency search process would be an excellent choice for a mentor. It is desirable to choose a mentor practicing within your specialty area(s) of interest, but it should not be the sole deciding factor. Many mentees ultimately decide to pursue a specialty focus different from their mentor.

The process of finding good mentors usually develops informally. You may find that assigned advisors whom you meet regularly with and get advice from become mentors. Or, you may find individuals whom you admire and seek them out for advice on career issues. Over time, these connections can develop into a mentoring relationship. Additionally, working on projects or being involved in organizations is a good way to build relationships with individuals who can serve as mentors. These connecting points often provide an informal mechanism to form a trusting relationship where you can regularly meet and feel comfortable discussing issues of concern. Because developing a mentor–mentee relationship takes time, it is often difficult to form these relationships by simply asking someone to be you mentor. You can start there, but you must also take time to build the relationship by seeking them out for a variety of needs. Along the way, you will find that you ask your mentor for certain things. Always be sure to be respectful and give them as much time as possible to help out with your requests.

Mentors can help refine your current goals and objectives. They help you to identify your strengths and weaknesses and can offer specific instructions or suggestions on how to work on areas needing improvement. Mentors play an excellent role in providing suggestions to perfect essential skills such as interviewing, time management, communication, and task prioritization. They also provide feedback on how to access additional resources. For example, an invested mentor might suggest pursuing specific rotations in specialized practice settings to help you decide on your interest in an area or round out your experience. Most importantly, the mentor can offer honest feedback necessary to strengthen your performance to help you achieve your professional goals and objectives.

Mentors can assist in the residency search process in many ways; one of the first steps is preparing for the ASHP MCM. Planning for ASHP MCM will require several months of preparation to complete multiple tasks. Your curriculum vitae (CV) should be completed and finalized before the meeting; mentors can help by offering templates and constructive review to improve this document. Discussing search strategies to narrow the choices of residencies and providing specific program recommendations are other ways mentors can help in the residency search process. Many mentors are willing to advocate for you by either helping introduce you to various programs or lending their support to your application with contacts they have. Since many pharmacy students will not have a professional network yet; a mentor can often help facilitate introductions and/or refer the mentees to residency programs of interest. While this text provides a wealth of information, a mentor can offer help by answering questions on residency program terminology, navigating the ASHP MCM or other meetings, and the structure of the match process and strategies for it. To prepare mentees, many mentors will meet and hold discussions prior to the ASHP MCM or other meetings to provide mentees with this information and assist with preparation for the meeting.

After ASHP MCM or other meetings, a mentor can continue to offer support in the preparation of your residency application materials and on-site residency interviews. They may help review your letter of intent to ensure that it accurately describes your motivation in pursuing a specific program and to highlight your strengths as a candidate. A mentor may also write a letters of recommendation. You should consider asking your mentor to write one of your letters; as this person is well positioned to be able to describe your abilities as a student and future pharmacist and comment on your growth observed over time.

One of the most important components during the residency search process is your performance during the on-site interview; and a mentor can help provide invaluable advice guiding you through this process. Generally speaking, residency interviews can be very demanding given the rigorous scheduling of residency interviews over a short period of time. The structure can differ significantly by the interview length, number of interviews, and the possibility of having multiple candidates during the same interview session. Many mentors have offered mock interviews as a way to provide simulated experiences. From these practice sessions, mentors can help refine your answers to interview questions so you articulate clearly your responses to questions and devise ways to handle difficult interview questions. A mentor is one of the best people to offer constructive criticism to help your interview performance. Perhaps you have some nervous behaviors such as lip smacking or playing with your hair or even something as simple as failing to blink one's eyes. You can imagine how some of these nervous behaviors can cause the interviewer to be uneasy, but might be difficult for your friends to tell you; a mentor can likely provide this for you. Even simple tips and reminders (e.g., dress, appearance, and making sure you don't have bad breath) can make a world of difference between an average versus great first impression. It is important to be mindful that all comments are meant to be constructive and not meant to demean or embarrass you.

After reading this section, the many benefits of having a mentor should be evident; however, there are some things that you should not expect a mentor to do for you. After all, it should be you who initiates these discussions and all of other tasks mentioned in previous sections. Keep in mind that your journey to postgraduate training is YOUR journey. Mentors will not assume responsibility for it. A mentor should not be in place of a few things. First, you should still evaluate your own abilities and skills, write or develop you own application materials, and, most importantly, make your own decisions. After all, you'll be the one in postgraduate training, so you should be the one to choose it. Self-reflection and evaluation is an important process for all health-care professionals; after all, it is you who will be your own strongest critic. Mentors can only critique on things they can observe and can't read your mind on what you are feeling or desire in your career. It is expected that you will critique your own abilities, determine your strengths and weaknesses, and decide your own goals and career path. Mentors should not be expected to write or develop any of your materials, but they can offer you templates and examples and provide guidance and critically evaluate your work so you can be adequately prepared. It is also not a reasonable expectation to have mentors access their personal contacts to ensure that you get an interview. Lastly, you should not expect mentors to be the final decision makers for you. The mentor's role is to provide you with guidance and advice throughout the process. These individuals have already chosen their unique career paths, have experienced similar trials and tribulations, and many are more than willing to offer their input and opinion on a specific situation. You should take all of the gathered information and make these decisions for yourself and determine your own path. A mentor will help guide you through the pursuit of a residency program, but it is essential to take ownership of your own responsibilities and obligations in this process.

A mentor plays an important role in the professional development of many pharmacists, especially during the pursuit of postgraduate training and navigating through the overwhelming nature of ASHP MCM. Getting advice on how to develop your CV and letter of intent, refine your search for the right residency program, and interview successfully can prove invaluable. A mentor's feedback and guidance can make the difference between an average and stellar residency application/interview and can subsequently improve your chances of a successful match between you and your desired program. A mentor and mentee relationship is a mutual investment where both sides will need to nurture it in order to reap the greatest benefit. To optimize your relationship with a mentor, it is important to touch base with them on a regular basis to set mutual expectations and discuss progress. Your relationship with your mentor can be a rewarding one and that carries over your future career.

Chapter Takeaways

▶ Identify a mentor who has advance practice skills that you admire and has the desire to motivate and guide you through your training process.

▶ Cultivate your mentor relationship by having regular contact with your mentor and being open about your needs and objectives.

FREQUENTLY ASKED QUESTIONS

Q: **How much time should I spend meeting with my mentor?**

A: This depends on how much time you need and your mentor's availability. It is important to be prepared for any meetings with your mentor and to communicate with your mentor what your needs are and to try and keep your discussions focused. Email is also an easy way to facilitate review of some of your materials, but keep in mind that it is often much easier to meet in person to have in-depth discussions. In-person meetings are most desirable but remain flexible and realize your mentor may have time constraints, so telephonic conversations may be a suitable alternative.

Q: **How much time should I give my mentor to complete a letter of recommendation?**

A: Typically, 4 weeks is sufficient especially when you know the submission deadline for the application materials. You want to ensure that your mentor has enough time to prepare and write you the best letter possible. In the post-match scramble, given the short time line and the urgency, it is reasonable to shorten this to 1 to 2 weeks. Your recommenders will understand the short time line.

Q: **How early should I begin when looking for a mentor?**

A: This will depend on a number of factors and will be highly individualized, but the earlier the better. You must consider whether you have the individuals before, determined what areas of pharmacy interests you, and if you have worked with individuals (i.e., IPPE or APPE preceptors) outside of the college of pharmacy. Typically, this can be sometime during the early rotations of the fourth pharmacy year, preferably no later than October. It is ideal to find a mentor as early as possible, and this can be helpful even in your P1 to 3 years of pharmacy school. They can be especially helpful in getting involved in scholarship activities or in helping you with rotation choices. Many colleges allow you to customize your APPE rotations so you can have faculty rotations, internal medicine, or specialty rotations.

ACKNOWLEDGMENTS

The editors thank the following individuals and institutions for providing sample materials for use in the text:

Individuals:

Jenna Foster—P4 Student, South Carolina College of Pharmacy, University of South Carolina Campus
Ashley E. Jones—P4 Student, University of Georgia
Megan Lawman—P4 Student, University of Florida, St. Petersburg Campus
Caitlin R. Musgrave—PGY-1 Resident, Medical University of South Carolina

Elizabeth C. Perry—Assistant Professor, University of Louisiana at Monroe College of Pharmacy

Caitlin L. Shamroe—P4 Student, South Carolina College of Pharmacy, University of South Carolina Campus

Institutions:

Palmetto Health Richland, Columbia, SC

Wake Forest University Health Sciences, Winston Salem, NC

III

Turn Left, Turn Right: Choosing the Postgraduate Pathway for You

- *Celeste R. Caulder and P. Brandon Bookstaver*

INTRODUCTION

Now that you've learned what residency training is, how to select a residency, and the necessary steps for applying to postgraduate training, it is time to discover a little more detail about the opportunities for both Postgraduate Year One (PGY-1) and Postgraduate Year Two (PGY-2) training. The opportunities are bountiful. That's where this section comes in. Use it as a guide to further your postgraduate training destination. In this section, you'll find the details on the PGY-1 residency year whether it is in a healthcare system or in community pharmacy. Following the PGY-1, PGY-2 residency options or other postgraduate training opportunities are numerous. Exactly what you do is up to you … mentors can advise you, but the decision is ultimately yours.

You'll start with an overview of the PGY-1 year in a healthcare system or the community. From there, you will be introduced to all the various specialty residencies, fellowships, and advanced degree programs. Each of these postgraduate training opportunities provides an overview of the programs including goals and objectives, application requirements, and career opportunities upon successful completion of such program.

Postgraduate Year One Pharmacy Residency 14

Colleen M. Terriff

WHAT THE YEAR IS ALL ABOUT

So you are thinking about a residency. It is a tough choice: secure a job after graduation or pursue additional training. The current, seemingly saturated job market and competitive residency environment is definitely making this decision more difficult. Many health-systems prefer, or even require, the hiring of a residency-trained pharmacist. For the first time in decades, many employers are cutting hours and even laying off pharmacists. So many soon-to-be graduate pharmacy students wonder if they should try to immediately accept a job offer or try for a residency position. We encourage you to consider a residency a wise investment in the future. And what is invested in that developmental, busy year will return 10-fold. It was an insightful resident who once informed me, "It's not just about what I will get out of a residency; but what I have to add ... to contribute ... to the program ... that is what the year is about!" It will be an exciting, and sometimes, challenging time. Yet, there will be many great opportunities to develop and enhance pharmaceutical care, leadership, and organizational skills; collaborate with a multitude of healthcare professions; and take valuable steps toward advancing your career. This chapter will review key concepts of Postgraduate Year One (PGY-1) programs, including the differing types, educational design and evaluation, resident responsibilities, and opportunities during the year and beyond.

> "Reflection and self-awareness are the cornerstones of choosing the right residency program."
>
> *Ohannes K. – Pharmacy Student, California*

PHARMACY GENERALIST

According to the American Society of Health-Systems Pharmacists (ASHP), the definition of postgraduate training is "an organized, directed, accredited program that builds upon knowledge, skills, attitudes, and abilities gained from an accredited professional pharmacy degree program."[1] The focus of this training should be on developing generalized skills in medication-use systems that foster "optimal medication therapy outcomes" in patients with a broad range of disease states.[1] Most PGY-1 residency programs are designed to provide the resident with a broad range of skills and experiences complimented with elective opportunities with more focused patient populations. For instance, you may be entering a hospital-based PGY-1 with rotations in general internal medicine, surgery, and intensive care, providing care to a variety of patients (with different age ranges, ethnicity, socioeconomic status, and immune status). You may then have a few electives in pediatrics or geriatrics, or specialty areas such as oncology. The overarching goal of all programs is to develop a well-rounded, competent, and "comfortably confident" professional clinician. Pharmacists are advocates for proper medication use and are also educators of patients, caregivers, family members, and other healthcare professionals. The residency year may incorporate a variety of educational opportunities to also improve communication skills, such as developing written newsletters and handouts, delivering in-services, facilitating medication discussions, and presenting formal lectures to a variety of audiences. Learning how to effectively educate different groups is an important skill set that will translate well into both a clinical setting and academic environment.

The American College of Clinical Pharmacy (ACCP) presented their vision for residencies to be a mandatory step before a pharmacist enters practice.[2] This vision is particularly important for pharmacists who provide or will be providing direct patient care. While we cannot always predict our future, most pharmacy careers involve patient care. This generalist training offers opportunities to gain more experience, exposure, and skills. In addition, this training dovetails nicely into subsequent specialized training (i.e., PGY-2). ACCP also states that nearly all pharmacists will provide this level of care by 2020.[2] With 2020 rapidly approaching, what other means than residency training could effectively achieve this end?

TYPES OF RESIDENCIES

According to ASHP, pharmacy residencies have been around since the 1930s and have undergone many evolutions. ASHP has collaborated with other pharmacy associations, such as ACCP, Academy of Managed Care Pharmacy (AMCP), and American Pharmacists Association (APhA), to develop current standards of PGY-1 and PGY-2 programs.[3] Specific program standards established through these organizations are available in Table 14-1.

There are approximately 76 community residencies, 36 managed care residencies, and 751 pharmacy practice PGY-1 residencies, of which over 100 are based within the Veterans Affair (VA) health-system and nearly 50 are associated within a college or school of pharmacy. While many residencies are based out of large academic medical centers, small- to medium-sized community-based hospitals seem to comprise the majority of training opportunities. Below are brief, general descriptions and features of the different settings of pharmacy residencies.

TABLE 14-1 • Residency Program Information

Organization	Web Site	Updated Lists
American College of Clinical Pharmacy (ACCP)	www.accp.com	Directory of residencies, fellowships and graduate programs (enter Students section, then click Career Development Resources)
Academy of Managed Care Pharmacy (AMCP)	www.amcp.org	Accredited and nonaccredited managed care PGY-1 and PGY-2 residencies (enter Professional Development section, then click Residency)
American Pharmacists Association (APhA)	www.pharmacist.com	Directory of all community pharmacy residency programs (enter Pharmacy Practice section, then click Residencies/Advanced Training)
American Society of Health-Systems Pharmacists (ASHP)	www.ashp.org	Residency Directory (enter Accreditation section, then click Residency Directory)

Academic Medical Center

Many pharmacy residency programs are located in institutions and health-systems that are affiliated with medical schools and are training sites for medical residents and medical, nursing, and pharmacy students. This "teaching environment" commonly creates many educational opportunities for the resident and by the resident. For example, many of the staff, including physicians, nurses, pharmacists, dietitians, and therapists, participate in precepting the students and residents. This is a common daily activity in addition to the provision of patient care. There may be rotations that involve rounding with a multidisciplinary team, comprised of faculty from nearby healthcare professional programs. In addition, within this "teaching environment" you may have the opportunity to be involved with journal clubs, case discussions, educational symposia, precepting and teaching students (at nearby healthcare professional programs).

Urban Community Hospital

PGY-1 residency programs may be located at hospitals based in urban communities or large cities. These facilitates often are very busy, treat a diverse patient population, and offer a variety of inpatient and outpatient services and specialties, including trauma, pediatrics, anticoagulation, and wound care. Many of these urban community hospitals are also academic medical centers, so they are also more likely to have medical residency programs and train other healthcare professional students. These programs may offer an on-call experience with other healthcare providers. You may be more likely to also work with pharmacists who have specialized in fields like oncology or infectious diseases. Like academic medical centers, residency programs in this setting most likely will have multiple pharmacy residency positions, including both PGY-1 and PGY-2 programs. There are some advantages in having a large residency group. You have many comrades and colleagues to bounce ideas off of, to offer support during the busy year, and to learn collaboration and negotiation skills and different work ethic or styles.

Smaller Community Hospital

Another setting for PGY-1 training is at a smaller hospital that serves a more rural population. While these smaller health-systems may not have a similar depth and variety of services, compared to larger medical facilities, programs in these environments are still able to offer a surprisingly large scope of experiences. While their urban or academic counterpart might provide care for a higher volume or level of complexity of patients and offer many specialties, programs within community hospitals commonly have a number of pharmacists who can work any shift, any floor, satellite or patient care area, any time. Interestingly, many of these pharmacists still gravitate toward a specialty, like critical care or nutrition, and as a resident you will gain great insight on how to effectively do both. In addition, smaller hospitals usually have fewer residency positions. For some PGY-1 candidates, this is appealing since they may feel like they can make a greater impact within this type of a program.

Veteran Affairs Medical Center

The VA is one of the largest health-systems in the United States with over 150 hospitals and 860 community-based clinics, providing inpatient care to half a million veterans and outpatient care to 50 million annually.[4] The VA pharmacy residency program trains well over 300 residents and has a variety of practice areas, including pharmacy practice, specialty residencies, and even research. The VA also offers pharmacy fellowships, as well. One of the areas the VA health-system is known for is the computerized system for clinical notes and orders including labs and prescriptions. In addition, while there are inpatient services within the VA system, their largest clinical area is outpatient clinics. You will have ample opportunity for experiences within ambulatory care services and to work with a potentially large geriatric patient population.

While many programs seem to offer similar overall experiences, figuring out which environment or setting might best fit your needs is crucial. Community pharmacy will have more ambulatory care and outpatient type service opportunities. Pharmacy residencies within a hospital environment may emphasize more acute care, inpatient rotations. All programs should have a management and project component. However, managed care programs would seemingly offer more opportunities in this arena and areas like formulary management. Regardless of the residency type and setting, developing a philosophy that you "will get out what you put into it" (and many times so much more!) should be an important motivator for your work effort and approach during your training year.

RESIDENCY EDUCATIONAL STANDARDS

ASHP has created accreditation standards for residencies, which encourage residency programs to design and implement an evaluation process of the resident and the program's ability to achieve certain required and elective educational outcomes, goals, objectives, and instructional objectives.[5] This can be one of the most important components of your residency program. Briefly, *educational outcomes* are broad categories of the residency graduate's capabilities, such as to not only manage but also to improve the medication-use progress. Subsequent *educational goals*, also broad, are additional statements of the resident's abilities. An example goal would be to design and implement changes to improve the quality of the organization's medication-use system. *Educational objectives* are more specific, follow Bloom's taxonomy (i.e., comprehension or evaluation) and types of learning (cognitive, affective, or psychomotor), and facilitate both teaching and assessment of the resident's performance. For instance, in order to demonstrate the above-mentioned goal, a program would foster the resident's learning and exposure to opportunities and then evaluate the resident's ability to explain a formulary system, create a medication-use policy after analyzing or critiquing a formulary review, develop and implement a protocol or guideline, and pilot an intervention geared toward quality improvement. Lastly, *instructional objectives* are a resource for preceptors to guide a resident struggling to achieve a particular educational objective. These contain further details and suggestions, such as having the resident draft a flowchart demonstrating medication-use process steps, and are not meant to be individually evaluated. Table 14-2 lists the required and elective PGY-1 educational outcome standards for pharmacy residency.

An important consideration is that it is up to the program to create an environment and experience to foster the achievement of these outcomes, goals, and objectives. In addition, the evaluation of the resident's performance with respect to the program should be through a competency-based approach.[1] Truly, most of the evaluation responsibility is shouldered by the resident. For instance, you will be self-assessing your own performance and providing preceptor and learning experience (e.g., rotation and project) feedback. The preceptor will be assessing you as well, and the residency program director should be reviewing and providing additional insight for all evaluations. Before you commence your training, having an understanding of how the evaluation process should work and how often evaluations will occur is important. During the year you should look for opportunities, even brief moments, for feedback about your performance, positive attributes, and needed improvements. Many times I would share my personal style and philosophy for evaluation with residents. I believed that we could together identify and move beyond areas of strong performance and then spend more time on areas needing additional

TABLE 14-2 • PGY-1 Pharmacy Residency Required and Elective Educational Outcomes[a]

Type	Outcome
Required	R1: Manage and improve the medication-use process
	R2: Provide evidence-based, patient-centered medication therapy management with interdisciplinary teams
	R3: Exercise leadership and practice management skills
	R4: Demonstrate project management skills
	R5: Provide medication and practice-related education/training
	R6: Utilize medical informatics
Elective	E1: Conduct pharmacy practice research
	E2: Exercise added leadership and practice management skills
	E3: Demonstrate knowledge and skills particular to generalist practice in the home care practice environment
	E4: Demonstrate knowledge and skills particular to generalist practice in the managed care practice environment
	E5: Participate in the management of medical emergencies
	E6: Provide drug information to healthcare professionals and/or the public
	E7: Demonstrate additional competencies that contribute to working successfully in the healthcare environment

[a]Community and managed care residency programs have similar outcomes.

development. Not only did I work with preceptors to provide more detailed, honest feedback, but also worked with the residents to specifically ask for both positive and constructive comments with ideas on how to improve.

RESIDENT RESPONSIBILITIES

While many joke that the term resident implies that one has "moved in," there is some truth to the name. Residents, with the training year commencing around July, will be expected to put in long hours, while not exceeding standards set forth by the Accreditation Council for Graduate Medical Education. For instance, you may start a rotation at 6 am and work on a clinical service until 3 pm. Then you may work on a project throughout the rest of the afternoon or staff in the pharmacy for a 4-hour shift. This "duty period" or time at the facility should not exceed 16 hours.[6] Also, over the course of a 4-week period, total duty hours, which include rotations, project time, and staffing, should not exceed 80 hours per week.[6] These standards are put in place for patient safety and residency burnout protection. While the overall hours spent within your residency year may seem like a lot, the time will go by fast. It should also be reassuring that responsibilities are linked to learning objectives, goals, and overall outcomes. Activities are not busy work; they have a purpose.

Staffing

Most programs, if not all, have a "staffing" component. This is viewed as valuable time spent learning what it is like to truly work as a pharmacist within the residency environment, whether a community hospital, managed care clinic, or community pharmacy. After receiving training and becoming licensed in a respective state, you may work "online" just as a pharmacist would and your responsibilities would evolve over time. For instance, during the first 2 months of the program, you would work initially within the roles and responsibilities of a technician, and then expand to shadowing pharmacists, focusing on the distribution function.

> "Utilize your staffing time to learn from the other pharmacists—they have spent quite some time in their position and can be great resources."
>
> *Chris H. – Pharmacy Resident, Tennessee*

This training may occur in a concentrated manner during the summer months. Time spent staffing would then become more clinically oriented, such as reviewing patient care reports and shadowing pharmacists working within specific patient care areas. At this time, the staffing requirement may be every other or third weekend or one day a week. The goal throughout the year is that you will then be able to independently staff certain care areas, which are usually predefined by the programs staffing preceptor. As an example, by the fall our residents were expected to staff within the main pharmacy. Only after completing rotations in specific care areas, like orthopedics and general surgery, oncology, and critical care, could the resident commence staffing within more specialized floors and the pharmacy satellites.

Project

From experience, the responsibility that seems to cause residents the most angst is completing a major project. Some of this anxiety maybe derived from the resident's lack of previous project experience, especially a longitudinal component that can span 12 months. Some of this stems from what seems like, to the resident, roadblocks in their progress. For example, residents may run into challenges with informatics or delays in obtaining key data, with getting essential departments together to discuss the project, with approval of protocols or procedures (such as through Institutional Review Board or P&T committees). These are usually great teaching moments to brainstorm solutions and continue pushing on, or to reevaluate the project and its objectives and make modifications. Some of the project "stress" is related to resident's organizational and multitasking skills, which can be alleviated through improvements in these strategies. Regardless, the purpose of the project is for the resident to gain experience with trying to find ways to improve a system or process and start implementing change. Some programs assign projects to the residents; some have residents select from a list; and some may ask the resident to design their own project. All programs should provide residents with guidance, time lines and expectations for certain steps and the final completion, which will most likely involve a presentation and a write-up. You should take great pride that you might help positively change patient care or patient safety either directly or indirectly through your project. An example project might be for the resident to evaluate and improve antibiotic surgical prophylaxis timing in orthopedic patients. Finally, the project experience will give you the great opportunities to develop and present a poster, deliver a podium presentation at a regional pharmacy residency conference or state pharmacy meeting, and submit findings for publication.

In addition to their major project requirement, residents may have other quality improvement projects or research opportunities throughout the year. These could include compiling, analyzing, and reporting adverse drug reaction data; writing up a case report for publication; or authoring a formulary review for P&T Committee.

Rotations

Rotations, whether they are block style (i.e., 4 or 6 weeks), concentrated (Advanced Cardiac Life Saving or emergency training), or longitudinal (i.e., 10 to 12 months) seem to be the part of the program in which residents are the most excited. There are required rotations or experiences and usually a few electives, which give the resident some creative freedom during their training. Examples of pharmacy residency rotations are nutrition, surgery, oncology, intensive care, respiratory care, general medicine, internal medicine, geriatrics, outpatient pharmacy, infectious diseases, pediatrics, drug information, management, teaching, or academia to name a few. Rotations should have a defined description, goals and objectives (see Table 14-2), expectations, and schedule. A resident, for example, may have to deliver a nursing in-service, facilitate a journal club, or lead a medication review class during some of their rotations, and should be aware of these responsibilities in advance. Rotation responsibilities can sometimes compete with other expectations, such as meeting attendance, completion of projects, and staffing. You will need to work with your rotation preceptor and residency director to find the most successful balance of your time and efforts.

Some experiences may overlap with training of other individuals. For example, a large hospital may have pharmacy interns, pharmacy students, and PGY-1 pharmacy residents working in the intensive care unit. It will be important for you to understand their expectations and how they will be different in some regards, and be the same in others. It also may be a great opportunity to work with your residency preceptor and coprecept a pharmacy student (IPPE or APPE). In addition, you may be asked to help educate others (e.g., nurses or medical staff) on how your role in patient care may be different than a pharmacy student or the pharmacist.

Management

While management seems like a general term, it is an important skill to foster as a resident. The definition implies using resources, including groups of people, in an efficient and effective manner to accomplish goals and objectives. During the PGY-1 this can pertain to project management, managing a medication process, or both. In addition, residency programs are encouraged to have components or experiences, which address areas such as meeting facilitation and agenda setting, budget and contract review, human resources, negotiations, interviews, and decision making. Residency projects could address pharmacy management issues. For example, you could develop and implement a way to measure and document clinical pharmacy services while working with informatics, medical and pharmacy staff, and both pharmacy and health-system administration.

Leadership

Many assume management and leadership are synonymous, but they can mean vastly different things. To lead is to inspire. William Zellmer shares with us how important leadership is to helping our profession bridge the gap between the vision of our profession (where we want to be in the future) and how our profession is practicing (where we are today).[7] ASHP, ACCP, AMCP, and APhA all hope that residency programs can offer opportunities to observe and experience leadership.

Surprisingly, many residency candidates come to programs with more leadership than management experience. Earlier in their pharmacy student career, residents seem to have been very active and involved as students and assumed positions of leadership within pharmacy student organizations, and related activities. Sadly, during their APPE rotations and continuing throughout their residency, the momentum seems to shift. Reasons for this decreased involvement might range from less abundant opportunities, busier schedules, decreased motivation and mentoring, and moving to a different city or state. Regardless, residency programs are obligated to try to reenergize their residents and inspire them to stay involved. Table 14-3 lists some ideas for you to continue your path of becoming pharmacy and community leaders.

Meetings

As a resident, you will have frequent meetings to attend throughout the year. Some of you will be a guest and just observe; while others of you may be asked to facilitate (part of management component of program) and/or present. The first general categories of meetings are those within your practice site. These include, but are not limited to, interdisciplinary (such as critical care and infection control), P&T Committee, department staff and faculty, preceptor, and program director meetings. The other types of meetings are those related to the profession, such as local, state, regional, or national pharmacy meetings. In addition, you may be expected to attend your related national pharmacy organization meeting (e.g., ACCP, ASHP, AMCP, and APhA) and present a poster of preliminary progress on your main residency project. Residency programs belong to certain regions within the country, and toward the end of your training year, you will attend a conference to present the final results of your

TABLE 14-3 • Leadership Opportunities[a]

Level	Organization or Group	Comments
Local	Pharmacy organization	• Serve as a board member • Observe governance if board meetings are open • Help plan a CE presentation or awards banquet
	College or school of pharmacy	• Serve as a judge for competitions (i.e., clinical skills, counseling, and business plan) • Lead a student discussion about postgraduate opportunities • Help students establish a local chapter of a national organization, if not available
	Charities and service groups	• Consider volunteering for organizations that serve vulnerable populations • Lead a medication review class or discussion
	Medical Reserve Corps	• Become a trained volunteer responder • Join planning committee to help strengthen local public health and emergency response
State	Pharmacy organization	• Serve as a board member • Observe governance (many board meetings are open and usually held before clinical meetings)
National	Pharmacy organizations	• Volunteer to serve on subcommittees, as a poster reviewer, or assist with student activities

[a]List is not all inclusive.

project. It is also a great time to reconnect with your former classmates completing residencies within the same region. Finally, remember you are an advocate and personal advertising for your program and profession! These gatherings are a great chance to start developing a solid professional reputation and a chance to expand your professional network.

With all these requirements and activities, the year can seem very full. It is important to have time set aside for stress-relief, relaxation, and fun. Many times this "down time" will get you reenergized to tackle your projects, staffing, meetings, and other responsibilities.

LOOKING AHEAD

Over a 38-year career, my father was a teacher and then a high school guidance counselor. It was amazing and inspiring how he guided the future steps and career paths of young, somewhat naïve, and relatively inexperienced, students. He helped them decide whether or not to pursue vocational school, the armed forces, or full-time or part-time employment or college. He helped them navigate complicated applications and entrance exams and decisions surrounding which programs or schools to apply. How was, say, a 17-year-old, to know what they wanted to do "when they grow up?"

> "Know the market. If you are in a region with a lot pharmacy schools, and you are not a competitive candidate (Rho Chi plus Phi Lambda Sigma plus research experience plus work experience) then consider applying to areas where the market isn't so saturated. Also, consider smaller programs and community hospitals. You will be surprised at the kind of experiences that can be obtained at community hospitals."
>
> *Kelly M. – Pharmacy Student, Tennessee*

Even after deciding you want to pursue pharmacy as a profession, and then a residency, how do you know if you then want to pursue additional training and specialize, and if so, in what area? Or decide which setting you want to practice: small community hospital, managed care setting, large academic medical center, or clinic? What about someday teaching, precepting, or both? My advice is to keep an open mind during your residency year. Some experiences may help solidify what you want to do over the next few years or decades. Yet, some experiences may help you decide what you might not want to do. That's okay. It helps narrow your choices. Also, try to take advantage of opportunities throughout the year. Partner with a community college, pharmacy school, or senior center to gain teaching and education experience. Be strategic about selecting your electives, if available. Take an elective in an area you never considered before. A few years ago one of our residents declared that she wanted someday to work in the field of psychiatry and mental health. Initially I was trying to line up some psychiatric electives for her; though, she stopped me, saying, "I know I will be a better pharmacist for my patients if I have experience in these other areas." However, some PGY-2 programs might want candidates to have some experience in their specialty area, like oncology or pediatrics. It might be wise to contact potential PGY-2 programs to gain their philosophy before you solidify your electives or experiences throughout your PGY-1 year.

Do not forget to balance taking on extra activities with your main responsibilities and performance standards and minimize potential "burn out." Ask for assistance from your residency director to help prioritize, if necessary. In addition, do not wait too long to consider a PGY-2. Time flies fast, especially when you are busy. The next thing you know it is December and applications and interviews are right around the corner. For additional information on PGY-2 residency training, please refer to Chapters 18 to 23.

Finally, my last piece of advice is to diversify your training and experience if you can! My father used to facetiously state, "Get your bachelor's degree from Harvard; your master's from Yale; and your doctorate from Stanford." His point—Diversify! Diversify! Diversify! If opportunities present themselves to give you a different way of thinking, a different approach, a different style, take it if you can!

Below are just a few professional development pathways, in addition to the above-mentioned PGY-2 training, which a resident could pursue. Although many residents may pursue a job similar to their residency experience and environment, some might consider these unique opportunities.

Fellowships

Fellowships are additional training, usually 2 years in length, following doctoral training. For example, one would obtain a bachelors, masters, and PhD degree, and complete a postdoc fellowship. These programs offer experience for the fellow to continue their research, publish articles, write grants, and lecture and/or precept. There are a few PhD clinical pharmacology-training programs through schools or colleges of pharmacy, which also offer subsequent fellowships. In addition, there are fellowships at many research associations, such as the Cancer Research Institute, Foundations, and pharmaceutical industry. In addition, there are clinical fellowship opportunities after one obtains a PharmD. While still including a research component, requiring the fellow to conduct clinical, laboratory, or both types of research projects, these fellowships are usually in a specific care area, like infectious diseases or geriatrics, and also have components of pharmacy student clinical training and teaching. A list of pharmacy fellowships can be found on ACCP's Web site (refer to Table 5-1 in Chapter 5). Fellowships are discussed in greater detail in Chapter 24.

Careers in Industry

Pharmaceutical industry (Pharma) is a dynamic field, which offers job opportunities to pharmacists, particularly with PharmD degrees and residency and/or fellowship training. In addition, Pharma offers fellowship training. For example, partnering with Pharma, Rutgers University offers 15 fellowship positions in drug development with a secondary specialty in pharmaceutical industry. Many graduates pursue a career in Pharma. Another option for PGY-1 graduates is to pursue clinical liaison positions. These individuals interact with healthcare professionals and provide resources, including drug information, and are able to interface with sales, marketing, and research within the industry.

Academia

As of March 2012, there are 121 colleges or schools of pharmacy recognized by the AACP in the United States and Puerto Rico.[8] Many schools are new and expanding, and therefore, actively seeking clinical faculty. Residency graduates with teaching experience are frequently considered for positions such as clinical instructor or clinical assistance professor. During your PGY-1 you should take advantage of opportunities to teach and precept, work on scholarly activities (such as posters and publications), and service and leadership (see Table 14-3), especially if you are considering becoming a future preceptor or faculty member (either adjunct or professor). If you are less interested in didactic lectures, you could consider volunteering as a preceptor for IPPE and/or APPE students, an evaluator for presentations, or facilitator for certain activities, like case discussions or journal club.

CONCLUSION

While your future is uncertain and where you practice is yet to be defined, your time and energy and the great opportunities during your PGY-1 training will be a wonderful career investment. You will find over the year you became a more confident and competent pharmacist, ready to help provide excellent pharmaceutical care to a variety of patients, in a range of settings. You will look back on all your accomplishments with pride and amazement; from all the tasks and opportunities, like completing a large project, staffing extra hours, and the variety of rotations and experiences, to the positive impact you made on medication systems, safety, and patient care. You made a wise choice!

Chapter Takeaways

► Residency year will be busy; full of a variety of responsibilities and opportunities.

► Main experiences include rotations, a multitude of projects, and staffing.

► Management and leadership opportunities are important components of the PGY-1 program.

► Electives are a great opportunity to reinforce a fondness for specialty area or try a new experience.

ROLE FOR THE MENTOR

Identify resident's strengths to continue developing and maintaining these areas.

Identify areas-to-improve for the resident and develop targeted activities to provide valuable experience and evaluation for resident.

Be encouraging and positive, yet honest, when necessary.

Be astute and quickly intervene when the resident experiences major roadblocks, frustrations, or potential burnout.

Find balance between providing opportunities for independence and knowing when to provide more specific guidance, parameters, suggestions, pearls of wisdom.

FREQUENTLY ASKED QUESTIONS

Q: What should the resident expect their year to be like?

A: The year should be busy, most likely much busier than the resident's former APPE experiences. They will be learning new systems, techniques, and be given opportunities, such as ACLS certification and code participation, teaching and even publishing. Also, residents should anticipate and plan for stressful, particularly busy times, like around December and January, with holidays, travel, meetings and potential PGY-2 applications and interviews, and toward the end of the year (June) with final project presentations, write-ups, evaluations, and end of year "clean up."

Q: How much creative freedom would I have to design my experiences?

A: This is a discussion to have with your residency program director and preceptors. If you stray too much from designed rotations, formats, and expectations, it may be challenging to evaluate your progress. Work together on deciding which areas to expand into and "spread your wings" and which areas to stick to the predesigned plan. You may have opportunities, like selecting your own project, giving extra in-services, and participating in elective rotations, which will give you a chance for more independence and creativity.

Q: Why are there some many different kinds of projects during the year?

A: There are a variety of projects throughout the year to give the resident exposure to many management and leadership opportunities. The largest amount of energy and time is usually devoted to the main residency project, which continues throughout the year. However, there will potentially be a multitude of smaller scale projects, many preplanned, but some will be sprung at the last minute. Smaller projects include developing a handout and presenting an in-service on a new drug, side effect, or protocol; gathering and analyzing medication utilization review data, facilitation journal club, or reviewing budget information.

Q: What type of qualities should a resident develop or foster to be successful in during their PGY-1 and beyond?

A: One of the most important attributes a resident can have during their busy year is effective time management skills. Residents are sometimes running from one thing to the next and it is important to preplan their day, week, and even month. Strong organizational skills are crucial, as well. Flexibility and keeping an open mind will also make the year more enjoyable. Finally, problem-solving and critical thinking are not only important for management of patients' pharmaceutical care management but also for resident's independence and maturity. These skills will help the resident identify and triage which issues (e.g., communication with other providers, project roadblocks, or staffing schedule) they can resolve on their own and for which ones they should ask for assistance.

References

1. ASHP Commission on Credentialing. ASHP accreditation standard for postgraduate year one (PGY1) pharmacy residency programs. [Online] http://www.ashp.org/DocLibrary/Accreditation/ASD-PGY1-Standard.aspx. Accessed February 6, 2012.

2. Murphy JE, et al. American College of Clinical Pharmacy's vision of the future: Postgraduate pharmacy residency training as a prerequisite for direct patient care practice. Pharmacother apy. 2006;26(5):722–733.

3. ASHP. History of Residency Training. [Online] http://www.ashp.org/menu/Residents/GeneralInfo/ResidencyHistory.aspx. Accessed February 18, 2012.

4. Korman N. The many roles of a VA pharmacist. Pharmacy Practice Perspective. January 26, 2007. http://www.pbm.va.gov/PharmacyResidencyProgram/The%20Many%20Roles%20of%20a%20VA%20Pharmacist.pdf. Accessed February 22, 2012.

5. Commission on Credentialing of the American Society of Health-System Pharmacists. Required and Elective Educational Outcomes, Goals, Objectives, and Instructional Objectives for Postgraduate Year One (PGY1) Pharmacy Residency Programs. 2nd ed.—effective July 2008. http://www.ashp.org/menu/Accreditation/ResidencyAccreditation.aspx. Accessed February 6, 2012.

6. ACGME. Common Program Requirements. Effective July 1, 2011. [Online] http://www.acgme-2010standards.org/pdf/Common_Program_Requirements_07012011.pdf. Accessed February 18, 2012.

7. Zellmer W. Pharmacy vision and leadership: Revisiting the fundamentals. Pharmacotherapy. 2008;28(12):1437–1442.

8. American Association of Colleges of Pharmacy. AACP Institutional Member. http://www.aacp.org/about/membership/institutionalmembership/Pages/usinstitutionalmember.aspx. Accessed February 4, 2012.

Postgraduate Year One Community Pharmacy Residency

15

Stefanie P. Ferreri

Postgraduate Year One (PGY-1) community pharmacy residency programs (CPRPs) strive to develop creative and innovative pharmacy practice leaders who will be able to meet the challenges presented by the rapidly changing healthcare system. The overarching goals for these programs are twofold. The programs aim to provide advanced training to pharmacists, enabling them to deliver patient care services in the community setting, while also translating innovative ideas and services into clinical practice.[1] These programs offer training in a more patient-focused, care-based practice that students may not otherwise have had exposure to if taking a job in a community setting immediately upon graduation. According to the 2011 PGY-1 Community Pharmacy Resident Exit Survey, residents reported the opportunity to develop pharmacy services and acquire management or ownership skills were important features of their residency experience. Most residents felt their experiences related to practice, business planning, financial management, and precepting were enhanced due to the additional training.[2] Ultimately, residents felt they have a jump start on their professional development in their careers. Benefits are also seen in community pharmacies that have residents embedded in the practice site. Through training residents, the companies have additional clinical pharmacy services, opportunities for pharmacy education and pharmacy staff development, and potential monetary benefits.[3] The current CPRPs are almost equally distributed among chain, supermarket, and independent pharmacies, and some university-based programs have practice sites.[4] PGY-1 community pharmacy residencies also have a presence in less traditional community pharmacy settings such as outpatient health-system pharmacies and community clinics.

RESIDENCY ACCREDITATION

Although CPRPs were established in 1986, it was not until 1999 that formal accreditation standards were adopted by a partnership with the American Society of Health-System Pharmacists (ASHP) and the American Pharmacists

TABLE 15-1 • Advantages of Community Pharmacy Residency Accreditation

- These programs are surveyed periodically to ascertain that the site is compliant with current accreditation standards.
- Future employers will feel confident about hiring pharmacists who have completed an accredited program because of the standardization that accreditation requires.
- Accreditation provides a benchmark for initial and ongoing program evaluation.
- Prospective residents often perceive accredited programs as being more desirable with the potential of greater impact on their future.
- Accredited programs have priority for a number of recruitment forums for residents, including the residency showcase at the ASHP Midyear Clinical Meeting.
- Accredited programs are listed in the ASHP Residency Directory and are eligible for inclusion in the national residency-matching program.

Association (APhA). The adoption of an accreditation standard was an important step in the development of PGY-1 CPRPs. Accreditation led to initial and ongoing program development, stronger perceptions of the value of community pharmacy residencies by students and employers, and eligibility for pharmacy students seeking these residencies to participate in the Residency Match Program. As of 2011, there were 82 CPRPs and 139 residency positions. Sixty-three of these programs were accredited or in the process of accreditation.[4]

Pharmacy students should consider whether the CPRP they are interested in is accredited or plans to become accredited. Table 15-1 lists advantages of accredited programs.

Accreditation gives programs credibility with potential residents and confers stability and commitment to the program by all collaborating parties. Still, there are various reasons a CPRP may not be accredited, so a more thorough investigation may be necessary when considering a nonaccredited program. Many programs do not apply for accreditation until the program has had time to develop fully in the first year. Accreditation, once granted, is retroactive to the date of application submission. Students considering a program that has a new site should understand it may not be accredited and they should ask whether or not it is the program's desire to become accredited.

> "I am the first resident to complete a residency at my practice site. When I applied, the site was unaccredited. It is a very challenging and rewarding endeavor to work through the creation and establishment of a CPRP. However, my program actively pursued accreditation which was conferred during my residency year."
>
> *Jill O. – Pharmacy Resident, Georgia*

The accreditation process for PGY-1 CPRPs is similar to that of PGY-1 residencies in health-systems.[5] Programs pursuing accreditation undergo a three-step process: application for accreditation, accreditation site visit, and action by the ASHP Commission on Credentialing. When a program seeks initial accreditation, the program will be reviewed by surveyors from both organizations (ASHP and APhA), as well as by a guest surveyor from an already accredited CPRP. The main difference in accreditation between a CPRP and a traditional PGY-1 in a health-system is the partnership between ASHP and APhA.

APPLICATION PROCESS

The recruitment and application process for CPRP is similar to that of most residencies. The main difference is the presence of a multisite CPRP, in which several sites are affiliated with one program. In a traditional PGY-1 health-system residency, you may apply to one site with multiple PGY-1 residents at that single site. In a multisite CPRP you may be applying to a single program with multiple different sites with one PGY-1 resident per site, which should be considered when applying. Alternately, one can be a single resident at a single CPRP.

There are several places in which a student interested in this type of residency can gather more information. Three organizations maintain residency directories that describe what community residency programs are available; they are as follows: the ASHP Online Residency Directory; the APhA Online Directory of Community Pharmacy Residency Programs; and the American College of Clinical Pharmacy (ACCP) Online Directory of Residencies, Fellowships, and Graduate Programs (refer to Chapter 5, Table 5-1).[4,6,7] These directories provide useful information about CPRPs and application requirements. Programs that are accredited by the partnership with ASHP and APhA are required to follow the National Matching Services (NMS) procedures. Candidates will need to register with NMS to successfully match with the program.

Figure 15-1 identifies strategies to be successful in pursuing a community pharmacy residency during your professional years in pharmacy school. Other helpful strategies can be found in Chapter 6.

Early in your pursuit, students are encouraged to attend the APhA residency showcase held during their annual meeting in the spring. This showcase is geared toward CPRPs allowing an intimate setting to meet with these

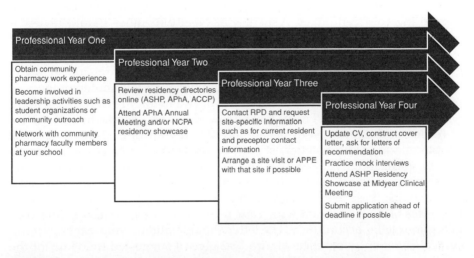

Figure 15-1: Strategies on Becoming a Quality Residency Applicant[a]

[a]Assumes a 4-year professional pharmacy curriculum.

programs. Students in their first, second, or third professional year will benefit from this meeting because they can ask informative questions about the different programs. The advantage of speaking with CPRPs at APhA annual meeting is preceptors and directors know these are students early in the decision-making process. The programs welcome questions to help guide students. Pharmacy students should speak to several programs in order to gain a good understanding of all the available opportunities. The National Community Pharmacists Association (NCPA) also holds a community pharmacy residency showcase at its annual meeting every fall. This is another great venue to meet and talk with residency directors and current residents. The NCPA showcase is valuable for all students, no matter what year you are in the professional program. Students early in their careers can use this venue to explore different programs. The most important meeting for final year professional students and graduates is the ASHP Midyear Clinical Meeting (MCM) held in December. All types of residencies are showcased and most community residencies are present. This showcase is the best opportunity for final professional year students and graduates to network and talk with current residents and preceptors. Students in their final year of the professional program should treat showcases as they would an interview. Students should have researched the different programs by this point in their career and they should be asking questions that are specific to the program's in which they are interested. It is not looked upon favorably if you are a final year student asking exploratory questions at the NCPA and ASHP showcases. Table 15-2 has useful tips for residency showcases. Detailed information on being successful at organizational meetings can be found in Chapter 8.

Once pharmacy students identify the programs they have the most interest in via the residency directories and the showcases, they should find out the application requirements and deadline. The deadline for most residencies is usually during the month of January. Most, if not all, programs require a cover letter or a letter of intent in the application materials. It is important to remember that this letter is the first impression you will give the program concerning your candidacy. A mentor or faculty member should review it prior to sending. It needs to be free of spelling and grammatical errors and should be customized to explain why you are interested in a particular program. For example, talk about the aspects of the program that appeal to you and what you think you can offer the program. Your CV is another important piece of the application. It is necessary to have a mentor review this in addition to your cover letter. Lastly, you will need to select people to write letters of recommendation on your behalf and obtain your official transcript. The people selected to write letters should understand your career goals and be able to speak about your work ethic, patient care activities, and leadership. These people should know what you want to get out of a community residency so that these features can be aligned with an appropriate CPRP. Share the fortes of each program with your recommendation writers so they can tailor your letter accordingly. The letter should validate your experiences in clinical community practice. Figure 15-2 gives a suggested time line for the application process for CPRP during your final year of pharmacy school.

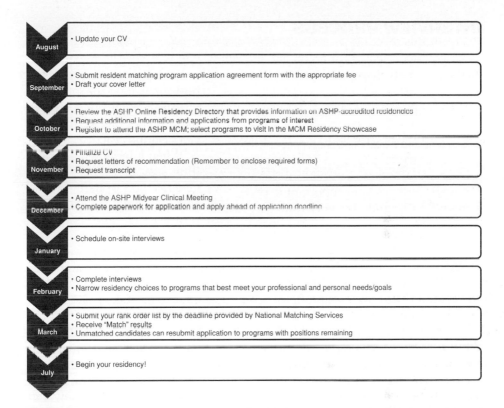

August
- Update your CV

September
- Submit resident matching program application agreement form with the appropriate fee
- Draft your cover letter

October
- Review the ASHP Online Residency Directory that provides information on ASHP-accredited residencies
- Request additional information and applications from programs of interest
- Register to attend the ASHP MCM; select programs to visit in the MCM Residency Showcase

November
- Finalize CV
- Request letters of recommendation (Remember to enclose required forms)
- Request transcript

December
- Attend the ASHP Midyear Clinical Meeting
- Complete paperwork for application and apply ahead of application deadline

January
- Schedule on-site interviews

February
- Complete interviews
- Narrow residency choices to programs that best meet your professional and personal needs/goals

March
- Submit your rank order list by the deadline provided by National Matching Services
- Receive "Match" results
- Unmatched candidates can resubmit application to programs with positions remaining

July
- Begin your residency!

Figure 15-2: Application Process for CPRP During Your Final Year of Pharmacy School

A web-based centralized application service is targeted for launch in Fall 2012 for students applying to residencies, PhORCAS.[8] This system will offer several advantages to students, such as single online submission with dissemination of several applications, notification of application progress, customization and consolidation of NMS, and Pharmacy Online Residency Centralized Application (PhORCAS) registration. Further details can be found in Chapters 9 and 27.

TABLE 15-2 • ASHP Residency Showcase Tips

Beginning in mid-November, print the Residency Showcase Listing

Determine which sites you want to visit during the showcase

Find out the date and time those sites will be at the showcase

Look at the diagram of the showcase and know where those sites will be located in the hall

Programs are listed by site, not by specific type of residency program offered

Adapted from American Society of Health-System Pharmacists.[9]

INTERVIEW PROCESS

Once you get selected for an on-site interview, you will need to make travel plans. If a multisite program invites you for an on-site interview, inquire as to how many days the interview will last. Some may require more than 1 day so that you can visit the practice sites.

> "My residency interview was separated into two separate days, one at the program site in South Carolina and another at my potential practice site in Georgia. Different programs organize interviews in various ways. It is important to remain flexible and plan very well."
>
> *Jill O. – Pharmacy Resident, Georgia*

When interviewing or visiting a program, observe the general atmosphere of the site. Observe if the staff seem professional and supportive when dealing with one another. Most community pharmacy residencies require you to be self-directed in your learning with oversight from a preceptor; therefore, you want to ask questions that will help you gain a better understanding of your support system. Ask specific questions as to which people at the practice site will serve as preceptors and how easy it is to contact directors when necessary. Ask preceptors and residents about a sense of team spirit throughout the program. Many residents learn and achieve more in a supportive environment. Conducting research about the practice sites and the preceptors before the interview will allow you to have a better idea about the answers to these questions. The interview can be used to confirm or deny your thoughts. Have a faculty member assist you with a mock interview. Table 15-3 lists potential interview questions at a CPRP interview.

It will be important to ask the same questions at the many sites you interview with so you can compare the answers. Additional tips for a successful interview can be found in Chapter 11.

On rank day, weigh your pros and cons carefully. Decide which program is the best fit for your long-term career goals. You will be working with the preceptors and directors for a year, so be sure that your personality meshes with them. Each residency site is different and each espouses a different philosophy. The objective is to find a residency where the philosophy of pharmacy practice best fits yours. Some programs are more competitive than others. Be thorough in your search and honest in your assessments, and you'll end up with a program that meets your needs.

LEARNING OUTCOMES AND OBJECTIVES

Table 15-4 lists the required outcomes for accredited CPRPs. Each outcome has a set of goals and objectives that each resident is required to complete in order to complete the residency. Because many CPRPs are longitudinal rather than concentrated, these learning objectives are evaluated throughout the year to demonstrate the resident's growth in a particular area. As a potential resident in the program, you will want to know the structure that facilitates

TABLE 15-3 • Common CPRP Interview Questions

What makes your program different from other CPRPs? What are the strengths and weaknesses of your program?

What percent of time will be spent dispensing?

What elective opportunities are available for the residents? Are there any special opportunities that exist (specialty pharmacy, long-term care pharmacy, consulting, etc.)?

Preceptor- and Director-Specific Questions

Are there opportunities to network with pharmacists in the area?

What are typical residency projects that past residents have done? What support is there for the residency project? What is the goal of the residency project?

Are there publication opportunities available to the resident?

How many residents does your program have? How often do they interact with one another?

How do the residency directors serve as mentors?

What teaching opportunities does your program offer? How much direct precepting will I obtain from your program?

What training/orientation do you provide your residents?

What positions did your past residents take after completing their residency with your CPRP?

Can you describe the mentors' roles and/or the availability of preceptors and directors?

What are the niche programs that the CPRP offers?

What is the experience/background of the CPRP director and preceptors?

What types of travel opportunities are offered through the CPRP?

Current-Resident-Specific Questions

How much time do I spend with the primary preceptor? How many preceptors will I have? What is the preceptor's teaching/management style?

What has surprised you about the residency that you may not have expected?

What will a typical week look like?

What is your residency project about? How did you come up with the idea for your project? What support is there for the residency project?

achievement of the program's educational goals and objectives. The structure should allow you to gain experience in diverse patient populations, a variety of disease states, and a range of complexity of patient problems as characterized by a generalist's practice. Accredited programs should have a description of learning experiences and a list of activities to be performed by residents in the learning experience. CPRPs may advertise the practice strengths they seek to develop as defined by their choice of program structure. If you are seeking entrepreneurship opportunities, look for programs with independent pharmacy practice partners. If you are seeking a more clinical track with the intention of pursuing a Postgraduate Year Two (PGY-2), look for long-standing programs with documented clinical outcomes.

TABLE 15-4 • Required Educational Outcomes for PGY-1 CPRPs

Outcome 1	Manage and improve the medication-use process
Outcome 2	Provide evidence-based, patient-centered care and collaborate with other healthcare professionals to optimize patient care
Outcome 3	Exercise leadership and practice management skills
Outcome 4	Demonstrate project management skills
Outcome 5	Provide medication and practice-related information, education, and/or training
Outcome 6	Utilize medical informatics

Adapted from American Society of Health-System Pharmacists.[10]

In addition to placing emphasis on longitudinal learning experiences, innovative clinical services are encouraged and business plan generation may be part of the program. Students should determine whether their long-term goals will be met by the preceptors and directors of the program. This will help you find the best fit for you. Business opportunities and entrepreneurship tend to be unique learning experiences for some CPRPs, so it will be extremely useful to conduct research about the site and ask about the types of experiences you will or could get. Some programs may also focus on leadership or teaching experience as well.

The program should have a method in which they evaluate the resident's performance of the program's educational goals and objectives. This evaluation process should include a resident self-assessment of their performance, resident evaluation of preceptor performance, and of the program.

This evaluation must be conducted at the conclusion of the learning experience (or at least quarterly for longitudinal learning experiences). It should reflect the resident's performance at that time, and be discussed by the preceptor with the resident and residency program director (RPD). The resident, preceptor, and RPD must document their review of the summative evaluations.

During the first month of the program, residents should be oriented to the program to include its purpose, the applicable accreditation regulations and standards, designated learning experiences, and the evaluation strategy. The RPD and, when applicable, preceptors conduct orientation activities. Preceptors orient residents to their learning experiences, including reviewing written copies of the learning experience educational goals and objectives, associated learning activities, and evaluation strategies.

Each resident should have a customized training plan based on an assessment of the resident's entering knowledge, skills, attitudes, abilities, and interests. Any discrepancies in assumed entering knowledge, skills, attitudes, or abilities will be accounted for in the resident's customized plan. Similarly, if a criteria-based assessment of the resident's performance of one or more of the required educational objectives is performed and judged to indicate full achievement of the objective(s), the program is encouraged to modify the resident's training plan accordingly. This would result in changes to both the resident's educational goals and objectives and to the schedule for assessment of those goals and objectives. The resulting customized plan should be consistent with the program's stated purpose and outcomes. Customization to account for specific interests should not interfere with achievement of the program's educational goals and objectives.

Preceptors in the program must have a record of contribution and commitment to community pharmacy practice. Pharmacy students should ask about preceptor contribution when interviewing to determine if it is a good fit for them. Some examples may be the following:

- Development and/or implementation of a new patient care service
- Improvements in management of the pharmacy
- Improvements in customer service
- Implementation of risk management or other patient safety programs
- Participation on a committee/task force resulting in practice improvement
- Development of treatment guidelines/protocols
- Leadership in advancing the profession of pharmacy through active service in professional organizations at the local, state, and/or national levels
- Effectiveness in teaching; appointments to appropriate work groups (e.g., medication safety, health coalitions, performance improvement, drug utilization review commissions, state pharmacy association, and P&T)
- Serving as a reviewer of contributed papers or manuscripts submitted for publication
- Formal recognition by peers as a model practitioner (e.g., awards, board certification, and fellow status)
- A record of contributing to the total body of knowledge in pharmacy practice through publications in professional journals and/or presentations at professional meetings.

ACTIVITIES UNIQUE TO A COMMUNITY RESIDENCY

The most commonly reported clinical services offered are immunizations (77%), medication therapy management (MTM) (70%), and smoking cessation services (35%). The most frequently reported disease states targeted included diabetes (85%), hyperlipidemia (66%), and hypertension (60%).[1,2] Some programs have a narrow focus of clinical services and others will offer broad services with multiple disease states. Be sure the programs you're considering have appropriate patient populations, pharmacy services, and staff to match your career goals; this will be the biggest influence in determining which site is the best fit for you. It will be important to know how long these services have been offered and what makes the services sustainable. You will also want to ask if the practice site tracks economic, clinical, and humanistic outcomes for these services to demonstrate the needs of society for improved therapeutic outcomes. Those with longevity and sustainability will offer better learning experiences. Community residencies also offer experience in business, finance, and management. Residents should have a much better understanding of pharmacy workflow including how to incorporate clinical services in the workflow or dispensing.

When visiting the practice site, ask questions concerning with whom the resident will collaborate. Many community residencies have collaborative practice agreements in place with other healthcare providers that allow the resident to be part of a medical model. The sites may also have contracts with employer groups in the area to offer clinical services. In addition to providing the patient care, pharmacy residents will also want to know if they will be able to see the establishment of these contracts. There are many business opportunities available to community residents, so it will be important to ask about your involvement in those opportunities.

Many programs also have a teaching commitment. Ask about teaching certificates and what is involved in that certificate. Determine ahead of time exactly what is expected in terms of teaching pharmacy students, and be sure you are comfortable with the amount of teaching that is expected. Most sites will require precepting at the practice site. As a resident you should have mentoring in this area. You will also want to know what staffing expectations are required. Ask about preceptor support when you are staffing. It is your responsibility to evaluate whether the type and amount of staffing is acceptable to you.

Residency projects are usually a requirement of the program. Residents develop many skills through the residency project. Ask about the projects of current or previous residents. Determine the expectation of the research project. For example, some programs require completion of the project before a certificate is issued; others require publication. You will also want to know how a resident decides upon a project, how much time is allocated for project work, and what the outcome of the research component is.

Other opportunities for residents may include community outreach and continuing education programs. Some programs may have numerous electives to choose from as well.

In addition to the information outlined above, many of the programs vary in size, number of preceptors, number of mentors, and number of co-residents. Ultimately all of the factors may vary from program to program. These differences will be important to consider as you apply and interview.

WHERE DO YOU GO AFTER SUCCESSFUL COMPLETION?

With a great number of pharmacists practicing in the community setting, PGY-1 CPRPs can transform the pharmacy profession. They represent a key component of the paradigm shift focusing on the patient-centered model of care. In the future, community pharmacy practice is going to be less product-focused and more service-driven. Those who have completed community pharmacy residencies will be better prepared for this change. When evaluating the quality of a program, it is important to consider where former residents have accepted positions post-residency. The best program is the one that most suits your needs and has a history of candidates whom also share your career goals. You can assess the quality of a program by examining the program's reputation, the pharmacy's clinical services, and information on previous residents (e.g., Where are they now?). Other sources of information include faculty, preceptors, alumni, and current residents. Be sure the program aligns with your career goals and patient population of interest, and that you are compatible with the preceptors.

Many former community residents have assumed patient care positions in chain pharmacy, independent pharmacy, and ambulatory care settings post-residency where they have been primarily responsible for generation and evaluation of a pharmacy services. Depending on the program the resident graduates from, they may pursue positions in state and professional associations, independent ownership, or other postgraduate opportunities such as PGY-2, fellowship, masters, or PhD programs.

Ultimately a community pharmacy residency can prepare you for a career rather than a job. After a short, 12-month experience, you will have had numerous opportunities for direct patient contact and to learn how to develop patient care services and hone patient care skills. A community residency program helps you prepare to become a leader and innovator in community pharmacy practice.

Chapter Takeaways

▶ A PGY-1 community pharmacy residency is a longitudinal experience, and at the end of the year you should feel confident taking care of patients.

▶ Community residencies also offer experience in business, finance, and management. Residents should have a much better understanding of pharmacy workflow including how to incorporate clinical services in the workflow or dispensing.

▶ Both single site and multisite CPRPs exist. It is important for you to know in which environment you will thrive. Finding a program that best fits your overall career goals will be vital during the recruitment process.

▶ Accreditation gives programs credibility and confers stability and commitment to the program by all collaborating parties.

▶ Most CPRPs allow customization for your goals to account for specific interests. As a result, your career goals must align with the program's educational goals and objectives.

ROLE OF THE MENTOR

Talk with your mentor to help identify career goals and strengths that will align with your interests. Your mentor should be able to help you identify what you want to get out of a community residency, so that these features can be aligned with an appropriate CPRP.

Speak with your mentor about environments in which you not just survive, but thrive. They should be able to help you look for a CPRP that fits accordingly. If you have a knack for entrepreneurship, look for a CPRP with strong independent pharmacy offerings. If you are slightly more clinically geared than community generally is, consider ambulatory care residencies or CPRPs that have long-standing clinical sites.

Seek help from your mentor regarding networking with any RPDs, preceptors in CPRPs, or past graduates of community residencies they may know. Your mentor should encourage you to look at and speak with several programs.

Work with your mentor to identify and obtain practice experiences with clinical community sites.

Utilize your mentor to review your curriculum vitae and cover letter, conduct a mock residency interview with you, and write a letter of recommendation that validates your pharmacy experiences in clinical community practice.

FREQUENTLY ASKED QUESTIONS

Q: **Where can I find more information about community pharmacy residency programs?**

A: General information about CPRPs can be found at www.pharmacist.com/residencies as well as online residency directories from the various pharmacy organizations.

Q: **What are some benefits of completing a CPRP?**

A: You will be able to practice at an advanced level of patient care, enhance your clinical skills, develop and implement patient care services, teach and conduct research, facilitate community outreach programs, foster leadership skills, develop management and marketing skills, work with innovative practitioners, enhance professional network and career opportunities, and earn a stipend with benefits.

Q: **What is the difference between a community residency and an ambulatory care residency?**

A: Both residencies enhance your clinical knowledge. Community residencies also offer experience in business, finance, and management. You are exposed to clinical service development and evaluation.

Q: **Should I be sure that the site received all my application materials?**

A: It is very important to follow up with the program to be sure that they received your completed application. At times the registrar may forget to send your transcripts. Alternatively, a letter of recommendation may be missing, making your application incomplete. This may impact your chances of being asked for an on-site interview. It is always important to make sure all materials have been received by the program.

Q: Should I write a thank you note to all the sites I interviewed with if it is a multisite program?

A: Yes, every preceptor, resident, and director should receive a thank you note after the interview. An email would be fine, but the personal thank you note leaves a great impression. If you really liked the site and plan to rank it high, then write a personal note.

Q: Should I take notes during the interview process?

A: Taking notes is a good way to remember what was discussed. You may want to let the interviewer know that you are taking notes and checking your list of questions so they understand why you may not be making eye contact. You should also take notes immediately after the interview.

References

1. Stolpe S, Adams A, Bradley-Baker L, Burns A, Owen J. Historical development and emerging trends of community pharmacy residencies. Am J Pharm Educ. 2011;75(8).160.

2. American Pharmacists Association. 2010–2011 Postgraduate Year 1 Community Pharmacy Resident Exit Survey. www.pharmacist.com/residencies/exitsurvey. Accessed March 30, 2012.

3. Schommer J, Bonnarens J, Brown L, Goode JV. Value of community pharmacy residency programs: College of pharmacy and practice site perspectives. J Am Pharm Assoc. 2010;50:e72–e88.

4. American Pharmacists Association. Postgraduate Year 1 Community Pharmacy Residency Program Directory. www.pharmacist.com/Residencies/Directory. Accessed March 30, 2012.

5. American Pharmacists Association. PGY-1 Community Accreditation Standard. www.pharmacist.com/residencies/standard. Accessed March 30, 2012.

6. American College of Clinical Pharmacy (ACCP) Online Directory of Residencies, Fellowships, and Graduate Programs. http://www.accp.com/resandfel/index.aspx. Accessed March 30, 2012.

7. ASHP Online Residency Directory. http://www.ashp.org/menu/Accreditation/Residency Directory.aspx. Accessed March 30, 2012.

8. American Society of Health-System Pharmacists and Commission on Credentialing Updates. http://www.ashp.org/DocLibrary/Accreditation/ASDMCMTownHall2011.aspx. Accessed March 30, 2012.

9. American Society of Health-System Pharmacists Tips for Prospective Residents. http://www.ashp.org/Midyear2011/ResidencyShowcase/Tips.aspx. Accessed March 30, 2012.

10. American Society of Health-System Pharmacists Accreditation Standard for Postgraduate Year One (PGY1) Community Pharmacy Residency Programs prepared jointly by the American Society of Health-System Pharmacists and the American Pharmacists Association, approved in 2006. www.pharmacist.com/residencies/goalsobjectives. Accessed March 30, 2012.

Managed Care Postgraduate Year One Pharmacy Residency 16

Jessica R. Daw

Managed care pharmacy is a healthcare delivery system that balances clinical and economic factors, including cost, quality, and access. The goal of managed care pharmacy is to administer the benefit in a way that creates the best clinical patient outcomes in a cost-effective manner. Traditionally, managed care organizations are considered to be health plans, including health maintenance organizations (HMOs) and preferred provider organizations (PPOs), and pharmacy benefit managers (PBMs). The concepts of managed care, however, can be learned in a variety of settings.

Many managed care pharmacy residency programs are newer as the interest level of pharmacy students continues to grow. Although these programs, like most pharmacy residencies, are typically 1 year in length, they are fairly specialized to the area of managed care. Pharmacy students do not need to complete a Postgraduate Year One (PGY-1) pharmacy practice residency before applying for a PGY-1 managed care pharmacy residency. Some pharmacy students who are undecided in their career path may choose to complete a PGY-1 pharmacy practice residency and then later decide to specialize in managed care. Depending on the PGY-1 managed care pharmacy residency program, completing a prior pharmacy practice residency may be helpful, but is typically not required. Completing the two residencies may also offer an advantage to a person who is looking to specialize in certain areas within managed care like medication therapy management programs. A majority of students complete their managed care residency in the first year out of school.

After the completion of the residency, most residents search for their first job in a managed care setting or related field. There are a few specialized second year managed care residency programs that are offered as well, although most of the programs currently available have a focus on pharmacoeconomics. Unless the resident has a desire to concentrate in this area, a second year residency in managed care is usually not necessary. If a PGY-1 managed care resident would be interested in completing a nonmanaged care Postgraduate Year Two (PGY-2) residency, it is advised to review the expectations and qualifications with the program director.

PGY-1 managed care pharmacy residency programs are designed to train pharmacists to deliver patient-centered care using three practice models that include (1) individual patient care in which the resident is responsible for managing the patient's treatment plan and communicating clearly to both the patient and the provider regarding the patient's progress; (2) designing, performing, monitoring, and evaluating the outcomes of clinical programs for targeted groups of patients; and (3) policy development based on population-based health management.[1]

ACCREDITATION PROCESS FOR MANAGED CARE PHARMACY RESIDENCIES

PGY-1 managed care pharmacy residency programs are accredited through a joint process between the American Society of Health-System Pharmacists (ASHP) and the Academy of Managed Care Pharmacy (AMCP). During the program's on-site accreditation review, representatives from both organizations are present to evaluate the program. The purpose of accreditation is to ensure a high-quality and comprehensive learning experience of the residency program. More managed care residency programs are applying and becoming accredited through the ASHP/AMCP process. Programs that are accredited have met certain standards in their programs, including the training site, design of the residency program, learning experiences, and preceptor and resident qualifications.

Additionally accredited programs have access to a Web-based electronic system called ResiTrak™ to evaluate residents' progress throughout the year. This system allows the program to keep all evaluations in one place. For most rotations, residents fill out a self-evaluation of the rotation, an evaluation of the learning experience, and an evaluation of the preceptor. The preceptor also completes an evaluation of the resident. This system facilitates the feedback process ensuring that both the resident and the program have the appropriate information leading to continued growth and improvement.

Not all programs, however, are able to meet the necessary outcomes, goals, and objectives to become an accredited managed care residency program. Even if a program is not accredited, it still may be a suitable fit for you. Some programs have more concentrated learning experiences in a certain area, like medication therapy management, and the organization sponsoring the program may not have the necessary opportunities for the candidates to meet all the requirements by ASHP/AMCP. As long as a nonaccredited program has robust learning experiences and opportunities, completing this program will allow you to meet your career goals. After residents complete a managed care pharmacy residency program, typically they are chosen for a job based on their training and skill set. Most organizations do not require that candidates complete an accredited residency in order to be a candidate for a managed care position. As a residency candidate, you should evaluate each program and the learning opportunities of that program to determine if it is right for you.

MANAGED CARE PHARMACY RESIDENCY APPLICATION PROCESS

For managed care pharmacy residencies, research is a requirement to understand what types of programs are available and which programs fit your interests. You should start with the AMCP Residency Web site (www.amcp.org/residencies) where you can find a listing of all accredited and nonaccredited managed care residency programs.[1] You may also be able to meet representatives from programs during the residency showcases at the AMCP Educational Conference in the fall and at ASHP MCM. It is recommended that you make yourself known as a candidate to programs either through one of these showcases, a local residency showcase that may be offered where you live, or by contacting the program to express your interest ahead of the application submission. You should also check to see if the program you are interested in requires you to interview at ASHP Midyear Clinical Meeting (MCM) through the Personal Placement Service (PPS). Even if this is not required by the program, it may be worthwhile to interview at PPS to express your interest to the program and to get some of your questions answered. Programs are more likely to offer interviews to candidates they have met previously.

Each managed care pharmacy residency program has its own application process. It is important to check the details of the process and ensure that you submit the proper materials in the appropriate format as requested by the program by the due date. Most programs require materials to be submitted sometime in January, but there are a few programs with deadlines in December. It is also necessary to check how the materials should be submitted—postal mail or electronic. It is important to follow directions as this reflects upon you as an applicant.

ASHP has announced that it will release a new online residency application process in Fall 2012. This centralized electronic application system will allow residents and programs to track the progress of applications.[2] You should check if the programs you are interested in are utilizing this new process.

Many managed care pharmacy residency programs require the same materials to be submitted for consideration of an on-site interview. A letter of intent will provide the program with an idea of your experiences relevant to the residency, your motivation for applying to this program, and your short- and long-term career goals. Programs may have a word count requirement for this letter. Two to three professional letters of recommendation are usually necessary. Some programs specify the types of people who should write these letters including clinical professors, rotation site preceptors, and/or previous or current employers. Official transcripts from your school of pharmacy will most likely also be necessary. Finally, most programs require that applicants submit a CV. This will provide the program with additional information on your work experience, rotations, presentations given, teaching experience, and organizational and community involvement. This should include any participation in national pharmacy associations as well as leadership positions held. See Chapter 9 for more details on residency applications.

In addition to these standard materials, some programs also have other requirements. There may be an application form to fill out or an online application process. A writing sample may be required. Also the program may request that you complete a certain task, for example, a drug therapy recommendation, to test your knowledge of a particular area. Some programs may also have a GPA requirement.

Programs typically require that you be licensed in the practicing state by a certain date. Ensure that you understand all licensing requirements and that you are able to meet them by the appropriate deadline. States differ in their licensing requirements so it is important to research this process through the State Board of Pharmacy before applying to a program.

Based on the written application materials submitted, a program may offer you an on-site or telephonic interview. Interview time slots usually start at the end of January and are completed by the beginning of March. Some factors programs use to determine whether to offer a candidate an interview include academic performance, extracurricular activities, leadership skills, how well your goals match to the program goals, and the competencies and behaviors discussed in the letters of recommendation. A telephonic screening interview may occur before an on-site interview is offered.

> "Be confident and be yourself during the interview. Always act professional, but don't be afraid to show some personality because this helps set you apart from other candidates!"
>
> *Nitha C. – Pharmacy Student, Massachusetts*

An on-site interview is typically one half day to one full day in length, and the candidate will meet with multiple employees of the organization, including preceptors of the residency program. On-site interview expenses are not always reimbursed by the program so you should be prepared for this cost. In preparation for the interview, practice answering questions. It may be helpful to rehearse verbally with a friend or mentor.

During the interview, you may also be asked to give a presentation 20 to 40 minutes in length. Candidates should be sure to ask what kind of topic is expected, make sure to tailor the presentation to the audience, and be ready to answer questions from the interviewers. Also, if you are using a presentation from a previous rotation, make sure the information is up to date. You should also find out if there will be a projector available or if you are expected to bring handouts or email the presentation ahead of time. A written presentation should always be available in case the equipment is not working. You should also prepare your own list of questions about the program to ask during the interview. See Chapter 10 for more tips on interviewing.

Candidates interested in an accredited managed care pharmacy residency program must sign up with NMS as all accredited residency programs must adhere to the residency match process (the Match). After programs interview all candidates, they will determine their rank order lists for the Match that is usually submitted to National Matching Service (NMS) in early March. The results of the NMS Match process are usually revealed by mid-March. Nonaccredited residencies follow a different time line so if you are applying to both accredited and nonaccredited residency programs, it is important to understand the expectations of the residencies as to when they plan to offer interviews and make decisions. Try to schedule your interviews in a way that will allow you to explore all programs you are interested in before making a final decision.

EDUCATIONAL OUTCOMES IN MANAGED CARE PHARMACY RESIDENCY PROGRAMS

The goal of managed care programs is to provide you with a comprehensive, unique learning experience in managed care pharmacy to help prepare you for your future career path. Although programs vary in their experiences and design, there are common learning objectives and outcomes that are required for ASHP/AMCP accreditation. These include seven required and nine elective outcomes for managed care programs as illustrated in Figure 16-1.

Under each of these educational outcomes are educational goals, educational objectives, and instructional objectives. Reading through the document "Required and Elective Educational Outcomes, Educational Goals, Educational Objectives, and Instructional Objectives for PGY-1 Managed Care Pharmacy Residency Programs" assembled by AMCP and ASHP will assist you in understanding how the outcomes will be met.[3] This document can be found on the AMCP and ASHP Web sites (www.amcp.org or www.ashp.org).

Required Outcomes	Elective Outcomes
• R1: Understand how to manage the drug distribution process for an organization's members.	• E1: Added knowledge and skills to manage the drug distribution process for the organization's members.
• R2: Design and implement clinical programs to enhance the efficacy of patient care.	• E2: Provide evidence-based, patient-centered medication therapy management with interdisciplinary teams.
• R3: Ensure the safety and quality of the medication-use system.	• E3: Added knowledge and skills to provide medication and practice-related information, education, and/or training.
• R4: Provide medication and practice-related information, education, and/or training.	• E4: Exercise added leadership and practice management skills.
• R5: Collaborate with plan sponsors to design effective benefit structures to service a specific population's needs.	• E5: Participate in the process by which managed care organizations contract with pharmaceutical manufactures.
• R6: Exercise leadership and practice management skills.	• E6: Conduct outcomes-based research.
• R7: Demonstrate project management skills.	• E7: Conduct pharmacy practice research.
	• E8: Participate in the management of business continuity.
	• E9: Demonstrate additional competencies that contribute to working successfully in the health care environment.

Figure 16-1: **Outcomes in Managed Care Pharmacy Programs.**[3]

SETTINGS FOR MANAGED CARE PHARMACY RESIDENCIES

Managed care concepts can be acquired in a variety of settings. The two most common settings for managed care residencies are health plans and PBMs. Within these organizations, the resident may report through clinical or operational areas. Therefore, the residency experience will be different depending on the program. Some examples of a program's focus include patient care activities, formulary management, and outcomes research. It is important for you as the candidate to ask the right questions during the recruiting process to ensure that the program matches your interests.

Other settings for managed care residencies include consulting firms, population health management companies that may focus on medication therapy management programs, and clinic-based settings. Programs where the primary site for the resident is a clinic typically also have a strong ambulatory care focus, along with learning managed care concepts. Programs may also have more than one setting depending on the rotation schedule. Many residency programs also have an affiliation with a university that may allow residents to attend various organized lecture series on topics such as research, teaching, and professional skills. With this relationship to the university, residents also may have the opportunity to teach both in a small group and large group lecture settings, as well as serve as preceptors for pharmacy students on rotation.

ACTIVITIES UNIQUE TO MANAGED CARE TRAINING

All accredited managed care programs are required to have resident exposure to certain managed care concepts, which drive the activities of the program. Rotations can either be in blocks of time such as 2 to 8 weeks in length or they can be longitudinal lasting up to the entire duration of the residency program.

As a managed care resident, there are both clinical and nonclinical managed care concepts to be learned. Pharmacy benefit management concepts that are nonclinical in nature include focusing on areas such as drug distribution and benefit structure. Activities include projects that focus on establishing and auditing pharmacy networks, including retail, mail order, and specialty pharmacies, as well as understanding the adjudication of claims in the processing system. Residents also have the opportunity to learn about benefit structures and how these affect the population utilizing the benefit. Residents may work with benefit options to understand the impact of changes to the plan design, such as the increase in copayments, a change to coinsurances, or the addition of mandatory mail order to a plan. They will work to identify suggestions for formulary and benefit design changes, as well as understand the clinical and regulatory requirements of plan sponsors.

A majority of the activities of a managed care resident are typically related to clinical concepts, such as formulary and utilization management and clinical program involvement. The resident will have the opportunity to track drugs in the pipeline and review medications for the Pharmacy and Therapeutics (P&T) committee, including the completion of a formulary monograph, therapeutic class review, and new policy development for utilization management, including prior authorization, step therapy, and quantity limits. Residents will need to utilize evidence-based literature, clinical guidelines, and physician feedback in developing recommendations. The resident will gain an understanding of the communication and implementation process for formulary changes. Typically residents also participate in the review of prior authorization requests by taking a protocol or policy and applying it to a particular patient case.

A second clinical area that is covered during the residency is disease state management and medication therapy management program development and implementation. Residents will work to develop a new clinical program by identifying an area of need and using evidence-based guidelines and literature to develop the program. The resident must then work to implement the program by developing the operational process, designing the patient and provider education, determining how to measure outcomes of the program, and deciding on a feedback process from stakeholders in the program.

Another clinical skill to be developed by the resident involves resolving medication-related problems for individual patients. This could take place at the site via telephonic intervention or off-site at a clinic or medical office setting. The resident will work to collect the patient's relevant clinical information and develop and then deliver the therapeutic care plan. The resident needs to determine how to monitor the patient progress and also ensure that all of the educational needs of the patient are met.

The resident will also be responsible for ensuring the safety and quality of the managed care processes by identifying problems and providing resolutions with a consideration to best practices in the healthcare industry. Problems can be identified by performing a drug utilization evaluation (DUE) on certain medications to determine current trends. Based on the results of this DUE, the resident will suggest a clinical program or process improvement that will lead to better quality of care. Residents will also gain an understanding of the quality organizations that play a role in managed care including the National Committee of Quality Assurance (NCQA), Utilization Review Accreditation Commission (URAC), and the Pharmacy Quality Alliance (PQA). Accreditation and regulatory standards of NCQA, URAC, Centers for Medicaid and Medicare Services (CMS), and state regulatory agencies are also discussed.

Residents will be required to demonstrate adequate communication and drug information skills. Creating patient and physician educational pieces is typically part of the residency program. In addition, the resident is required to utilize appropriate literature and references to complete responses to drug information requests.

Most programs typically also offer research projects as well as teaching experiences. Residents will work on the research project throughout the year developing the background, methodology, analyzing the data for results, and drawing conclusions. Residents usually present their research project in the form of a poster at the AMCP Spring Conference or at another conference, such as the regional residency conference. Many residents will also complete a manuscript that may be submitted for publication. Research projects are required for accredited managed care pharmacy residency programs; however, teaching experiences may vary depending on the program. Most residents are involved in teaching by serving as a preceptor for student rotations, but the amount of time dedicated to this depends on the programs and the interest level of the resident. Residents may also have the opportunity to facilitate small group or large group lectures. Some programs also offer a teaching program in which residents can earn a certificate.

Additionally, depending on the residency programs, other activities may be part of the learning experience. Rotations that focus around specialty medications and specialty pharmacies are becoming more common in programs as this area of managed care continues to grow. Residencies may offer opportunities in benefit configuration and call center management, including projects to assess the speed of answering calls and the quality of the customer service provided. Another elective learning option is rebates and understanding the strategy and negotiations between the managed care organization and pharmaceutical manufacturers. Other programs may have additional and more detailed electives in industry, strategy, direct patient care, clinical consulting services, and outcomes research.

Managed care residencies offer a wide variety of experiences. It is important for you as a candidate to ask questions of each program to understand what opportunities are available in comparison to your interests.

CAREER OPTIONS AND OPPORTUNITIES AVAILABLE AFTER SUCCESSFULLY COMPLETING A MANAGED CARE RESIDENCY

Depending on the focus of the managed care pharmacy residency program you complete, there are a wide range of career options and opportunities. You can utilize contacts that you make during the residency year to assist you in finding a job. Additionally, the program that you completed may have resources available for career planning.

Pharmacist positions in managed care can have a varying degree of clinical involvement in a health plan or PBM. Positions that are more clinical in focus include concentrations in formulary and/or utilization management, clinical strategy, or clinical program development and implementation, including disease state management and medication therapy management programs. Clinical pharmacists may also be involved with outcomes research, academic detailing (providing clinical information to physicians), quality improvement activities, specialty pharmacy management, and/or have a drug information focus.

Pharmacists may also have jobs that are less clinical in nature within a health plan or PBM. These include concentrations in client management, network development and auditing, marketing and sales, and/or more operational areas, such as call center or mail order. Pharmacists may also be involved with a range of product development activities like creating new benefit designs, such as a value-based benefit that would promote the use of preventive medications, or working on benefit configuration to make sure clinical decisions are translated into the claims processing system and medications pay correctly at the point of sale. Pharmacists in both clinical and nonclinical roles may also be involved in the administration or management of a department.

Depending on the program, residents may also be able to translate skills learned to other job settings. These could include positions with a pharmaceutical manufacturer/industry, ambulatory care clinics, consultation services, or academic settings, such as universities.

Some pharmacists may have a more specialized focus in some of the areas listed above and others may have a more generalized position that covers multiple areas. The job description will depend on each organization and how the job responsibilities are divided within a department or organization.

Chapter Takeaways

▶ Managed care pharmacy residency programs are specialized in their focus.

▶ You should ensure that you adequately research managed care pharmacy residency programs as each program offers different learning experiences and areas of concentration.

▶ Make sure to understand the application process for each program and what the requirements are for applying, including licensure in different states.

▶ There are a variety of settings in which a managed care residency program can be provided and also where managed care pharmacists work.

▶ Search for a program that matches your interests for your future career.

ROLE OF THE MENTOR

Mentors can provide insight into the managed care field and what types of residency programs may fit your interests.

Mentors may be able to point out rotations, internships, or shadowing experiences within managed care organizations.

Mentors should provide feedback on application materials to be submitted, including CV, letter of intent, and who to ask for letters of recommendation.

Mentors will be helpful in discussing what to expect for the on-site interview, including how to present yourself and how to prepare for questions that may be asked.

FREQUENTLY ASKED QUESTIONS

Q: **How do I choose a managed care residency program that is the best fit for me?**

A: You should be sure to do the appropriate research by attending residency showcases and asking many questions throughout the recruitment process. Some considerations include whether the program is accredited, the location, number of residency positions offered, and whether the learning experiences are best suited for your future career path. Additionally, you should consider the qualifications of the preceptors of the program and its reputation. Also the work environment and other coworkers should be a consideration. Talking to the preceptors of the program as well as past and current residents can help you to answer some of these questions.

Q: **What should I ask when speaking with the stakeholders in the managed care residency program?**

A: After your own research, you may still have questions that will help you to clarify how well the program fits with your interests. You should gain a better understanding of the rotations in the program and how they are administered (longitudinal versus block). You should understand the purpose of the learning experiences in the program and which rotations are required and which are elective and also ask what makes the program unique. Depending on your goals of a residency program, you may want to ask about the ability to customize the program or rotations to fit your needs. Additionally, you should ask where past residents are in their career and what some of the past projects were, including research that was completed by these residents. You should also ask about the qualifications of the preceptors of the program and what the process is for the program to provide feedback to the resident. The answers to these questions will give you a better idea of what the program has to offer.

Q: **Who should write my letters of recommendations for managed care residency programs?**

A: You should ensure that you have a good relationship with the people who will write your letters of recommendation and that you are confident they will provide a strong recommendation for you. It is important that the person know enough about you to detail your positive attributes that make you stand out from other pharmacy students. If you are able to, it is also a good idea to get letters from a variety of settings, including professors, preceptors of clinical rotations, and previous or current employers. This can demonstrate that you excel in multiple settings. It is also important to ensure your letter authors have a general understanding of the programs you are applying for so that they can tailor the letter appropriately.

Q: **What do managed care programs look for in a candidate?**

A: Typically, programs are looking for candidates with some managed care experience or some experience that can be tied to managed care concepts. Programs also typically look at academic performance (some may have GPA requirements), extracurricular activities (including involvement and leadership positions within organizations and in the community), how well your goals match to the program offering, and competencies and behaviors derived from your interview answers and your letters of recommendation. Programs also typically ask for examples of projects you have done on rotations and how you can tie them to managed care. They may also be looking at previous teaching experiences, direct patient care, and presentations given both during rotations and at national conferences. Your actions and the answers you give to questions during the on-site interview are typically weighted the heaviest.

References

1. Residencies. http://www.amcp.org/Residencies/. Accessed January 29, 2012.
2. Managed care residencies to be included in ASHP's new online residency application process. *AMCP Monthly News.* February 2012;24:8.
3. AMCP and ASHP. Required and Elective Educational Outcomes, Educational Goals, Educational Objectives, and Instructional Objectives for Postgraduate Year One (PGY-1) Managed Care Pharmacy Residency Programs. http://www.amcp.org/WorkArea/DownloadAsset.aspx?id=9565. Accessed February 19, 2012.

Unique Postgraduate Year One Residency Opportunities and Settings

17

Michael D. Hogue

You may be thinking, "I know I need to complete a residency to give myself a competitive advantage in the job market, but I just don't think a traditional hospital-based, or even a community-pharmacy residency is right for me." It might be that you want the skills of a traditional residency, but want to gain these skills in a unique setting. The great news is that there are many unique opportunities available to build your practice credentials while gaining valuable experience in a more focused or specialized area of practice. Whether it is association management, public health, military service, focused medication therapy management (MTM), or even international pharmacy practice, chances are pretty good that there is an opportunity out there that will fit your professional and personal needs.

FINDING UNIQUE PROGRAMS

Unique programs are, by their very nature, outside of the norm in their design. Because of this, in some cases they do not and/or cannot meet defined accreditation standards set by American Society of Health-System Pharmacists (ASHP) for Postgraduate Year One (PGY-1) or Postgraduate Year Two (PGY-2) residency training. For example, Principle 7 of the ASHP standards for PGY-1 programs relate to the organization of a pharmacy and provision of safe and effective services.[1] However, a residency in association management may not be able to meet this outcome due to the lack of patient contact in a pharmacy association. This doesn't make the program less valuable—only different! Thus, there are times when selecting a residency program that is *not* accredited would be in your best interest.

Why would you even consider a unique residency program outside of the framework of a standardized PGY-1 experience? Don't get me wrong: accredited programs are great, and are certainly the gold standard for quality in our profession. However, a nonaccredited residency might be appropriate, especially if the program can make you competitive for a job category or career track. In the case of association management residencies, having completed one of these programs equips the pharmacist with a unique skill set that would make one more competitive for jobs in this segment of the pharmacist market. In the case of a military or armed forces residency, regardless of whether the program is accredited or not, you can count your service time as a resident toward rank and retirement in the uniformed service—definitely an advantage if you think you might be interested in a career with the U.S. government. As MTM becomes increasingly the mantra of our profession, especially in these early days of adoption of new care models, an MTM residency, regardless of its accreditation status, may be seen by employers as providing a specific and desired skill set and give you that edge up in the job market.

So how do you find a unique residency program opportunity? While there are many ways to search for residencies, the largest repository for nonaccredited and accredited unique pharmacy residencies is an online database maintained by the American College of Clinical Pharmacy (ACCP) (http://www.accp.com/resandfel/index.aspx). Another way to learn about unique residency programs is through attendance at state and national professional association meetings (such as the American Pharmacists Association (APhA), the National Community Pharmacists Association (NCPA), the Academy of Managed Care Pharmacy (AMCP), the American Association of Colleges of Pharmacy (AACP), and the ASHP; see Table 5-1 in Chapter 5). Many of these organizations now offer residency showcase times, residency round table discussions, or have sections in their exhibit halls for residency programs to exhibit. A number of the unique programs that exist are offered in conjunction with schools and colleges of pharmacy. You might consider visiting Web sites of individual schools in the geographic area where you are interested in completing a residency. New, unique residency programs are often announced by the schools using press releases, many of which will appear on AACP's Web site. In addition, Table 17-1 provides a listing of several unique programs discussed in this chapter.

TABLE 17-1 • Selected Resources, Unique Residency Programs[a]

American Association of Colleges of Pharmacy	http://www.accp.com/resandfel/index.aspx *Provides a searchable online database of both accredited and nonaccredited programs.*
Public Health Emphasis Residency Programs	Samford University McWhorter School of Pharmacy[b] http://pharmacy.samford.edu/Public-Health-Residency.aspx St. Louis College of Pharmacy http://www.stlcop.edu/academics/residencydescription.asp?id=2 University of Missouri-Kansas City http://pharmacy.umkc.edu/academic-divisions/residencies/public-health/

TABLE 17-1 • Selected Resources, Unique Residency Programs[a] (*continued*)

Nontraditional Federal Government Residency Programs	Federal Bureau of Prisons http://www.usphs.gov/corpslinks/pharmacy/bop/Residency%20 Training%20Program%20Flyer.pdf Indian Health Services http://www.ihs.gov/medicalprograms/pharmacy/resident/index. cfm?module=faqs U.S. Army Medical Service Corps http://www.bamc.amedd.army.mil/staff/education/allied-health/ pharmacy/ National Capital Consortium (Navy, Army, Air Force Collaborative) at Walter Reed National Military Medical Center http://www.bethesda.med.navy.mil/careers/graduate_medical_ education/gme_residencies/pharmacy/index.aspx U.S. Navy http://www.navy.com/careers/healthcare/clinical-care/pharmacy.html U.S. Air Force *Contact the local Air Force recruiter or the pharmacy department a local Air Force base for more information.*
Global Health Emphasis Residency Programs	Purdue Pharmacy http://ampath.pharmacy.purdue.edu/residency/information.pdf University of Pittsburgh School of Pharmacy http://www.pharmacy.pitt.edu/programs/residency/underserved.html
Association Management Residency Programs	American Pharmacists Association Foundation http://www.pharmacist.com/AM/Template. cfm?Section=Executive_Residency&Template=/CM/ HTMLDisplay.cfm&ContentID=27109 National Association of Chain Drug Stores Foundation http://www.nacdsfoundation.org/WHATWEDO/ SCHOLARSHIPSANDSTUDENTOPPORTUNITIES/ NACDSFoundationExecutiveResidency.aspx National Alliance of State Pharmacy Associations http://cop-stage.cws.oregonstate.edu/sites/default/files/ NASPAResidency2011_2012.pdf National Community Pharmacists Association http://www.ncpanet.org/pdf/students/exec_res_brochure.pdf
Medication Therapy Management Emphasis Residencies	Outcomes Pharmaceutical Health Care http://www.getoutcomes.com/aspx/pressroom/ internshipresidencypositions.aspx PharmMD Solutions, LLC http://www.pharmmd.com/residency-program/ University of Florida College of Pharmacy http://www.cop.ufl.edu/wp-content/uploads/2012-Residency-Flyer.pdf

[a]*The above listing is not intended to be comprehensive. Because these programs are unique, often in emerging areas of pharmacy practice, program availability and information changes rapidly. Do your homework by conducting regular Internet searches for keywords related to your area of interest!*

[b]*In addition to the above, there are an increasing number of PGY-2 residencies in ambulatory care that are offered in conjunction with county and state departments of public health and/or community health centers.*

RESIDENCIES WITH EMPHASIS ON PUBLIC HEALTH

The role of the pharmacist in public health has evolved tremendously over the past 20 years. Largely spurred by the pharmacy-based immunization movement that started in 1996, pharmacists have been increasingly engaged at disease prevention and health promotion activities, as well as mitigation of chronic disease.[2] In addition, pharmacists have stepped up to the plate in a huge way as the nation and world has faced a number of natural disasters.[3-5] These high-impact public health activities have created new demand in the marketplace for pharmacists who have greater insight and training in public health concepts. While some pharmacy schools have developed dual PharmD-Masters in Public Health (MPH) programs, this option may not be within reach of many pharmacy students for time and money reasons (it typically takes 1 to 2 years beyond the normal time frame of the PharmD to finish a dual PharmD-MPH degree program).

Given the emerging need for public health trained pharmacists, PGY-1 residencies with emphasis on public health were developed. The first of these programs was accredited by ASHP in 2007.[6] Since that time, a number of schools and colleges of pharmacy have teamed up with local public health departments and community health centers to launch public health-emphasis residency programs. The vast majority of these programs strongly resembles ambulatory care practice and typically occurs in outpatient ambulatory care clinics; however, the opportunities for provision of indigent care, engagement in epidemiologic surveillance, emergency preparedness and disaster response, and public health education and outreach efforts are unique to this setting. For example, a resident in a public health program may have specific learning objectives in the area of infectious diseases surveillance, working with public health officials to track disease outbreaks and stop their spread. Additionally, the resident may be responsible for working together with emergency preparedness staff to conduct training exercises and develop plans for points of dispensing or immunization during a disaster situation—and many residents have been able to participate in actual disaster response during their residency programs. These are activities you won't typically be involved with in a traditional ambulatory care program.

What are the career options in this area of residency training? Schools and colleges of pharmacy are placing increased emphasis on public health training. There is currently a lack of well-qualified, public health trained pharmacists in academia, thus you'll find a host of career opportunities with the schools and colleges of pharmacy. In addition, agencies such as state and county health departments and the Centers for Disease Control and Prevention are often looking for healthcare providers with a deeper knowledge and experience in public health. Ambulatory care clinics will also find your kill set of tremendous value, as will health systems in general.

ASSOCIATION MANAGEMENT RESIDENCIES

If you've ever dreamed of being right in the thick of things related to shaping public policy and advocacy in pharmacy, perhaps you should consider a residency in association management. Several national pharmacy organizations currently offer 1-year executive management programs, many of which have been in place for decades (ASHP's program is the oldest; however, the association has suspended their program at present). These programs provide pharmacists with skill-building opportunities related to budget and finance, public policy and government affairs, professional affairs, executive office operations, publishing and professional writing, continuing education development, meeting and event planning, media outreach, industry relations, and a host of other association-specific activities. With most of the 50 state pharmacy associations and state societies of health-system pharmacy being run by a CEO pharmacist, as well as the dozens of pharmacists employed by the major national pharmacy associations, there is without question a job market for well-qualified pharmacists in association management. However, there are also very few residency programs available for advanced training in this area, so you'll need to be sure you've done your homework and be well prepared for your interview! It will be of tremendous benefit to you if you actively engage in professional associations as a leader at your school or college of pharmacy while you are a student. Professional associations will be looking for individuals with a demonstrated commitment to the profession. You might even consider completing an APPE course at the association you believe you are most interested in applying for residency placement. Talk with your experiential program director about these opportunities.

One of the serendipities of completing an association management residency is that all but one of these programs exists in Washington, DC. This author found that the cultural and professional opportunities outside of the structure of the residency program were often just as enriching as the program itself. Being in the heart of the nation's capital can be exhilarating, and you definitely will feel as though you are "in the know" when it comes to our profession. The downside to Washington is that the cost of living, pace and intensity of daily living, and transportation challenges may require quite an adjustment!

What are the career options in this area of practice? You'll definitely be in demand with pharmacy associations and pharmacy foundations. What you might be surprised to know is that some former association management residents have found themselves in positions with the FDA, the pharmaceutical industry, and even in nonpharmacy, healthcare-related associations and foundations. A few are even in academia! Your skill set in executive management and business management learned through these programs definitely will open doors.

UNIFORMED SERVICES RESIDENCIES

The United States has seven uniformed services. In addition to the armed services (Army, Navy, Air Force, Marines and Coast Guard), there is the U.S. Public Health Service (PHS) and the National Oceanographic and Atmospheric Administration (NOAA). All of these services employ pharmacists except NOAA.

For well over 40 years, the U.S. PHS has engaged pharmacists in high levels of direct patient care.[7] For many residency directors, preceptors, and even current students, the U.S. PHS model of patient counseling served as the basis for how we learned communication skills and patient interviewing. It's not surprising that such an innovative organization would also innovate when it comes to residency training. Most PHS residencies are accredited through ASHP as either PGY-1 general practice residencies or as PGY-2 ambulatory care or primary care. Of course, because PHS facilities are federal government entities, pharmacists are not bound by state pharmacy practice acts, and are capable of practicing as they were trained and fully capable of practicing. In addition, historically the PHS in particular has offered a generous student loan repayment program for residents who then stay on with PHS for an extended service commitment.

The U.S. military service offers an even more unique opportunity to experience pharmacy practice. The U.S. military pharmacists, like PHS pharmacists, are not bound by state pharmacy practice acts, and are asked to engage in a wide variety of patient care services, including primary care. You do not have to be in the military reserves (i.e., Army or Air Force) as a pharmacy student to be considered for a military branch residency program, although this may provide some advantage in the application process. However, you do need to be a person with flexibility in your geographical location, and you have to be willing to serve your country in both peacetime and wartime situations. Most military branch residency programs are accredited by ASHP as PGY-1 residencies, although Walter Reed National Military Medical Center in Bethesda, MD, has offered selected accredited PGY-2 opportunities in the past. All current military residency programs are centered in a hospital/health-system environment at domestic military bases. One additional note: the U.S. government requires that you hold a license in good standing in at least one of the 50 U.S. states; however, you do not necessarily have to be licensed in the state in which you are practicing. This is very unique to federal programs!

What are your career options in this area of practice? Beyond the obvious with the respective uniformed services, a residency with PHS or the military will position you very well to assume a clinical faculty position at a school or college of pharmacy. You'll also be quite competitive for pharmacy positions in health systems and hospitals, as well as ambulatory care clinics. You'll have a leg-up on your colleagues seeking positions in community pharmacy practice as well!

MEDICATION THERAPY MANAGEMENT RESIDENCIES

All of us expect that MTM skills could be honed during any patient care residency program. Many PGY-1 and PGY-2 programs will specifically highlight the opportunities in MTM on their Web sites. However, a few new MTM-centric residency programs have been birthed in recent years.

These programs engage the resident in the provision of MTM almost exclusively. The setting for some of the early programs is based on patient call-centers/managed care office practices. These programs tend to be a mixture of the components of a managed care residency and a direct patient care experience. You'll definitely spend lots of time doing pharmacoeconomic impact analysis of MTM interventions, as well as crafting and performing benefit analysis of MTM for employers and health plans. But you'll also engage in telephonic and less frequently face-to-face, direct patient care interventions. Some of the organizations offering these residencies primarily employ their own full-time pharmacists to provide MTM services to patients telephonically, while others administer a community pharmacy-based network as their primary mechanism for delivering direct patient care. Regardless, even in those that administer a network, the residency positions currently known to be available are largely based in the headquarters facility of a MTM benefit management firm and have very little opportunity for face-to-face patient contact. These programs are not for everyone, but if you are truly interested in a focused experience with MTM, these programs can offer an enriching, focused, in-depth experience unlike any other.

What are your career options related to this area of residency training? You'd certainly be equipped to work in a managed care organization administering an MTM benefit for the firm. You'd also have possible career paths with chain pharmacy organizations in developing corporate MTM services and in executing MTM services at the pharmacy level. Independent pharmacies may be interested in your skill set and knowledge of the workings of MTM management companies to better position them for this market opportunity. Finally, schools and colleges may find your skills useful in teaching students about MTM.

EVALUATING EMERGING RESIDENCY TRAINING

Let's face it: in today's world employers have some pretty tough choices to make in terms of their pharmacists. Every school of pharmacy graduating pharmacists today is accredited by ACPE. Assuming the applicants pass their boards, there is really not much other than perhaps university and professional leadership and service, intern/extern work experience, or maybe relevance of APPE coursework that will differentiate you from your peers entering the job market. How do you ensure that your resume and application really stand out with that most desired employer? Schools and colleges of pharmacy especially are beginning to think out of the box and innovate in their residency program offerings. Even some health-systems are finding that there are emerging trends in informatics, accountable care organizations, pharmacogenomics, medical home practices, executive hospital management, and more for which they would like to grow their own leaders through residency training. Think about it: if you are an employer, residencies are a great way to mentor people as pipeline for future employment in your health-system. However, there are some cautions. While unique and specialty residencies can certainly have their place, you need to carefully consider a few factors:

- Is the scope of the training so narrow that what you learn won't be applicable outside of the health-system offering the residency? Put another way; be sure you'll gain fully transferable skills.

- Is the residency accredited? Is this important to you? In some cases, accreditation is not relevant (e.g., association management), but in the case of direct patient care residencies, you need to carefully evaluate the "why" behind a program making the decision to *not* pursue accreditation. Ask tough questions such as "Did you ever pursue accreditation and were denied or had your accreditation revoked?"

- Is the unique program you are pursuing truly providing an educational/training opportunity? Sometimes, upstarts and innovators may see the creation of a residency position as a way to get adequate staffing for a task set for a lower salary commitment, without ever really thinking through the educational components necessary to ensure it is truly a residency program. No one wants to get to the end of a year in residency to look back and feel as though they were simply cheap labor. You should be able to clearly document what you have learned and how you have grown over the course of the year! Ask your potential unique program director what they envision being the key opportunities for learning before you move forward in the process.

- Will there be jobs available in the area in which I am pursuing a unique residency training? For the unique programs highlighted in this chapter, there is a clear employment path that is fairly well established. However, as more unique programs emerge in the future, it is important to consider the employment horizon. For example, some hospitals have policies that they will only hire pharmacists who complete ASHP-accredited residencies. You may have had an awesome experience in your nonaccredited program, and you may well be just as highly qualified, but if your dream institution for future employment won't recognize your residency program, you might need to rethink your options.

Chapter Takeaways

▶ Nontraditional or unique residency programs can provide an enriching, life-changing experience for pharmacy graduates. Many of these programs have been around for a very long time and provide excellent training. Others are emerging and you will want to use an appropriate level of inquiry and honest skepticism in your evaluative approach to find a program that is right for you.

▶ Association management residencies have been around for decades and provide training for a well-established niche in pharmacy. These programs are of high quality and meet a real need in the profession. However, there are very few positions available and you will need to do all that you can as a student to position yourself to be competitive for these positions (e.g., actively engage in professional organizations).

▶ Public health focused residency programs are relatively new, but are probably here to stay. The pharmacist's role in disease prevention, wellness, and health promotion seems to have taken strong root in our society, and there will be an increasing need in the future for pharmacists to have even more training in public health.

▶ Residencies in the uniformed services offer the opportunity for pharmacists to practice at the very top of their license. Many of these pharmacists are considered primary care providers within the health system. These programs offer excellent clinical skill development in a very unique environment.

▶ MTM residency programs are very new and it is yet to be seen if they will gain traction as a major national movement. Certainly every residency program should provide some training in MTM, but the unique programs that have emerged early on seem to provide exposure to both managed care and direct patient care. These won't be for everyone, but might be just perfect for you!

ROLE OF THE MENTOR

Discuss your short-term goals, as well as your long-term career horizon goals with your mentor. Get their feedback on whether or not the specific unique residency program is likely to provide you with the skills to be successful given these career goals.

Identify graduates from unique residency programs who can mentor you and discuss the ins and outs of their experiences in a candid way. Select people who have gone on to work for the same organization residency, but also seek out some program graduates who've wound up in an alternate career path to determine how the residency prepared them for this path. There truly is wisdom in a multitude of counselors!

FREQUENTLY ASKED QUESTIONS

Q: **Should I pursue a unique residency program in a setting outside of a typical health-system setting?**

A: Depending on your career goals and the skills you wish to develop, a unique residency program in a nontraditional setting may be the very best choice for you to consider in pursuing postgraduate training. Consider carefully what you want to achieve, and all of your options in achieving your goals, before settling in on any one option in particular.

Q: **How do I identify unique or emerging residency options?**

A: The ACCP maintains the largest database of both accredited and nonaccredited residencies with unique focus and/or in nontraditional practice settings. In addition, a variety of resources are shown in Table 17-1 which may help you in finding a program that is right for you!

Q: Should I disclose to a program director of a unique program that I have also applied for a more traditional PGY-1 residency program?

A: Honesty is always the best policy. If you are asked directly about what types of residencies you've applied for, answer the question honestly. Let the interviewer know why you chose to apply for their program. Express what interests you most about the position, but also let them know of any worries or concerns you have about their program. An open dialogue at the interview will provide you with the best information possible to make decisions for your future.

Q: Do unique and emerging residency programs go through the National Matching Service ("The Match")?

A: Typically new and unique programs do not go through the match in the first year of their existence. Only programs accredited or seeking accreditation from ASHP participate in the match. Therefore, the time frame for applications, interviews, and decisions in unique programs may vary from the process in accredited PGY-1 programs.

References

1. ASHP PGY-1 Residency Standards Page. ASHP website. http://www.ashp.org/DocLibrary/Accreditation/ASD-PGY1-Standard.aspx. Accessed February 21, 2012.

2. Hogue MD, Grabenstein JG, Foster SL, Rothholz MC. Pharmacist involvement with immunizations: A decade of professional advancement. J Am Pharm Assoc. 2006;46:189–203.

3. Velazquez L, et al. A PHS pharmacist team response to Hurricane Katrina. Am J Health Syst Pharm. 2006;63:1332–1335.

4. Hogue MD, Hogue HB, Lander RD, Avent K, Fleenor M. The nontraditional role of pharmacists after hurricane Katrina: Process description and lessons learned. Public Health Rep. 2009;124:217–223.

5. Veltri K, Yaghdjian V, Morgan-Joseph T, Prlesi L, Rudnick E. Hospital emergency preparedness: Push-POD operation and pharmacists as immunizers. J Am Pharm Assoc. 2012;52(1):81–85.

6. Pharmacy, Public Health Intersect in Alabama Disaster Plans webpage. American Society of Health-System Pharmacists site. http://www.ashp.org/menu/News/PharmacyNews/NewsArticle.aspx?id=2653. Accessed February 23, 2012.

7. Giberson S, Yoder S, Lee MP. Improving patient and health system outcomes through advanced pharmacy practice. A report to the U.S. Surgeon General. Office of the Chief Pharmacist. U.S. Public Health Service, December 2011.

Excerpt

III

Further Your Training into PGY-2, Fellowships, and/or Advanced Degrees

- *Elizabeth A. Coyle*
- *Anne M. Tucker*
- *P. Brandon Bookstaver*

The remaining chapters in Section III focus on pharmacy post-graduate training beyond the Postgraduate Year One (PGY-1) year. Chapters 18 through 23 specifically highlight Postgraduate Year Two (PGY-2) opportunities describing the patient care activities, residency expectations, and future career options available upon completion of this specialized training. Although the process for pursuing and obtaining a second year residency or fellowship is similar, the training and experience obtained in the daily activities and career opportunities are quite different.

Why would one want to pursue a PGY-2 residency?

There are various reasons one chooses to pursue a second year of specialty residency training. As educators and residency directors, students and pharmacy residents frequently ask us why they should pursue a second year residency. Often the individual has expressed a desire to practice or has an interest in a particular area such as infectious diseases, cardiology, or oncology. On the other hand, many students cannot fathom doing more than 1 year of residency training as "an additional year after 4 years of pharmacy school is just too much." Yet some of these individuals ultimately end up pursuing specialty training. So what is it that leads a person to pursue a PGY-2 residency?

The desire to practice or work in a particular specialty of pharmacy is usually the attraction for doing a PGY-2 residency. Many individuals have known since they started pharmacy school or even before that they had an interest in a particular area of practice. Others develop an interest in a specialized area during their schooling or PGY-1 residency. Many pharmacists do specialty training in order to become more marketable or to make sure they have the credentials to practice in a certain area. For instance, with regard to infectious diseases pharmacists, according to the Society of Infectious Diseases Pharmacists (SIDP) and ID Practice and Research Network (PRN) of the ACCP Joint Opinion paper written in 2009, pharmacists wishing to obtain a clinical position as an infectious diseases trained pharmacist should complete a PGY-1 and an infectious diseases PGY-2 residency (reference 1, Chapter 20). Other individuals may pursue PGY-2 training to prepare them for their ultimate goal of going into academia to teach, practice, and conduct scholarship/research in their specialty area. Whatever the reason for pursuing specialty training, second year residencies provide a year of focused training in a concentrated area. You will find first-hand information from RPDs, preceptors, and current residents in the proceeding chapters to help direct your course in choosing postgraduate training beyond a PGY-1. Additional information on fellowships and advanced degrees will conclude the section in Chapters 24 and 25.

PGY-2–Ambulatory Care and General Internal Medicine 18

Daniel M. Riche and Lena M. Maynor

The overreaching goals of a Postgraduate Year Two (PGY-2) Internal Medicine or Ambulatory Care resident are to become an autonomous expert in delivering pharmacy care to a large cohort of patients, develop the interpersonal skills needed to become an effective leader and educator, and develop practical research skills that can be translated into clinical research. Residency outcomes are outlined below for PGY-2 Ambulatory Care and General Internal Medicine.

AMBULATORY CARE

The ambulatory care specialty in pharmacy has evolved since the adoption of the PGY-1/2 residency model. Previously, ambulatory care could be separated into "Primary Care" and "Family Medicine" specialties. These programs could be completed as either a first or second year residency, dependent on the program application criteria.

Family medicine pharmacy residency programs were structured as a hybrid between internal medicine and ambulatory care. Typically, a resident would be expected to perform 50% to 70% outpatient duties and 30% to 50% inpatient duties. This model allowed for flexibility in interest and diversity of disease state management from birth to death. Unfortunately, the family medicine hybrid model programs were a poor fit in the structure of primary care accreditation from the American Society of Health-System Pharmacists (ASHP).[1] Switching to the PGY-1/2 residency model has increased the emphasis on accreditation, despite little change in ASHP's residency structure. As such, family medicine programs have decreased in number and only a few remain as PGY-2 Ambulatory Care residency programs with an emphasis on family medicine. Certainly, there still remains an opportunity to participate in a family medicine practice as a dedicated or longitudinal experience in most PGY-2 Ambulatory Care residency programs.

Primary care programs were also impacted significantly with the shift to the PGY-1/2 residency model. Many primary care programs adjusted their criteria to match the 2007 PGY-1 standards. Some of these programs maintained their ambulatory care interest by listing as a PGY-1 Pharmacy Practice residency with emphasis on ambulatory care. Initially, this type of training was sufficient for post-residency employment. Unfortunately, an increase in PGY-1 Pharmacy Practice residents and more uniform PGY-1 program structure have decreased the competitiveness for external employment of a PGY-1 residency trained candidate in the absence of PGY-2 experience. Thus, PGY-2 Ambulatory Care programs are becoming more prominent and sought-after by both candidates and employers.

ASHP has outlined six required outcomes for PGY-2 Ambulatory Care residents[2]:

1. Establish a collaborative interdisciplinary practice.

2. In a collaborative interdisciplinary ambulatory practice provide efficient, effective evidence-based, patient-centered treatment for chronic, and/or acute illnesses in all degrees of complexity.

3. Demonstrate leadership and practice management skills.

4. Promote health improvement, wellness, and disease prevention.

5. Demonstrate excellence in the provision of training or educational activities for healthcare professionals in training.

6. Serve as an authoritative resource on the optimal use of medications.

GENERAL INTERNAL MEDICINE

The specialty of internal medicine focuses on the health care of the adult patient. Patients may be seen by internal medicine physicians, also known as internists, in either the inpatient or outpatient setting. Physicians completing a 3-year internal medicine residency receive training related to multiple complex disease states in the various subspecialties of internal medicine including cardiology, nephrology, neurology, endocrinology, infectious diseases, and pulmonology. Internists are not trained to treat pediatric patients. Many physicians completing internal medicine residencies choose to become further specialized and will subsequently complete fellowships in one of the subspecialties of internal medicine. Given the expansive nature of internal medicine as a specialty, pharmacists completing a PGY-2 Internal Medicine residency must develop pharmacy expertise over a very wide range of disease states and mastery level skill in the management of complex patients with multiple comorbidities.

ASHP has outlined six required outcomes for PGY-2 Internal Medicine residents[2]:

1. Serve as an authoritative resource on the optimal use of medications.

2. Optimize the outcomes of internal medicine patients by providing evidence-based, patient-centered medication therapy as an integral part of an interdisciplinary team.

3. Demonstrate excellence in the provision of training and educational activities for health care professionals in training.

4. Demonstrate leadership and practice management skills.

5. Contribute to the body of pharmacy knowledge in internal medicine.
6. Evaluate, manage, and improve the medication-use process.

UNIQUE ASPECTS OF PGY-2 AMBULATORY CARE AND GENERAL MEDICINE RESIDENCIES

Several aspects of any PGY-2 residency should be consistent including progressive growth in knowledge, skills, and attitudes, but there are specific components unique to PGY-2 Ambulatory Care and Internal Medicine residency programs.

Ambulatory Care

Ambulatory Care residency programs are similarly structured in terms of goals and outcomes to a PGY-2 Internal Medicine residency, but the responsibilities predominately incorporate multiple components of the outpatient setting. There is a general approach taken to a resident's education, especially in the first few months of the year. Specialization is more common in the latter half of the year and can vary greatly based on an individual program's strength. There are two primary differences between these types of PGY-2 programs.

First, ambulatory care programs are required to focus on promoting health improvement, wellness, and disease prevention. There are many ways a program can interpret this requirement, but the opportunity should exist for a resident to initiate their own clinical and educational services. Establishing independent services helps foster growth on the resident and increase competitiveness for external employment following program completion.

Second, while internal medicine program models can focus on improving the medication-use process and contributing to the body of pharmacy knowledge, ambulatory care programs concentrate on long-term patient-centered care.

The ambulatory care model includes an integrated and interrelated stepwise progression (similar to the internal medicine model). However, the design of patient-care activities including patient education as well as long-term follow-up differentiates these two programs.

General Internal Medicine

Most PGY-2 Internal Medicine residency programs focus on the inpatient aspect of internal medicine as a specialty. Many residencies will also include an ambulatory care component in the residency year. While it is easy to think of internal medicine pharmacists as "jacks of all trades," the reality is that you must become an expert for a wide breadth of subspecialty topics. Depending on the structure of your institution's internal medicine service, you may also have the opportunity to complete rotations in multiple internal medicine subspecialties such as cardiology, nephrology, infectious diseases, psychiatry, pulmonology, or gastrointestinal services.

Unlike some other specialties of clinical pharmacy that may work with health-care providers as part of a consult service specific for that specialty, internal medicine pharmacists are generally members of the primary service caring for the patient. As a resident, this gives you the opportunity to have an enormous impact on the pharmacy care of each patient across multiple disease states.

Some PGY-2 Internal Medicine residencies incorporate an area of emphasis into their program, such as cardiology or nephrology. Pharmacists completing a PGY-2 Internal Medicine residency with an area of emphasis generally complete all internal medicine requirements, with elective experiences and longitudinal projects focused on the specific subspecialty in question.

RESPONSIBILITIES

Ambulatory Care

Currently, an ambulatory service can vary greatly in the type of patients and disease states treated, but this was not always the case in the United States. For many years, pharmacists only saw patients with four specific chronic diseases (diabetes dyslipidemia, anticoagulation, and hypertension), unless the ambulatory care service was family medicine based. Over the past decade, ambulatory care pharmacy has grown to include numerous other diseases including human immunodeficiency virus (HIV) associated complications, heart failure adherence, complex medication administration clinics (such as teriparatide use in osteoporosis), men's health (including benign prostatic hyperplasia and testosterone deficiency), and women's health (particularly hormone replacement therapy). While some clinical services, especially anticoagulation services, will still concentrate on a single disease, many now incorporate several disease management protocols with a wide range of patients. The state of ambulatory care pharmacy has never been more inclusive, and it is continuing to grow!

General Internal Medicine

The mix of patients on an internal medicine service is very broad. Most patients present with multiple comorbidities, each requiring careful consideration. Common diagnoses include acute coronary syndrome, exacerbations of chronic obstructive pulmonary disease and chronic heart failure, pneumonia, urinary tract infection, atrial fibrillation, decompensated liver disease, acute kidney injury, diabetic ketoacidosis, and altered mental status. Patients who present with medical problems that are not well determined, but are not critically ill or do not require surgery, will often be admitted to the internal medicine service. Because of this, as a PGY-2 Internal Medicine resident, you will be exposed to some unusual or rare presentations of illness as well.

POST-RESIDENCY OPPORTUNITIES

Ambulatory Care

As previously mentioned, PGY-1 Pharmacy Practice residents are increasing in number and decreasing in post-residency position competitiveness versus PGY-2 trained candidates. Frequently, full-time faculty positions will at least encourage (if not require) PGY-2 training for their ambulatory candidates. These positions are the most commonly sought out following residency graduation. Nonfaculty clinical positions are also available to PGY-2 trained individuals, but may rely on grants or other dependent funding source. Federal funding is available for career development (K awards) and should be considered early in a new practitioner's career. Experiences, such as establishing clinical services or outstanding residency research, in PGY-2 Ambulatory Care residency can more rapidly progress a career into a clinical coordinator or tenure-track position. Board certification, particularly Board Certified Ambulatory Care Pharmacist (BCACP), should be pursued immediately following completion of a PGY-2 Ambulatory Care residency program. Other certifications (e.g., Certified Diabetes Educator [CDE], Board Certified-Advanced Diabetes Manager [BC-ADM], Certified Geriatric Pharmacist [CGP], Certified Anticoagulation Care Provider [CACP], Clinical Lipid Specialist [CLS], HIV Pharmacist™ [AAHIVP]) can be considered with more independent and targeted clinical experience.

General Internal Medicine

PGY-2 Internal Medicine residencies train pharmacists primarily to provide clinical services to internal medicine patients. The depth and breadth of the training make graduates of these residencies uniquely qualified for several roles within health care. After residency, many pharmacists obtain positions as internal medicine clinical specialists, providing primarily cognitive services in inpatient settings. Others will accept faculty positions in schools of pharmacy, which generally involve teaching any number of internal medicine topics, maintaining an internal medicine practice site, and precepting Advanced Pharmacy Practice Experience (APPE) students. These faculty positions are sometimes funded fully through the school of pharmacy and place more emphasis on teaching or research responsibilities. Other faculty positions are cofunded, where a hospital provides some of the pharmacist's salary in exchange for increased time spent providing clinical services at the hospital. Because of the wide scope of their knowledge, pharmacists with PGY-2 Internal Medicine training may also be well suited for clinical coordinator positions, especially in smaller community hospitals with very few clinical specialists.

Chapter Takeaways

▶ Graduates of PGY-2 Internal Medicine residencies acquire expertise over a wide range of diseases and are uniquely qualified for inpatient clinical specialist positions in internal medicine, faculty positions, or clinical coordinator positions.

▶ PGY-2 Ambulatory Care trained individuals have a large opportunity for clinical service development and acquire expertise over a wide range of chronic diseases.

▶ Research is an integral component of a PGY-2 program and should incorporate a stepwise progression in development from the resident's PGY-1 research experience.

ROLE FOR THE MENTOR

Concentrate on resident competitiveness for external opportunities. The career path of a resident is a reflection of the residency program; therefore, resident career success should be an area of focus throughout the year.

Frequently revisit learning and career goals with residents to ensure that elective rotations as well as longitudinal projects are targeted toward achievement of those goals.

Undergo consistent self-development, including advocacy, leadership, and mentorship seminars. Activity in specialized areas of professional organizations (ACCP PRNs or ASHP sections) should be encouraged for residents.

FREQUENTLY ASKED QUESTIONS

Q: **What specific characteristics should I be looking for in a PGY-2 (internal medicine or ambulatory care) program?**

A: The program characteristics that you look for should really depend on your long-term career goals. If you are interested in becoming a clinical specialist at a large academic medical facility, then it is a good idea to apply to programs that are also in that particular type of environment. If you are interested in academia, then it is beneficial to train at a program that is affiliated with a school or college of pharmacy or that provides various teaching opportunities, including a teaching certificate. If you are unsure of what you would like to do, then applying to programs that are well rounded and offer a lot of different opportunities for career growth can be the way to go.

Q: **Should I plan on taking the board certification exam in pharmacotherapy (BCPS) during or after my PGY-2 internal medicine residency?**

A: This really depends on personal preference. There are certain residents who successfully obtain BCPS certification during the fall of their PGY-2 residency. Having your BCPS certification can give you a competitive edge when applying for your first post-residency position; however, some residents feel that the added pressure of preparing for the examination in addition to beginning their PGY-2 residency is overburdening. A PGY-2 Internal Medicine residency itself provides excellent training and preparation for the BCPS examination, which is also an important consideration when making this decision.

Q: **Should I apply to PGY-1 programs that include my PGY-2 interest (internal medicine or ambulatory care)?**

A: Given the competitive environment of the match process, PGY-1 residents at programs with a PGY-2 program may choose to commit early and forgo the requirement of matching. For PY-4 students who are quite confident that PGY-2 training is a strong interest, then consideration for programs with an early commit PGY-2 option should be given.

Q: In terms of ambulatory services, does it matter what the Pharmacy Practice Act for an individual state says?

A: Absolutely! Pharmacy Practice Acts are extremely variable. Some states are so limited in terms of ambulatory care that a program may not be able to offer experiences that are best for certain individuals. Federal programs (e.g., Veteran Affairs Medical Centers) are not restricted by state law and can practice under the same regulations regardless of location. In general, the more progressive the Pharmacy Practice Act, the better for a PGY 2 program.

References

1. Marrs JC. Family medicine pharmacy residency programs. Am J Health Syst Pharm. 2006;63(19): 1803–1805.

2. American Society of Health-System Pharmacists. Educational Outcomes, Goals, and Objectives for Postgraduate Year Two (PGY2) Pharmacy Residencies in Internal Medicine. http:// www.ashp.org/menu/Accreditation/ResidencyAccreditation.aspx#RegulationsandStandard. Accessed March 12, 2012.

PGY-2–Acute Care Medicine 19

Asad F. Patanwala

At some point during your pharmacy education, perhaps while learning therapeutics in the classroom or while practicing patient care on your rotations, you will learn something very important about yourself. Either you will decide that you belong in a primary care setting (e.g., clinic and outpatient pharmacy) or that your calling is in the acute care environment (e.g., inpatient hospital and emergency department [ED]). Of course, there are some students who are not inclined either way and others who make this decision during their Postgraduate Year One (PGY-1) residency or later in their career. Nonetheless, if you prefer a fast paced environment, thrive under stressful conditions, or if you consider yourself to be an "adrenaline junkie," then your passions likely fall into the acute care category.

> "Choosing a PGY1 residency program with a broad selection of rotations is one of the most common recommendations that I give to students inquiring about and candidates interviewing for residency."
>
> *Kara G. – Pharmacy Resident, Georgia*

The term acute care is rather broad and incorporates a variety of disciplines within the hospital setting. However, in this chapter we will discuss three specific areas of pharmacy practice, in which patients require a very high acuity of care. These specialties are critical care, emergency medicine, and nutrition support.

CRITICAL CARE

When you conjure up images of a hospital setting in which you see a healthcare team, what do you see? Well, perhaps because of subtle biases that may have crept into my psyche during my training or maybe because of watching too many movies and television shows, I usually see professionals wearing white coats, standing in a circle next to a patient, while contemplating life or death decisions. Most of them look very serious. One of them is older than the rest, and appears to be listening intently to a younger doctor explaining the situation at hand. In my mind, I also see a pharmacist providing drug-related suggestions. It is possible that you may dream differently, but if there is one place in the hospital where you will see a scene like this, it is in the intensive care unit (ICU).

The value of pharmacists on the critical care team in the ICU is well studied. In fact, in one landmark study published in the *Journal of the American Medical Association* (*JAMA*) in 1999,[1] the presence of a pharmacist on patient care rounds in the ICU decreased preventable adverse drug events by 66%, compared to a time period when there was no pharmacist. Also, a historic moment for critical care pharmacists was when a pharmacist (Dr. Judith Jacobi) was elected as the president of the Society of Critical Care Medicine (SCCM) in 2010. In addition, the Critical Care PRN is one of the largest groups of all sections in the American College of Clinical Pharmacy (ACCP). When you look globally at the literature showing the value of pharmacists, leadership that extends beyond the pharmacy profession, or the volume of membership in pharmacy organizations, the specialty of critical care certainly has a lot to be proud of. You may be wondering, "What does this mean for me?" It means that if you do become a critical care pharmacist, with a few exceptions, your role will generally be well delineated, and the utility of your presence will certainly not be foreign to other healthcare professionals or hospital administrators.

Patient Case Mix

It is safe to say that the sickest patients in the hospital are in the ICU. Many of these patients require mechanical ventilation or cardiovascular support and may have varying degrees of organ dysfunction. These patients need intensive monitoring using sophisticated equipment. Although the patient case mix in critical care can vary greatly, there are some similarities in this patient population. Picture a patient in an ICU with an endotracheal tube, nasoduodenal tube, central intravenous line, multiple peripheral lines, arterial line, bilateral chest tubes, and Foley catheter. There is basically a device for every human orifice. Imagine that this patient was recently in a high-speed motorcycle collision and has multiple injuries. If you were this patient, it is likely that you would want adequate analgesia and sedation. Even in patients with no injuries, the presence of invasive devices can be painful. Therefore, critical care pharmacists should be proficient with regard to the management of pain, agitation, and delirium. Pharmacists in this setting must also be knowledgeable about antimicrobials and the management of sepsis. Patients in the ICU often develop complications such as infections, which are primarily caused by resistant organisms. In addition, the provision of adequate nutrition in these patients is a critical concern managed by the pharmacist and dietician on the ICU team. While these are just some of the more common issues pharmacists are involved with, there are myriads of drug therapy topics that will require your competence.

Because of obvious reasons, patient survival is lowest in the ICU compared to any other area of the hospital. Larger institutions may have specific ICUs for certain patient populations. These include medical, surgical, neurosurgical, cardiac, burn, pediatric, and neonatal ICUs. For instance, a patient with acute respiratory distress syndrome secondary to pneumonia is likely to be in the medical ICU, whereas a patient with multiple injuries after a motor vehicle collision may be admitted to the surgical ICU postoperatively. Therefore, the patient case mix will depend on the type of ICU.

Responsibilities

Before discussing the details of patient care in the ICU, I want to give you some references for future reading. A position paper describing critical care pharmacy services, published jointly by ACCP and SCCM, serves as an excellent starting point for any pharmacy student interested in critical care.[2] The paper comprehensively elucidates the activities of a pharmacist in this setting. Recently, an article published in *Pharmacotherapy* has made recommendations for the training, credentialing, documenting, and justifying of critical care pharmacy services. This paper is another important article for future critical care pharmacists.[3] Now that those readings are on your "to-do" list, let us discuss what a typical day is like for critical care pharmacists in many ICUs in the United States. Daily activities will typically start by touching base with the inpatient pharmacists with regard to any pertinent or time-sensitive patient care issues that need to be addressed. Such hand-off communication is vital to maintain continuity in care and to ensure patient safety. Once pertinent issues have been addressed, you can start preparing for patient care rounds in the ICU.

Ideally, patient care rounds are multidisciplinary, involving physicians, nurses, respiratory therapists, dietitians, social workers, and pharmacists. In most academic institutions, it is likely that the critical care team will consist of a variety of resident physicians from different specialties such as surgery, anesthesiology, pulmonology, emergency medicine, and internal medicine. The flow of rounding is meant to be systematic and inclusive, so that members of the team are able to contribute to the patient's care based on their area of expertise. Within this format, drug therapy issues fall within the pharmacist's domain. As a critical care pharmacist, you are expected to be knowledgeable about the patient's medication plan, to make recommendations, and to provide information that will help the team make evidence-based decisions. Depending on the pharmacy practice model at your institution, you may be involved with entering or verifying medication orders so that they can be processed and administered to the patient in a timely manner. Both patient rounding and medication order review serve as opportunities to intercept medication errors and prevent patient harm.

The length of patient care rounds can vary depending on the number of patients on the team. Typically, rounds can last from a few hours to several hours. However, it should not be assumed that all ICUs conduct patient care rounds in such a format. Some hospitals may have individual attending physicians or admitting teams caring for select patients within the ICU. This results in a potpourri of physicians responsible for some patients within the ICU rather than the entire ICU. This is referred to as an "open-ICU model." There is no clear consensus regarding what is a better model for patient care. However, the open-ICU model can be challenging from a pharmacist's perspective, since it may not be logistically possible to round with all teams simultaneously.

Some institutions may not have any patient care rounds in the traditional sense and the pharmacist will spend a lot of his or her time reviewing patient charts to obtain needed information. Chart review activities in the ICU have also been shown to be effective in preventing adverse drug events.

As the morning hours rapidly fly by, the rest of the day may be spent in a variety of different patient care activities. The pharmacist may need to follow up with important patient care issues discussed during rounds, query drug information requests, process pending medication orders, and conduct student and resident teaching. At any time of the day, the critical care pharmacist may also be needed to respond to cardiac arrests and other medical emergencies. Since cardiac arrest in the hospital is most likely to occur in the ICU, the critical care pharmacist is well positioned to be responsible for this function. Finally, the critical care pharmacist may be involved in a variety of other activities such as medication utilization evaluations, reporting and review of adverse drug event data, research, and other quality improvement initiatives.

EMERGENCY MEDICINE

Imagine a medical specialty in which you will (1) see patients no matter what time of day or night, any day of the week; (2) see the very old, the very young, the rich, and the poor; (3) see people you have never met, who will tell you the most intimate details of their lives, and then you will never see them again; (4) never know who or what you will see next; (5) develop big adrenal glands from all the excitement and maintain an average heart rate of 100 beats per minute while you respond to medical or traumatic emergencies; (6) go home each day with the thought that you have contributed to saving a life; and (7) be mentally and physically exhausted at times and yet will be enriched by your appreciation for life and your loved ones. That specialty is emergency medicine.

Although emergency medicine pharmacy services have existed in a few institutions in the United States for decades, it is only in the last few years that there has been an exponential growth in this specialty of pharmacy practice. For instance between 2008 and 2009, the number of EDs in the United States that used emergency medicine pharmacists increased from 6.8% to 28.6%. This number is likely higher in larger academic institutions. In 2010, a prospective, multicenter observational study showed that pharmacists in the ED were able to intercept medication errors to prevent patient harm.[4] More recently, another multicenter study involving almost 16,000 patients showed that pharmacists were most likely to intercept errors when directly consulting with ED staff, rather than simply reviewing medication orders on a computer terminal.[5] This study highlights the value of pharmacists being at the bedside and interacting with the healthcare team. In one survey, ED nurses and physicians highly valued the presence of a pharmacist in the ED and believed that the pharmacist improved patient safety.[6] The career outlook for Postgraduate Year Two (PGY-2) trained emergency medicine pharmacists is very positive given the continued expansion of this service by institutions.

Patient Case Mix

There is no single way to describe the type of patients that the emergency medicine pharmacist will encounter. First, let us address some misconceptions about the specialty. Contrary to popular belief, the ED does not contain only critically ill patients. In fact, many patients are considered to be ambulatory, whereas some could likely be seen in a primary care clinic rather than an ED. Some students may walk into the ED on their first day expecting to see chest compressions on every other patient. Although this will probably occur during the rotation, you are more likely to spend your time talking to patients about their home medications, than pounding on their chests.

Patients in the ED are extremely diverse. For instance, you may be involved in the care of a 90-year-old with pneumonia, then a moment later answer drug therapy questions about a neonate. Therefore, you must be knowledgeable about geriatrics and pediatrics, as well as everything in between.

There is also great variation in the severity of illness of patients who present to the ED. You may be resuscitating a critically ill trauma patient, and then a moment later perform discharge counseling with a patient prescribed oral antibiotics for a sore throat. Of course, if you are at a tertiary care Level 1 Trauma Center in a big city, you are likely to see a lot more of the former rather than the latter. The disease states you will encounter will vary greatly and will include almost anything that you can imagine. Pick up the big pharmacotherapy book on your shelf, randomly open a page, and there will be someone in the ED with that issue. Although emergency medicine is considered to be a specialty with a unique skill set, including expertise in resuscitation, the emergency medicine pharmacist in many ways has to be the "jack of all trades."

Responsibilities

There are two articles developed by ASHP that pertain to the practice of pharmacy in the ED. The first is a position statement that describes pharmacy services which should be provided to the ED.[7] This provides some insight at an institutional level and identifies how the pharmacy department can best serve patients in this setting. The second is a guideline document from the perspective of the emergency medicine pharmacist.[8] It expands on the previous position statement and focuses on services that emergency medicine pharmacists should provide. These articles serve as an important starting point for any pharmacy student interested in pursuing a career in emergency medicine.

The responsibilities of the emergency medicine pharmacist are institution specific. In fact, prior to implementing pharmacy services in the ED, it is critical to perform a needs assessment at each institution. The needs of a large Level 1 Trauma Center could be considerably different than a small community ED. As previously described, the patient case mix can vary based on the institution. Therefore, the pharmacist's responsibilities will also be different based on the setting.

Similar to the critical care pharmacist, the typical day of the emergency medicine pharmacist also starts with a brief discussion with the inpatient pharmacist to maintain continuity of care. In the ED, the high patient volume times are generally in the afternoon and evening. Therefore, in many institutions with just one emergency medicine pharmacist, the pharmacist's shift will mirror times when the ED is busy. So, expect to start in the late morning or afternoon and end your shift in the late evening or close to midnight. Some institutions with 24×7 pharmacist coverage in the ED will also include overnight shifts.

Unlike the ICU, most EDs do not have formal multidisciplinary patient care rounds. The rapid turnover of patients and relatively brief encounters do not make rounding conducive to this setting. However, the emergency medicine pharmacist is frequently consulted by physicians and nurses and others regarding drug therapy issues. In most cases, the pharmacist is present at the patient's bedside, directly interacting with the patient and other healthcare providers. Depending on the number of available beds in the ED, the pharmacist may be responsible for a large volume of patients (exceeding 100 patients in some EDs). Therefore, it is important for the pharmacist to be able to triage patients based on the pharmaceutical care they may require. For instance, a patient with pneumonia and septic shock requiring early goal directed therapy would require immediate attention of the pharmacist. However, a stable patient with a small soft tissue abscess would not require immediate pharmacologic management.

Work in the ED can be highly variable and sporadic. On some occasions, the pharmacist may receive several consultations simultaneously, have to respond to a patient experiencing cardiac arrest or a patient with major trauma, and be required to participate in a procedural sedation all at the same time. On other occasions, the ED census may be very low with relatively low acuity patients. This fluctuating course during the day enables administrative functions to be performed when the ED is not busy. This is also an opportunity to interview patients to obtain their medication histories and facilitate their transition to the inpatient ward. Furthermore, the pharmacist may be responsible for performing culture follow-up calls for patients who were previously discharged from the ED. This entails evaluating culture results for patients discharged on antimicrobial therapy, following up on the appropriateness of those therapies, and confirming clinical cure by calling patients. As the specialty of emergency medicine pharmacy practice evolves, the opportunities for involvement in different aspects of patient care in the ED will continue to increase in the future.

NUTRITION SUPPORT

Nutrition support was one of the first "clinical" pharmacy services to be provided in the acute care setting. At any given time in large hospitals, there could be dozens of patients who are unable to receive nutrition orally. Many of these patients require placement of a feeding tube and are given nutrition via the enteral route. The enteral formulas and dietary supplements for these patients are usually managed by dieticians. You have probably heard the phrase, "if the gut works, use it." But if the gut does not work, and enteral nutrition is not possible, then nutrition has to be provided via the intravenous route. This is called parenteral nutrition (PN). The primary role of pharmacists with regard to nutrition support in the hospital is managing patients who need PN. There are few pharmacy services in the hospital that allow the pharmacist as much autonomy as in this specialty. This is likely because the issues related to PN largely fall within the pharmacists area of expertise. For instance, stability of macro- and micronutrients, as well as drug and nutrient compatibility in PN, is unique to the pharmacy profession. Physicians, dieticians, or nurses may not have adequate knowledge or training to optimally formulate PNs. On the contrary, this is routinely taught at most colleges of pharmacy. In many specialties of pharmacy practice, there are also equally specialized and qualified physicians and other healthcare professionals. For example, if you are a pharmacist working with the infectious diseases team, it is likely that the infectious diseases fellowship trained physician, in some cases, knows as much or even more about antibiotics than you might as a pharmacist. We could say that situations like this exist in virtually any medical specialty. However, when it comes to PN services, it is safe to assume that a PGY-2 trained nutrition support pharmacist is likely to have a lot more expertise, since similar programs rarely exist for physicians and other healthcare providers.

Patient Case Mix

Unlike critical care and emergency medicine, in which the patient case mix total parenteral nutrition (TPN) are located throughout the institution. Patients may be in the ICU or in the medical or surgical wards. So, who are the patients in the acute care environment who do not have a functioning gut and require PN? One of the most common populations includes those who have had surgery or complications involving the bowel anatomy. For instance, consider a patient who developed a bowel obstruction because of opioid use, which ultimately resulted in part of his/her bowel requiring surgical resection. This type of scenario could result in a remaining bowel that is too short to absorb the required nutrients. In addition, this patient could have poor bowel recovery or develop a fistula. These complications may require temporary or long-term PN. Another common patient population that utilizes the nutrition support service is the oncology patient population. For example, some chemotherapy regimens can result in severe inflammation or ulceration of mucous membranes lining the gastrointestinal tract. In these circumstances, oral or enteral nutrition intake can be very painful and patients may require the use of PN until their mucous membranes heal. Finally, critically ill patients in the ICU may require PN. The need for PN may be due to reasons as described above or due to the use of high-dose vasopressors. This is based on the theoretical rationale that the provision of large volumes of enteral feeds to unstable patients who are on high-dose vasopressors could increase oxygen requirements of the gut. Increased oxygen demand could lead to alterations in gut perfusion leading to mesenteric infarction. Therefore, the nutrition support pharmacist should have a sound understanding of bowel anatomy while also being well versed in the clinical course and drug therapy issues in critical care, surgery, and oncology patients.

Responsibilities

The American Society of Enteral and Parenteral Nutrition has developed standards of practice for nutrition support pharmacists.[9] This is a valuable resource for students interested in this specialty of pharmacy practice. The primary responsibility of the nutrition support pharmacist is to coordinate the care of patients who require PN. This coordination of care usually occurs using a consultation-based model. The pharmacist's day starts with acquiring the list of patients who are currently on PN, along with list of new consultations to initiate PN. Consultations can be requested by any physician or team in the hospital. However, it is important to remember that the role of the nutrition support pharmacist is not to simply start new PNs but to ensure that PN is appropriate for each patient. It is not uncommon that the nutrition support pharmacist may recommend against initiation of PN and to use enteral nutrition instead. Once the patient is deemed to be a candidate for PN, a nutritional assessment is conducted to determine calorie, protein, fluid, electrolyte, and other nutrient requirements. A formal assessment should be extremely thorough and include pertinent patient-specific information relating to nutrition support. An appropriate patient-specific PN is then formulated, approved by the consulting team, and subsequently compounded for administration to the patient.

The pharmacist also collects data on each patient who is currently on PN in the hospital in order to determine if changes need to be made to the formulation each day. This includes following serum electrolyte and other laboratory values, acid–base status, renal and hepatic function, fluid intake and output, and evaluating the use of medications that could influence any of these parameters. Information related to the progress and clinical course of the patient is also evaluated. The continued need for PN is assessed daily by evaluating the resolution of conditions that resulted in the initiation of PN. The pharmacist plays an important role in facilitating the transition from PN to enteral or oral nutrition. In some cases, the patient may need to be discharged to a long-term care facility or require home care. In these circumstances, the pharmacist may communicate and transmit details regarding the patient's in-hospital nutritional care to the outside facility. This communication is essential to make sure there is no disruption or error in the PN during this important transition.

There are different models by which PN services can function. Some institutions provide the nutrition support pharmacist with greater autonomy compared to others. For instance, at our institution the nutrition support pharmacist independently conducts patient assessments, formulates new PNs, and manages existing PNs. All of this is done with or without involvement from dieticians, depending on patient-specific requirements. The consulting team then approves any PN-related changes that need to be made. At other institutions, the PN service may have more direct physician involvement. As previously discussed, there is no single physician specialty that is likely to be involved with nutrition support. However, physicians commonly involved include those from surgery, internal medicine, and gastroenterology.

LEARNING OBJECTIVES AND OUTCOMES

ASHP has developed standardized learning objectives and outcomes for both PGY-2 residencies in critical care and nutrition support.[10] The objectives and outcomes for emergency medicine are currently under development.

> "It is important to read the ASHP published objectives and outcomes about each pharmacy residency practice area that you are interested in before you apply and complete residency interviews."
>
> *Jessica S. – Pharmacy Student, Texas*

These documents serve as requirements for each of these residency programs. As a resident your progress will be continually assessed with respect to these objectives and outcomes. There are certain themes that are common to each of these specialties and likely also apply to other areas of pharmacy practice, including (1) demonstrating leadership and practice management skills, (2) optimizing patient outcomes by providing evidence-based medication or nutrition therapy, (3) conducting clinical pharmacy research, (4) developing excellence in teaching and providing educational programs, and (5) performing administrative functions such as quality improvement and patient safety initiatives. It is important to familiarize yourself with these documents prior to your residency. This will help you establish your baseline competency, identify areas of improvement, and track your progress during residency. Imagine you matched for your residency at a large institution that offered PGY-2 residencies in critical care, emergency medicine, and nutrition support. Table 19-1 is a hypothetical example of a typical rotation schedule for the PGY-2 residents who will start in July. Notice the overlap between programs and how rotations are scheduled so that all three residents receive the training they need.

TABLE 19-1 • Typical Rotation Schedule

Month	Critical Care	Emergency Medicine	Nutrition Support
July	Orientation/Medical ICU	Orientation/EM	Orientation/Nutrition
August	Surgical ICU	EM	Nutrition
September	EM	Toxicology	Surgical ICU
October	*Elective*	EM	Oncology
November	Pediatric ICU	EM	Enteral nutrition
December	Burn ICU	Pre-hospital EMS	*Elective*
January	Cardiac ICU	*Elective*	Nutrition
February	EM	Medical ICU	Home care
March	*Elective*	EM	Nutrition
April	Academia/Research	Pediatric ICU	Medical ICU
May	Medical ICU	Surgical ICU	*Elective*
June	Surgical ICU	*Elective*	Nutrition

ICU, intensive care unit; EM, emergency medicine; EMS, emergency medical services.

CAREER OPPORTUNITIES

If you were to ask most PGY-2 trained residents in critical care, emergency medicine, or nutrition support what they would like to do after they complete their residency, almost all will respond that they would like to work as a clinical specialist in a hospital in the area of their training and expertise. Depending on their training and exposure to academia, many will be inclined to develop formal relationships with colleges of pharmacy. Others will work for colleges of pharmacy and yet have clinical responsibilities in an ICU or ED.

It is important to mention that there is also some overlap between training in these PGY-2 programs, which may enable flexibility with regard to career options. For instance, a PGY-2 resident in critical care may end up primarily working in an ED, and vice versa. This is provided he/she has had enough exposure and rotations in each setting during the PGY-2 program. There is also considerable overlap between critical care and nutrition support, which may enable similar flexibility. However, there is very little similarity between nutrition support and emergency medicine. To think of an emergency medicine resident working as a full-time nutrition support pharmacist is hard to fathom.

CRITICAL CARE

After completing a PGY-2 residency in critical care, most graduates will work in an ICU setting. However, as previously mentioned, ICUs may be subspecialized. For instance, you may be specifically recruited to work in a cardiac ICU. Thus, as you seek a residency program, make sure that the program is able to offer you experiences in variety of different ICU settings. Other job opportunities may be nonspecific to a particular ICU setting, especially in smaller hospitals. In these circumstances, you should be prepared to rotate between different ICUs, such as medical, surgical, and cardiac.

EMERGENCY MEDICINE

PGY-2 trained emergency medicine pharmacists will usually practice in an ED setting. However, there can be great differences between institutions. Some community EDs are small (~20 beds) and other academic EDs are large (>100 beds). As previously discussed, variations in job functions can be large depending on the needs of the institution. Pharmacy practice in the ED setting is still evolving and relatively new. It is possible that you may be the very first emergency medicine pharmacist at your institution given the task of developing, refining, and justifying pharmacy services in the ED. So, be prepared to be a "trail blazer," shaping your own path, molding your own destiny, and being a pioneer for all those who follow you. Furthermore, training in emergency medicine also offers the opportunity for practicing in EDs dedicated to the care of pediatric patients. Thus, it is important to have sufficient exposure to this patient population during your training.

NUTRITION SUPPORT

Nutrition support trained PGY-2 residents typically seek positions in institutions that have large critically ill, surgical, or oncology populations. Because of the nature of their condition, these patients are most likely to require PN. You may be recruited to lead the nutrition support team or be in charge of nutrition-related endeavors at such institutions. In addition, you may have the opportunity to work with home care departments of hospitals or home care companies that compound or manage PN on an outpatient basis. Finally, it is worth mentioning that PGY-2 trained residents in any of these specialties may be suitable candidates to work for pharmaceutical companies that manufacture and market medications used in these settings.

Chapter Takeaways

▶ The sickest patients in the hospital are in the ICU, and many of these patients need treatment for pain, agitation, and delirium.

▶ Ideally, patient care rounds in the ICU are multidisciplinary, involving physicians, nurses, respiratory therapists, dietitians, social workers, and pharmacists.

▶ The emergency medicine pharmacist needs to have a broad pharmacotherapy knowledge base. In many ways, a pharmacist in this setting has to be the "jack of all trades."

▶ The role of the emergency medicine pharmacist is diverse and will depend on the type (academic versus community), size, and specific needs of each ED.

▶ The primary role of the nutrition support pharmacist is managing patients who need PN.

ROLE FOR THE MENTOR

Choose the right acute care specialty for you: critical care, emergency medicine, or nutrition support.

Select a PGY-1 program with exposure to the right rotations and preceptors so that you are a competitive candidate for a PGY-2 residency.

Tailor your PGY-2 residency so that you are competent in a variety of settings that will enable you to have some career flexibility.

FREQUENTLY ASKED QUESTIONS

Q: Should I specialize in critical care or emergency medicine?
A: The answer depends on what you enjoy doing. You cannot truly make an informed decision until you have completed a rotation in each one of these

specialties. Although there are similarities between these two areas of pharmacy practice, the differences are vast. The emergency medicine pharmacist must also enjoy the ambulatory care setting, since many patients in the ED are not critically ill. You may need to obtain patient medication histories and even counsel patients about their medications on discharge. If you thrive in an environment where decisions are made rather quickly and there is no traditional rounding, then emergency medicine may be something you would prefer. Also, in the ED you will generally have a greater role in drug distribution, preparation, and administration. However, if you really enjoy traditional patient care rounds, then critical care may suit you better. Not all ICU pharmacists are necessarily fond of working with syringes, manipulating vials, or routinely obtaining medications from controlled access cabinets, which is a big part of the pharmacists role in the ED as previously described.

Q: Are there more job opportunities in emergency medicine than critical care?

A: Emergency medicine has seen exponential growth in the last few years. Yet, a majority of hospitals in the United States do not have emergency medicine pharmacists. So, there is great potential for future job opportunities as hospitals continue to embrace this service. However, critical care has always been and remains a very promising area of pharmacy practice. For instance, when hospitals start to incorporate clinical pharmacy services, one of the top areas in the hospital to receive these resources is the ICU. This is because of the complexity of these patients' drug regimens, impact on drug costs, and patient safety implications. Also, from an evidence-based standpoint, some of the best evidence for pharmacy services with regard to patient safety is in the ICU setting. Therefore, both specialties offer good job opportunities.

Q: Does specialization in nutrition support limit future career options?

A: The short answer is no. First, if you love nutrition support, then that is what you should do. However, it is understandable to be pragmatic so that you can maximize the flexibility of your future career path. Therefore, it is important that the rotations you have during your PGY-2 residency prepare to be competent in other areas as well. For instance, some programs allow the nutrition support resident to spend a considerable amount of time in the ICU setting. Thus, a PGY-2 resident in nutrition may be well suited to work as a critical care pharmacist if needed. Also, some programs may offer several rotations in oncology, because these patients commonly require this service. It is possible that a nutrition support trained pharmacist may end up working primarily with this patient population. Hence, future career options are not limited.

References

1. Leape LL, et al. Pharmacist participation on physician rounds and adverse drug events in the intensive care unit. JAMA. 1999;282:267–270.

2. Rudis MI, Brandl KM. Position paper on critical care pharmacy services. Society of Critical Care Medicine and American College of Clinical Pharmacy Task Force on Critical Care Pharmacy Services. Crit Care Med. 2000;28:3746–3750.

3. Dager W, et al. An opinion paper outlining recommendations for training, credentialing, and documenting and justifying critical care pharmacy services. Pharmacotherapy. 2011;31: 135e–175e.

4. Rothschild JM, et al. Medication errors recovered by emergency department pharmacists. Ann Emerg Med. 2010;55:513–521.

5. Patanwala AE, et al. A prospective, multicenter study of pharmacist activities resulting in medication error interception in the emergency department. Ann Emerg Med. 2012;59(5): 369–373.

6. Fairbanks RJ, Hildebrand JM, Kolstee KE, Schneider SM, Shah MN. Medical and nursing staff highly value clinical pharmacists in the emergency department. Emerg Med J. 2007;24: 716–718.

7. ASHP Statement on Pharmacy Services to the Emergency Department. http://www.ashp. org/DocLibrary/BestPractices/SpecificStEmergDept.aspx. Accessed February 10, 2012.

8. Eppert HD, Reznek AJ. ASHP guidelines on emergency medicine pharmacist services. Am J Health Syst Pharm. 2011;68:e81–e95.

9. Rollins C, et al. Standards of practice for nutrition support pharmacists. Nutr Clin Pract. 2008;23:189–194.

10. American Society of Health-System Pharmacists. Residency Accreditation. http://www.ashp. org/menu/Accreditation/ResidencyAccreditation.aspx. Accessed February 10, 2012.

PGY-2 Medicine Subspecialties– Infectious Diseases (Including HIV), Cardiology, Oncology, Psychiatry, and Nephrology

20

Elizabeth A. Coyle and Anne M. Tucker

This chapter will focus on the medicine specialties of infectious diseases (ID) (including human immunodeficiency virus [HIV]), cardiology, oncology, psychiatry, and nephrology. Many individuals find it hard to decide which specialty they want to pursue. In fact, quite a few find themselves at a crossroads wanting to train in more than one specialty. When making the final decision on which specialty to train, the candidate must fully evaluate what their interests are and which type of practice would be the best fit for their personality and passions. For instance, if one enjoys psychology, is intrigued by people, and is patient, psychiatry may be a good option for them. If one gets satisfaction from seeing drug effects work quickly or likes to solve complex problems and mysteries, ID or cardiology may be an ideal specialty choice. Someone who likes internal medicine and managing complex comorbidities, HIV or nephrology may be the right choice. As with Postgraduate Year One (PGY-1) residencies, the American Society of Health-System Pharmacists (ASHP) has a global set of standards for accreditation in Postgraduate Year Two (PGY-2) specialty residencies in general, as well as specific standards for a select number of specialties. In contrast to PGY-1 residencies, not all PGY-2 residencies are accredited. This is typically not a problem because the majority of nonaccredited PGY-2 programs follow the ASHP guidelines and standards. In whatever PGY-2 specialty one decides to pursue, it is very important that they properly research the specialty area to become familiar with the various areas and options for practice, the different patient populations, and the variety of opportunities to expand one's knowledge, skills attitudes, and abilities.

INFECTIOUS DISEASES

In microbiology did you like the grape smelling *Pseudomonas* spp or the mothball smell of *Escherichia coli*? Do you like solving mysteries and are you intrigued by grotesque looking wounds and strange organisms? If any of these things captivate your interests, ID could be right for you. Specialty training in ID should provide a clinician with the foundation to practice in a plethora of clinical settings. The opportunities for ID trained pharmacists are constantly growing. In the past 5 to 10 years, the ID pharmacist has become an integral part of the practice of antimicrobial stewardship in healthcare organizations.[1] In the 2007 Society for Healthcare Epidemiology of America (SHEA) antimicrobial stewardship guidelines, it is stated that an ID pharmacist should be part of the multidisciplinary stewardship team.[2] Since stewardship has become such a main focus of ID practice, it can be misconstrued that being a stewardship pharmacist or the "antibiotic police" is all that an ID pharmacist does. Although it is a very important part of overall practice to prevent the development and spread of antibiotic resistance, stewardship is not the sole practice of someone in ID. Most ID clinical pharmacists are part of the ID team, and in the inpatient setting, are part of the day-to-day activity of patient care participating in daily rounds with the ID consult team. Many also play an essential role in education of physician trainees (residents and fellows), nursing, respiratory therapy, and other pharmacists in the guidelines and ID information. The development of treatment protocols, formulary decisions, and outcomes research can also be a large part of the practitioner's duties. Calculating patient-specific pharmacokinetics and optimizing antimicrobial therapy based on pharmacodynamics are a few of the day-to-day challenges. ID pharmacists can also practice in a variety of settings and with various patient populations. Inpatient ID pharmacists may be in the general ward of an acute care hospital, in the ICU, oncology, geriatric, or pediatric units of an institution. They may also be based in a specialty hospital that focuses on a specific patient population such as the immunocompromised as seen at Memorial Sloan Kettering in New York, The University of Texas MD Anderson Cancer Center in Houston, or St. Jude's Hospital in Memphis. ID pharmacists may also be part of the outpatient clinic practices, especially in HIV-specialized clinics. Although there is not a specific board certification for the ID pharmacist, many ID pharmacy clinicians are Board Certified Pharmacotherapy Specialist with added qualification in infectious diseases (BCPS AQ-ID).

A PGY-2 in ID should offer a variety of learning experiences for the resident. The residency should be able to offer experience in microbiology and infection control. There should be a role for the pharmacist in the ID consult team, an opportunity to practice with a variety of patient populations such as the critically ill, oncology, transplantation (solid organ and stem cell transplant), and to see a range of different ID issues (see Table 20-1).

The residency should provide opportunities to apply pharmacokinetic and pharmacodynamic principles when caring for patients being treated

TABLE 20-1 • Example of Selected Diseases Seen or Discussed in Medicine Specialty Residency

Infectious Diseases (ID)	Infectious Diseases— HIV Focus	Cardiology	Oncology	Psychiatry	Nephrology
Osteomyelitis/ Septic arthritis	Opportunistic infections	Acute coronary syndrome	Breast cancer	Schizophrenia	Chronic kidney disease
Endocarditis	Endocrine disorders	Heart failure	Colorectal cancer	Bipolar disorder	Acute kidney injury
Central nervous system (CNS) infections	Psychiatric issues	Advanced cardiac life support (ACLS)	Gynecologic cancers	Depression	End-stage renal disease
Fungal infections	Pharmacokinetics/Pharmacodynamics (PK/PD)	Cerebrovascular disease	Prostate cancer	Anxiety	Peritoneal dialysis
Intra-abdominal infections	Cardiovascular (CV) disease	Arrhythmias	Lung cancer	Sleep disorders	Hemodialysis
Pneumonias	General ID topics	Hypertension	Brain cancer	Personality disorders	Hemofiltration
Sepsis		Peripheral vascular disease	Sarcomas	Substance abuse	Heart disease
Sexually transmitted diseases (STDs)		Cardiac devices	Leukemias	Developmental disorders	Diabetes
Skin and soft-tissue infections		Cardiovascular tests	Lymphomas	Neurological disorders	Drug-induced kidney injury
Tuberculosis and other mycobacteria		Transplantation	Myeloma	Pharmacokinetics/ Pharmacodynamics (PK/PD)	Inherited kidney disease
Urinary tract infections (UTIs)		Cardiomyopathy	Stem cell transplantation		Renal drug clearance
Viral infections		Cardiogenic shock	Chemotherapy		Anemia
Pharmacokinetics / Pharmacodynamics (PK/PD)		Hemodynamic monitoring	Cancer- and chemotherapy- related disorders		Nutrition

(*continued*)

TABLE 20-1 • **Example of Selected Diseases Seen or Discussed in Medicine Specialty Residency** (*continued*)

Infectious Diseases (ID)	Infectious Diseases— HIV Focus	Cardiology	Oncology	Psychiatry	Nephrology
Human immuno- deficiency virus (HIV)		Acid/base disorders	Tumor lysis syndrome		Electrolyte disorders
		Anticoagula- tion	Myelosuppres- sion		Acid/base disorders
			Infections		Vitamin and mineral deficiencies
			Pain manage- ment		Renal trans- plantation
					CV disease manage- ment

with antimicrobials. The resident should help provide antimicrobial and microbiology surveillance for the institution, even if there is not a formal antimicrobial stewardship program at the training site. Residency training should also provide opportunities to gain experience in tracking or optimizing clinical and pharmacoeconomic outcomes, as well as formulary management. ID residencies should also introduce residents to clinical or basic research in ID. For completeness, there should be the opportunity to work with an HIV patient population, as per the ASHP accreditation standards.[3]

The clinical practice for an ID clinician that focuses on HIV can be very different than the practitioner in general ID. A large percentage of practice in HIV is done in the outpatient setting; therefore, a PGY-2 ID residency that focuses on HIV will place the majority of the resident's practice in the HIV clinics. HIV practice is an ever changing and exciting clinical practice. The practitioner must be very good at keeping up with the guidelines and trends in therapy. The PGY-2 should become part of the healthcare team in managing the patients' HIV antiretroviral regimens, as well as the associated comorbidities. The residency should offer the resident the possibility to learn about the social and psychological issues associated with the HIV patient. Although the HIV-focused ID residency is mainly in the outpatient setting, the experience of caring for inpatient HIV patients should be provided to see disease states such as acute opportunistic infections (see Table 20-1). Currently, there are no specific standards for HIV residencies, and as a result these residencies will be listed as an ID PGY-2 residency with a focus on HIV.

CARDIOLOGY

Are you an individual who likes to get to the "heart of the matter?" Did the anatomy and physiology of the heart really intrigue you in pharmacy school? Were you the one in class that understood arrhythmias and liked reading the ECGs? Well a PGY-2 in cardiology may be what's best for you. Cardiology, much like ID, offers a variety of practice opportunities in both the inpatient and outpatient practice settings. A cardiology PGY-2 residency should establish a foundation for a trainee to practice in any such settings. In the acute care setting, a cardiology clinical pharmacist will be part of the multidisciplinary cardiology team taking care of patients with many different cardiology issues. They may be involved in the acute and/or chronic treatment of acute coronary syndromes, congestive heart failure, cerebral vascular diseases, and arrhythmias. A cardiology pharmacist may specialize in surgical or critical care patient populations managing bypass surgical patients, decompensated heart failure, arrhythmias, cardiogenic shock, left ventricular assist device (LVAD) patients, and cardiac transplantation. The clinical pharmacist is well versed in cardiovascular drugs as well as the many cormorbidities associated with cardiovascular disease. The pharmacist will also play a major role in the development of evidence-based treatment guidelines and protocols. As with HIV, the literature and treatment guidelines rapidly change, and it is very important that the pharmacist is committed in keeping up with the newest evidence. As with ID, there is not a specific board certification for the cardiology pharmacist. Many cardiology pharmacy clinicians are Board Certified Pharmacotherapy Specialist and with added qualification in Cardiology (BCPS AQ Cardiology).

There are also a variety of opportunities for pharmacists trained in cardiology to get involved in outpatient clinics, both multidisciplinary and stand-alone. Primary and secondary prevention, anticoagulation, and other cardiology clinics are a great way for the pharmacist to play a central role in the management of cardiovascular issues. Many of these types of clinics offer an opportunity for a pharmacy run clinic under collaborative practice agreements.

A PGY-2 in cardiology should be based in an institution where the resident can be exposed to a variety of cardiology patients in both the inpatient and outpatient settings. Although there are cardiology residencies offered in specific cardiology hospitals, it is not necessary to be in a specialty cardiology hospital. The resident should be able to build a knowledge base in experiences such as handling acute coronary issues regularly, and can practice with an established cardiology team. Exposure to procedures such as a cardiac catheterization and electrophysiology ablation is important. The resident should become part of the cardiology team and practice in both the inpatient and outpatient settings. Areas that should be covered in the residency either through experiences or discussions are listed in Table 20-1, and specific standards exist for ASHP accreditation for PGY-2 residencies in cardiology.[4]

ONCOLOGY

Is your passion to find the cure for cancer? Do you go to poetry readings reciting the hemato"poetic" stem cell line? Have you had the cell cycle memorized since physiology? A PGY-2 in oncology may be the specialty you pursue. Oncology is a specialty practice that has a large variety of opportunities and practice settings for pharmacists to get involved. There are a number of large medical centers that specialize solely in oncology, numerous hospitals that have dedicated oncology centers, as well as the majority of hospitals that work with oncology patients on a daily basis. In addition, there are outpatient clinics and outpatient infusion centers where oncology pharmacists routinely get involved with patient care. The practice opportunities for clinically trained oncology specialists are abundant. One can specialize in a particular type of cancer such as breast cancer, lung cancer, leukemia, or stem cell transplantation and specifically practice in that area on a daily basis. At The University of Texas MD Anderson Cancer Center, clinical pharmacy specialists are dedicated to a specific service and are considered experts in their oncology specialty. For example, the pharmacist, specialized in leukemia or breast cancer, will round with the multidisciplinary team in their specific specialty daily, helping to fully manage the patient's medical profile, medication therapy, chemotherapy, and cancer complications. In addition, they help design appropriate chemotherapy dosing and work with investigational agents and protocols. An oncology pharmacist who practices in a more general oncology patient population will do the same things as previously described, but will work with a variety of different malignancies and patients on a day-to-day basis. Whatever the practice setting, the oncology pharmacist is an integral part of the oncology team and has many interactions with patients and families as they go through cancer treatment. They may take part in a patient's care in the ambulatory care setting, general medical floor, and/or ICU. Pharmacists who specialize in outpatient chemotherapy infusion clinics help manage daily chemotherapy regimens, side effects, and complications. As with ID and cardiology, clinical oncology pharmacists participate in clinical protocol development, investigational therapies, formulary management, and drug information as it pertains to their specialty. Other opportunities for trained oncology pharmacists are in highly specialized groups such as US Oncology, where protocols are developed for specific institutions and assistance is given in their implementation. There is a specific board certification for oncology, Board Certified Oncology Pharmacists (BCOP).

A PGY-2 oncology residency can be offered in a variety of settings and institutions and should offer the resident a good foundation in a variety of oncology patients. The residency can be focused on adult or pediatric patients or can give exposure to both. In adult-focused residencies, experiences should incorporate the common adult malignancies including breast, colorectal, leukemia, lung, lymphomas, ovarian, and prostate cancers. Pediatric-based residencies should include common pediatric malignancies such as brain, leukemia, lymphoma, neuroblastoma, retinoblastoma, and sarcomas. The residency should include direct patient care experiences and engage the resident in the management of chemotherapy and cancer-related disorders such as fatigue, infections, mucositis, myelosuppression, alopecia, anorexia, tumor lysis syndromes, spinal compression, pain, and nutrition (see Table 20-1). Residents should also have experience in the management of hematopoietic stem cell transplant patients. For a more detailed description of an oncology specialty resident, specific standards for ASHP accreditation have been published.[5]

PSYCHIATRY

Do you find yourself constantly analyzing people for personality disorders? Is your favorite drink a Haldol® cocktail? Do you love the movie "The One Who Flew Over the Cuckoo's Nest?" Well maybe you should consider a PGY-2 with a focus on psychiatry. Years ago, psychiatry was an area where there was more psychotherapy than pharmacotherapy, but with increased understanding of the pathophysiology of psychiatric diseases as well as the increase in pharmacotherapeutic agents, this is a great area for pharmacists to get involved. In addition, psychiatry trained pharmacists are also highly involved in treating patients with neurological disorders. Clinical practice in psychiatry includes working with multidisciplinary teams in treating patients in acute inpatient psychiatric situations, step-down units/institutions, and outpatient clinics. Psychiatry provides the clinician an opportunity to interact with diverse patient populations working on patient-centered medication management. The abundance of psychiatric medications, drug interactions, and pharmacokinetic issues requires the pharmacist to play a central role in providing and monitoring patients for safe and effective therapy. The importance of compliance and medication adherence is imperative for this patient population, and the pharmacist is integral in working with and educating patients. In the inpatient setting, clinical pharmacists help in the initiation of medication therapy and monitoring for side effects and drug interactions. Psychiatric disorders they may be involved with managing include acute psychotic episodes, epileptic seizures, and drug overdoses. There are a variety of specialty outpatient clinics too. These include clozapine, movement disorders, psychiatric issues in HIV, mood disorders, eating disorders, and pain disorders to name a few. Regardless of the setting, the pharmacist serves as a resource for pharmacotherapy information and education in psychiatry and neuropsychiatry for the institution, helping in efforts such as legal and accreditation issues, outcomes, clinical research, and guideline/protocol development. There is a specific board certification for psychiatry, Board Certified Psychopharmacotherapy Pharmacists (BCPP).

A PGY-2 in psychiatry and neuropsychiatry should provide the resident with experiences in both the inpatient and outpatient settings. The residency should provide the foundation in treating patients with schizophrenia, depression, bipolar disorders, anxiety, substance abuse, and other psychiatric disorders. Residents should be exposed to adult, child, adolescent, and geriatric patient populations. Experience should also be gained with neurologic problems such as movement disorders, headaches, and pain disorders, as well as other neuropsychiatric issues (see Table 20-1). There are specific standards for ASHP accreditation for PGY-2 residencies in psychiatry.[6]

NEPHROLOGY

Do you have a drawing or a poster of the nephron on your wall? Did you love pharmacokinetics primarily for the renal clearance of drugs? Do you find yourself using the Cockcroft–Gault equation on everyone you meet? A specialty residency with a focus on nephrology may be right up your alley! With the number of patients with chronic kidney disease exponentially growing, there is a very large opportunity for a clinical pharmacy specialist to make an impact in caring for this patient population. Although there are a limited number of residencies with a focus on nephrology, the evaluation of renal function and drug clearance is an everyday part of any clinical pharmacist's daily patient care activities.[7] The role for a pharmacist with specialty training in nephrology is imperative in patient care. A nephrology pharmacist can work as part of the multidisciplinary renal team to manage patients with acute kidney injury, chronic kidney disease, and end-stage renal disease requiring dialysis and/or renal transplantation. The clinical responsibilities may be in both the inpatient and outpatient settings. In the inpatient setting, as stated before they can be part of a multidisciplinary team or they may be part of a clinical pharmacy team that is consulted for management of drug therapy in patients with renal dysfunction to ensure appropriate dosing and to optimize outcomes. Think of how many times on your Introductory Pharmacy Practice Experiences (IPPEs) and Advance Pharmacy Practice Experiences (APPEs) you had to adjust medication regimens due to changes in renal function! The nephrology pharmacist will work with a variety of patients in various clinical settings such as the diabetic admitted for pneumonia, the chronic hemodialysis patient admitted for a procedure, the septic patient acutely started on continuous renal replacement therapy in the ICU, or the renal transplant patient. The nephrology pharmacist can also play a central role in the transition of care and medication reconciliation between clinical settings to ensure appropriate dosing and prevent medication errors. In the outpatient setting, the pharmacist may work in specialty clinics such as diabetes, dialysis, or transplantation.

A PGY-2 in nephrology should provide a solid foundation and education in kidney disease and kidney-related issues from acute kidney injury to end-stage renal disease and transplantation. The residency should foster the ability to manage and educate patients and other healthcare providers on chronic kidney disease, hemodialysis, peritoneal dialysis, and continuous renal replacement therapy. The resident will also be exposed to kidney-related issues such as acid/base disorders, electrolyte imbalances, anemia, and others as found in Table 20-1. As stated before, there are not an abundant number of nephrology PGY-2 residencies as compared with the other medicine specialty residencies. Therefore, there is not a specific accreditation standard for nephrology. In addition, there is no specific board certification, so most nephrology clinical pharmacists seek recognition as a BCPS.

CAREER OPTIONS

Postgraduate training in a PGY-2 specialty should build a foundation for you to pursue a variety of options in your career. As highlighted in the specific sections, most of the specialties have the opportunities to work in inpatient and outpatient environments or a mixture of both. Administration is also an opportunity to get involved with as policy makers for an institution. Your PGY-2 training should help you build a solid foundation as a specialist to be able to work in a given area. Academia is also a viable option after completion of a PGY-2. We often hear from residents that they do not necessarily feel ready to work in academia until they get more experience in practice. However, the roles in academia are expanding, and many faculty positions are clinically based or have split (50/50, 40/60) positions with the college and hospital. The majority of residencies have prepared you well for academia through student precepting and academic teaching certificate programs. There are so many opportunities for jobs and career options after completing a PGY-2 residency. As we often tell our students and residents, PGY-2 training gives you the "magic ticket" to practice or be considered in a number of positions you would not have the opportunity for with just a PGY-1 residency.

Chapter Takeaways

▶ There are many reasons one decides to do a specialized PGY-2 residency, but mainly to gain the knowledge and skills to practice in a concentrated clinical area.

▶ The decision on what type of PGY-2 residency to pursue is built off of an interest and passion as well as career opportunities in a particular specialty.

▶ There are a variety of clinical pharmacy opportunities to work with a variety of patient populations in the area ID, HIV, cardiology, oncology, psychiatry, and nephrology.

▶ When deciding on where to do a PGY-2 residency, one should evaluate the opportunities, site, and preceptors to determine if the training site is right for what they want to pursue.

"The earlier you find your mentor in pharmacy school the better. They will not only help you with the residency application process, but also in developing skills that will ensure you are a successful resident."

Caitlin S. – Pharmacy Student, South Carolina

ROLE OF MENTOR

Talk with your mentor on why they decided to specialize in a particular area. They probably went through the same decision process at one time as you are going through now.

Speak with your mentor regarding the particular institutions, people, and specialties you are looking at, as pharmacy is a small world and your mentor may be able to offer you insight and how you in particular would do in that program.

Work with your mentor on your strengths and weaknesses as a student and/or PGY-1 resident, and get guidance on what things you can do to better prepare yourself for PGY-2 training.

Make sure you utilize your mentor and/or director in PGY-1 training to help you utilize your electives to help you better determine what specialty you want to pursue. Make sure to get opportunities and exposure in those areas you are interested in before interviewing for your PGY-2.

Talk to your mentors about what they enjoy about their specialty, and why they have practiced in this area for so long.

Most importantly, utilize someone as a mentor that you connect with and feel comfortable asking for questions or advice. Many times these mentor relationships will last a lifetime.

FREQUENTLY ASKED QUESTIONS

Q: Should I focus my attention toward a program that contains a PGY-1 and the PGY-2 programs that I desire?

A: If you know there is a particular area that you want to pursue for PGY-2 training and there are programs that offer both a PGY-1 and that PGY-2 specialty, then it is fine to look at those types of programs, but do not limit yourself to those programs only. Yes, residencies have become very competitive and you would like to have a better chance of getting your PGY-2 of choice and you would not have to change institutions during residency training. However, you need to make sure the PGY-1 you are pursuing offers a wide variety of options in all your areas of interest, as you will be surprised to learn how many residents change their mind of what they want to do during their PGY-1. We always encourage residents to search for a good variety of experience and exposure, and train in places they have not been educated at before in order to develop and expand their knowledge base. Unless you are restricted geographically, expose yourself to other institutions and areas of the country to gain as many experiences you can. As you mature professionally, you can build upon those experiences to make yourself a well-rounded, open-minded practitioner. Training in different places definitely helps expand that professional growth.

Q: What is an early PGY-2 commit?

A: An early commit is when a PGY-2 program takes a current PGY-1 resident from their program and formally agrees (commits) to them being the PGY-2 resident for the next year in advance of the match or interview process. The resident (PGY-1) must be in the same affiliation/organization as the PGY-2 they are early committing. The early commit process usually happens in October/November of the PGY-1 residency after the PGY-1 resident has had enough experiences to be able to determine/decide on what they want to do for their PGY-2 training. In other cases, institutions may choose to interview outside candidates at ASHP Midyear before taking an internal candidate.

Q: Should I look at or apply to PGY-2 programs that do not participate in the match or are not ASHP accredited?

A: First, for a program to enter the match, it must be ASHP-accredited or have submitted for accreditation (be in preaccreditation status). It is not as imperative for a PGY-2 residency to be ASHP-accredited as it is for a PGY-1. A PGY-1 must assure those residents get an equivalent general learning experience and residency foundation for future training, and accreditation verifies the equivalence in learning opportunities. PGY-2 residencies are more focused and specific and ASHP accreditation will ensure the education is appropriate for the specialty. However, the money for funding of some PGY-2 residencies is not as easy to come by as PGY-1 funding, so the investment in accreditation may take a few years until funds are more solidified. Overall, if you are looking at a program that is not accredited, look to see if there are established and reputable directors and preceptors in the specialty area. Also look at the credibility of the training site and if there is ample opportunity for training. Make sure the program is designed based off of the accreditation standards, and ask why the program is not accredited. Many nonaccredited programs are valuable places to train, and at this time there are no specific job requirements for ASHP accredited PGY-2 training. Remember that once a program is accredited, all past residents will be considered coming through an accredited program. The takehome message is do your homework, assure that it is a reputable site and past residents have acquired clinical specialty positions.

References

1. Ernst EJ, et al. Recommendations for training and certification for pharmacists practicing, mentoring and educating in Infectious Diseases Pharmacotherapy. Joint Opinion of Society of Infectious Diseases Pharmacists and Infectious Diseases Practice and Research Network of the American Colleges of Clinical Pharmacy. Pharmacotherapy. 2009;29(4):482–488.

2. Dellit TH, et al. Infectious Diseases Society of America and Society for Healthcare Epidemiology of America Guidelines for Developing an Institutional Program to Enhance Antimicrobial Stewardship. Clin Infect Dis. 2007;44:159–177.

3. American Society of Health-System Pharmacists, Society of Infectious Diseases Pharmacists. Required and Elective Educational Outcomes, Goals and Instructional Objectives for Postgraduate Year Two (PGY2) Pharmacy Residency in Infectious Diseases, 2007. http://www.ashp.org/import/ACCREDITATION/residency/RegulationStandards.aspx. Accessed January 29, 2012.

4. American Society of Health-System Pharmacists. Educational Outcomes, Goals and Objectives for Postgraduate Year Two (PGY2) Pharmacy Residency in Cardiology, 2008. http://www.ashp.org/import/ACCREDITATION/residency/RegulationStandards.aspx. Accessed January 29, 2012.

5. American Society of Health-System Pharmacists, Prepared Jointly with the Hematology/Oncology Pharmacists Association. Required and Elective Educational Outcomes, Goals and Objectives for Postgraduate Year Two (PGY2) Pharmacy Residency in Oncology, 2007. http://www.ashp.org/import/ACCREDITATION/residency/RegulationStandards.aspx. Accessed January 29, 2012.

6. American Society of Health-System Pharmacists Prepared Jointly with College of Psychiatric and Neurologic Pharmacists. Educational outcomes, Goals and Objectives for Postgraduate Year Two (PGY2) Pharmacy Residency in Psychiatry, 2007. http://www.ashp.org/import/ACCREDITATION/residency/RegulationStandards.aspx. Accessed January 29, 2012.

7. Matzke GR, Joy MS. Nephrology pharmacy: Historical reflections and future challenges. Ann Pharmacother. 2007;41:1884–1886.

PGY-2 in Special Patient Populations: Pediatrics, Solid Organ Transplantation, Geriatrics and Palliative Care/Pain Management

21

Lea S. Eiland, Pamela R. Maxwell, and Sharon Jung Tschirhart

As you have likely discovered throughout this section, a Postgraduate Year Two (PGY-2) residency is designed to build upon the skills achieved in the Postgraduate Year One (PGY-1) pharmacy residency program while focusing on a specific area of pharmacy practice.[1] The resident will gain experience in medication therapy managment (MTM) and clinical leadership skills that are necessary when practicing in a particular subspecialty area. Some PGY-2 programs focus on the care of a specific patient population; therefore, these programs may have different goals and objectives that correspond to the population. This chapter will focus on PGY-2 residency programs in special patient populations.

PEDIATRICS (INCLUDING PEDIATRIC HEMATOLOGY/ONCOLOGY)

The PGY-2 pediatric residency is focused to transform a generalist who has completed a PGY-1 residency to become a specialist in the pediatric population.[2] The six required and three elective outcomes set by American Society of Health-System Pharmacists (ASHP) are provided in Table 21-1.[2]

A PGY-2 pediatric residency program must provide the resident with direct patient care opportunities in both the inpatient and outpatient setting. Pediatric pharmacy residents will be exposed to patients of all levels of acuity. This can range from a maintenance visit in an outpatient clinic, a patient in critical condition in an intensive care unit (ICU), or someone in respiratory arrest in the emergency department (ED). This allows the resident to develop into a well-rounded practitioner who has experience in providing various levels of patient care.

TABLE 21-1 • PGY-2 Pediatric Residency Outcomes[2]

Core	Elective
Demonstrate leadership and practice management skills	Demonstrate added skills for functioning effectively in the pediatric pharmacy practice environment
Optimize the care of inpatient and outpatient pediatric patients by providing evidence-based, patient-centered medication therapy as an integral part of an interdisciplinary team	Conduct outcomes research
Serve as an authoritative resource on the optimal use of medications used to treat pediatric patients	Demonstrate skills required to function in the academic setting
Evaluate, manage, and improve the medication use process	
Demonstrate excellence in the provision of training or educational activities for pediatric healthcare professionals, healthcare professionals in training, and the public	
Conduct pediatric pharmacy research	

Participating in the care of pediatric patients is a unique and challenging opportunity for pharmacists. Infants and young children are unable to verbalize their symptoms and feelings, thus there is a lack of direct subjective patient information available. Caregivers are relied upon to provide information to assist with developing the patient's differential diagnoses. Pediatric practice also teaches practitioners to include the patient's caregivers in the patient's care plan. Pediatric pharmacy practice differs significantly from that in adults due to weight-based dosing of medications, age-based laboratory parameters, differing pharmacokinetic and pharmacodynamic principles, and unique fluid and nutrition requirements. In addition, the limited data on safety and efficacy of medications in the pediatric population and the lack of pediatric-friendly dosage forms make clinical decisions more challenging in the pediatric population. The PGY-2 pediatric resident will learn how to handle these issues as they become a pediatric medication expert. They will also develop experience in creating order sets or protocols and making formulary decisions for pediatric patients. As with PGY-1 programs, many PGY-2 pediatric pharmacy residencies are associated with colleges and schools of pharmacy. This provides the pharmacy resident the opportunity to teach in didactic pediatric classes and precept pharmacy students on rotation, which can be an enriching learning experience for the new practitioner.

Throughout the PGY-2 pediatric residency experience, pharmacy residents will be exposed to a variety of patients in different settings. Required rotations may include the neonatal ICU, general pediatrics, pediatric ICU, and pediatric ED. The neonatal ICU provides care for preterm (infants born <37 weeks gestation) or severely ill neonates. This population has very different pharmacokinetic and pharmacodynamic parameters due to immature organ systems, resulting in specialized drug therapy. The well-baby nursery provides care for newly born, full-term, infants. The general pediatric service cares for patients ranging in age from newborns who were discharged from the hospital but return needing medical care to patients who are 18 years of age with any disease state or illness. General pediatrics services provide the most variety of patient ages and disease states. It would not be unusual for patients such as a 2-week-old neonate with a fever, a 1-year-old with respiratory syncytial virus, a 5-year-old with abdominal pain, a 14-year-old with mild diabetic ketoacidosis, and a 16-year-old with a urinary tract infection to all be on the same service. The pediatric ICU admits pediatric patients who require critical care due to reasons such as trauma, respiratory failure from an asthma attack, or a child post-surgery. The pediatric ED not only provides services to stabilize critically ill children but also provides treatment of acute injuries and illnesses for ages of the pediatric population.

Other examples of core or elective rotations during a PGY-2 pediatric residency include hematology/oncology, infectious diseases, pulmonary, endocrinology, psychiatry, nutrition, neurology, poison center, administration, investigational drug services, and medication safety. Pediatric pharmacists are heavily utilized in the hematology/oncology setting, where patients with diseases such as sickle cell anemia, hemophilia, leukemia, or lymphoma are provided care. Some pediatric hospitals may also provide specialty pediatric care to cardiac or solid organ transplant recipients, thus allowing rotations in these areas. Residencies may provide pediatric ambulatory care rotation opportunities in general or specialty clinics. General pediatric clinics care for patients of all ages for well-child checks, vaccinations, infections (such as acute otitis media, cellulitis, or tinea capitis), and maintenance of chronic childhood disease states (such as asthma, diabetes, and attention-deficit/hyperactivity disorder). Experiences in specialty pediatric clinics in broad areas such as neurology or hematology/oncology, or for specific disease states such as asthma or sickle cell anemia, may also be available.

Multiple career opportunities are available for practitioners who complete a PGY-2 pediatric residency program. Practitioners may seek positions in hospitals that care for pediatric patients, whether it is a stand-alone pediatric hospital, a large academic teaching hospital, or a community hospital with pediatric beds. For hospitals with a small census of pediatric patients, the pediatric specialist may be responsible for all types of pediatric patients. In an institution with a large number of pediatric beds, practice may be focused on general pediatrics, pediatric ICU, neonatal ICU, hematology/oncology, or the ED. Large children's hospitals may have additional specialist positions in cardiology or solid organ transplant. The institution may also be focused on a specific disease state, such as St. Jude Children's Research Hospital, which is focused on hematology and oncology. Institutions that have pediatric ambulatory services may also seek pediatric pharmacists. Academia is an option for practitioners with a PGY-2 in pediatric pharmacy, as colleges and schools of pharmacy often develop relationships with a hospital or clinic that cares for pediatric patients to provide a practice site for the faculty member. Unique positions available to pediatric specialty practitioners include working for a medication management or pharmacy benefit company that require a pharmacist with knowledge of this unique patient population. Pediatric pharmacy continues to be a growing area in the profession. Seeing a newborn go home with proud new parents, a child recover from trauma or an illness, or celebrating when a child becomes a cancer survivor are all highlights in a pharmacist's day. Working with children is very rewarding as their smiles and laughter are contagious!

WOMEN'S HEALTH

Currently, an ASHP-accredited PGY-2 women's health residency is not available; however, practitioners can gain experience with this patient population during a PGY-1 or PGY-2 residency. Residency programs may incorporate women's care if they are associated with a women and children's hospital or provide women's specialty services such as labor and delivery, ante-partum, and post-partum care. Other specific areas include a women's surgery floor, special procedures unit (i.e., endoscopy), or an outpatient surgery unit. These types of services may also be found in academic, community, and specialized hospitals for women's services. Specialized hospitals may include a focus on high-risk pregnancies, breast cancer, or gynecologic cancer. Practitioners with extensive experience in women's health may obtain positions caring for this patient population in a general hospital or specialized hospital setting.

SOLID ORGAN TRANSPLANTATION

The PGY-2 solid organ transplant residency is intended to build upon generalist skills acquired during a PGY-1 residency and to allow the practitioner to develop expertise in the care of solid organ transplant recipients and, in some programs, living organ donors.[3] Desirable prerequisites for a transplant residency include a strong foundation of knowledge in internal medicine, critical care, infectious diseases, and ambulatory care. The six required and six elective outcomes of the PGY-2 solid organ transplant residency are listed in Table 21-2.[3]

Transplant residency graduates develop proficiency in the care of patients through all phases of their transplant. Pharmacists are essential members of the interdisciplinary transplant team as patients are selected, listed, and prepared to receive a transplant, during the acute inpatient peri-transplant hospitalization, and after transplant in the ambulatory care setting. Each transplanted organ, whether from a living or a deceased donor, is regarded as a precious commodity whose demand far exceeds the supply. Therefore, the ultimate goal of the interdisciplinary team is to work with the patient to maximize the survival of each transplanted organ, while optimizing the patient's quality of life after transplant.

Envision a patient who just received a renal transplant for chronic renal insufficiency secondary to diabetes. The patient's medical history also includes GERD, hypertension, hyperlipidemia, secondary hyperparathyroidism, and impaired vision from diabetic retinopathy. The patient will now begin a complex oral medication regimen consisting of three immunosuppressants, two prophylactic anti-infectives, two antihypertensives, a statin, a proton pump inhibitor, a long-acting and a rapid-acting insulin, a pain reliever, a laxative, a multivitamin, and a calcium supplement. Adverse effects of the immunosuppressive regimen include nephrotoxicity, hypertension, hyperlipidemia, hyperglycemia, nausea and vomiting, and bone marrow suppression. Do you

TABLE 21-2 • PGY-2 Solid Organ Transplant Residency Outcomes[3]

Core	Elective
Serve as an authoritative resource on optimal medication use in solid organ transplant recipients	Demonstrate additional leadership and practice management skills
Optimize the outcomes of transplant patients by promoting and/or providing evidence-based medication therapy as an integral member of an interdisciplinary team in acute and ambulatory care settings	Contribute to formulary decisions regarding transplant-related medications
Demonstrate excellence in the provision of training or educational activities about transplant-related medications for healthcare professionals and healthcare professionals in training	Demonstrating additional skills for managing and improving the medication-use process in transplant patient care areas
Demonstrate leadership and practice management skills	Publish on transplant-related topics
Demonstrate excellence in education and training activities about transplant-related medications for healthcare professionals and those in training	Function effectively in transplant settings that participate in clinical investigations
Conduct transplant research	Demonstrate the skills required to function in an academic setting

foresee any issues with this patient? This scenario is rather typical for a post-transplant recipient, and only the beginning of many unique challenges with which a transplant pharmacist is presented daily to ensure continued adherence with a complex medication regimen.

Pharmaceutical care in solid organ transplantation is individualized based on a recipient's risk for organ rejection, the etiology of end-organ disease, and preexisting comorbidities. Each patient is on a multifarious medication regimen after transplant that typically includes multiple immunosuppressants and anti-infective agents. Additionally, the regimen often includes numerous medications to prevent or treat surgical complications or adverse effects of the immunosuppressants, or to treat preexisting conditions unrelated to the transplant. Most immunosuppressive regimens require therapeutic drug monitoring and intense management of multiple drug interactions and adverse effects. The overall goal is to maintain a fine balance between preventing organ rejection and serious complications of immunosuppression, including but not limited to nephrotoxicity, infections, malignancy, and cardiovascular disease. The PGY-2 solid organ transplant resident will learn how to fine-tune this balance as they become a transplant medication specialist by building an extensive knowledge base in the disease states leading to organ transplant, transplant immunology and immunosuppression, mechanisms of organ rejection, and post-transplant complications.

In addition to direct patient care responsibilities, transplant residency graduates are equipped to serve as experts within the health system on the optimal use of medications in transplant recipients. Transplant specialists can play a lead role in the development and implementation of medication-related guidelines, protocols, and order sets for transplant patient care, formulary decisions for transplant medications, the interpretation of

> "When trying to decide on your interest area for a PGY-2 residency, sometimes it isn't a bad thing to go with your gut! My very first APPE as a pharmacy student was on a solid organ transplant surgery service, and I was hooked. I kept an open mind throughout the rest of my rotations as a pharmacy student as well as in the first months of my PGY-1 residency, but I knew all along that transplant was my passion. Next year, I'll be completing my PGY-2 solid organ transplant residency at the very institution where I completed that first rotation, and I couldn't be more happy that I trusted my instincts!"
>
> *Caitlin M. – Pharmacy Resident, South Carolina*

transplant-related drug information, and provision of the transplant pharmacy perspective for organizational technology and automation decisions. Graduates are highly trained in the design and delivery of transplant-related education and training for a wide variety of audiences, including healthcare professionals as well as patients and their caregivers. As members of such a dynamic field, transplant residency graduates are also skilled in conducting and supporting transplant research and outcomes analyses.

PGY-2 solid organ transplant pharmacy residencies may vary based on the types of organ transplants performed by the center's transplant program. A transplant pharmacy residency should provide direct acute and ambulatory clinical practice experiences in a minimum of two types of transplantation (heart, intestine, kidney, liver, lung, or pancreas/islet).[3] Other learning experiences may be customized for the specific needs and interests of the pharmacy resident and may include core or elective rotations in areas such as advanced critical care, bone marrow/stem cell transplant, transplant infectious diseases, and pediatric transplant.

Numerous career opportunities are available after completing a PGY-2 solid organ transplant residency. As the role of the pharmacist on the multidisciplinary transplant team has been justified and expanded by the United Network for Organ Sharing (UNOS) bylaws and Centers for Medicare and Medicaid Services (CMS) accreditation standards for transplant centers, the demand for transplant pharmacists has increased dramatically.[4] Therefore, the most common and visible career option is that of a clinical transplant pharmacist in a transplant center. A transplant clinical pharmacist may practice in the acute care setting, the ambulatory care setting, or a combination of the two. A transplant pharmacist may specialize in a particular type of organ transplant population or may work with a variety of organ transplants, depending on the size of the transplant center and the number of transplant pharmacists on the team. Another opportunity for a PGY-2 solid organ transplant residency graduate is a career in academia. A college of pharmacy may be affiliated with a health system that supports a transplant center to provide a practice site for the faculty member. The pharmaceutical industry provides an alternative career option for a PGY-2 transplant residency graduate, usually as a medical science liaison in the field of transplantation or related discipline. Lastly, many centers have adopted transplant pharmacists as their directors or leaders of clinical research within the transplant program.[4] For pharmacists interested specifically in research, a transplant fellowship provides additional specialized training with a focus on research after completion of a PGY-2 transplant residency. Solid organ transplant pharmacy is an expanding specialty, with many opportunities for practice. The greatest reward of practicing in this specialty area is being part of a team that can provide a cure for many diseases with a newly transplanted organ, and a support system that can sustain the life of the organ and improve the quality of life for a patient!

GERIATRICS/LONG-TERM CARE

The PGY-2 geriatric pharmacy residency will transition a graduate of a PGY-1 pharmacy residency into a specialist in geriatrics who is able to provide care to geriatric patients across a wide range of healthcare settings. The six required and nine elective outcomes of the PGY-2 geriatric pharmacy residency are listed in Table 21-3.[5]

The PGY-2 geriatric pharmacy residency is a comprehensive, postdoctoral clinical pharmacy training program designed to produce a clinician demonstrating skills necessary to provide comprehensive pharmaceutical care to geriatric patients in a variety of healthcare settings including geriatric primary care, long-term care, home-based primary care, and acute care. Intended outcomes of geriatric residency programs usually include the ability to function as a member of interdisciplinary and multidisciplinary treatment teams providing care to geriatric patients and serve as an educator for geriatric patients, family members, and healthcare trainees and providers. Graduates of the residency display characteristics of professional and personal self-growth as a geriatric practitioner and demonstrate the ability to proactively identify and meet opportunities available in the provision of pharmaceutical care to our aging population.

Pharmacy residents have many unique responsibilities in geriatric pharmacy residency programs. A resident utilizes their internal medicine knowledge and skills and then goes a step further to apply these principles to elderly patients, taking into account pharmacokinetic and pharmacodynamic changes that occur with aging. The care of geriatric patients requires a team approach. Pharmacy residents learn to interact as members of interdisciplinary and multidisciplinary treatment teams. Patients, caregivers, and family members require education and psychosocial support. When evaluating pharmacotherapeutic regimens or conducting MTM, the pharmacy resident must address issues such as polypharmacy, medication adherence, adverse drug reactions, drug–drug interactions, medications without an appropriate indication, therapeutic duplication, regimen complexity, and lack of benefit from a medication. Regimens must be individualized based on evidence-based medicine, comorbidities, ethical issues, and quality-of-life considerations. Geriatric pharmacy is a specialized area, but encompasses a variety of disease states and disorders in areas such as cardiology, hematology, neurology, oncology, psychiatry, renal, and urology. Falls/gait

TABLE 21-3 • **PGY-2 Geriatric Residency Outcomes[5]**

Core	Elective
Serve as an authoritative resource on the optimal use of medications used with geriatric patients	Demonstrate knowledge particular to geriatric pharmacy practice in the long-term care environment
Optimize the continuum of care for geriatric patients; recognizing diseases, disorders, syndromes, and psychosocial needs unique to this population; by providing evidence-based[a], patient-centered therapy as an integral part of an interdisciplinary team	Demonstrate knowledge particular to geriatric pharmacy practice in the home care environment
Manage and improve medication-use systems across the continuum of care for geriatric patients	Conduct outcomes research
Demonstrate leadership and practice management skills	Where the geriatric pharmacy practice is within a setting that allows pharmacist credentialing, successfully apply for credentialing.
Demonstrate excellence in the provision of training and educational activities for healthcare professionals, healthcare professionals in training, and the public	Demonstrate skills required to function in an academic setting
Contribute to the body of geriatric pharmacotherapy knowledge	Contribute to the management of medical emergencies for geriatric patients
	Demonstrate additional skills for the management and improvement in medication-use systems across the continuum of care for geriatric patients
	Demonstrate additional skills for contributing to the body of geriatric pharmacotherapy literature
	Demonstrate additional leadership and practice management skills

disorders, incontinence, cognitive decline, syncope, frailty, and behavioral and psychological symptoms of dementia are examples of some syndromes geriatric residents learn to manage.[6]

The population in a PGY-2 geriatric pharmacy residency must comprise "a majority of patients with advanced old age."[5] Examples of patient groups encountered during the residency include persons of advanced old age who have cognitive impairment and/or physical disability, medical and/or functional problems requiring assessment, multiple disease states, difficulties managing activities of daily living and who have the potential to benefit from a geriatric trained interdisciplinary healthcare team, and individuals in residential care.[5]

Numerous career options are available after successfully completing a PGY-2 geriatric pharmacy residency. Opportunities are available in areas such as long-term care/consultant pharmacy, academia, assisted living, primary care, internal medicine, home care, and research. Many geriatric specialists are employed by the Veteran's Association in hospital or ambulatory clinics. Upon completion of their geriatric pharmacy residency, many graduates pursue certification as a Board Certified Pharmacotherapy Specialist and/or Certified Geriatric Pharmacist (CGP). Graduates of PGY-2 geriatric pharmacy residencies are sure to be competitive in today's job market as the elderly population grows. Geriatrics is a challenging career path, and pharmacy residents will find that working with the geriatric population is extremely rewarding.

PALLIATIVE CARE/PAIN MANAGEMENT

PGY-2 pain management and palliative care pharmacy residencies will transition a graduate of a PGY-1 pharmacy residency into a specialist focused on the palliative care needs and pain management of patients. The five required and five elective outcomes of the PGY-2 pharmacy residencies in pain management and palliative care are provided in Table 21-4.[7]

Outcomes are designed to allow the resident to develop the ability to function as a vital member of interdisciplinary palliative care and pain

---

TABLE 21-4 • PGY-2 Pain Management and Palliative Care Residency Outcomes[7]

Core	Elective
Demonstrate leadership and practice management skills in pain management and palliative care	Demonstrate skills required to function in an academic setting
Optimize the outcomes of pain management and palliative care patients through the expert provision of evidence-based patient-centered medication therapy as an integral part of an interdisciplinary team	Demonstrate additional leadership and practice management skills
Serve as an authoritative resource on the optimal use of medications in pain management and palliative care	Manage and improve the medication-use process in patient care settings
Demonstrate excellence in the provision of training and educational activities for healthcare professionals, healthcare professionals in training, and the public in pain management and palliative care	Write additional articles on pain management and palliative-care-related topics for publication
Contribute to the body of pain management and palliative care knowledge	Function effectively in pain management and palliative care settings participating in clinical investigations

management teams in a variety of practice settings and to serve as an educator for patients and/or caregivers, family members, and healthcare trainees and providers. Resident graduates have the ability and skills to design and implement therapeutic guidelines and protocols related to pain management and palliative care and to be proficient in conducting clinical research and analyses.

Pain management and palliative care pharmacy residents will gain experience serving as the resource for the optimal use of medications on palliative care and pain management teams. Learning to understand factors that consider a patient as a candidate for hospice/end-of-life care versus palliative care/pain management is a unique aspect the resident will gain during this residency. They will assist in developing an individualized patient plan based on evidence-based medicine, comorbidities, ethical issues, and quality-of-life considerations. Pharmacy residents become experts in evaluating, designing, and monitoring pharmacotherapeutic regimens for palliative care and hospice patients, while gaining exposure to nontraditional therapies, alternative routes of medication administration, nonpharmacological treatments, use of devices for pain management/palliative care, and pain management complicated by tolerance and addiction.[7]

Pain management and palliative care knowledge and skills are applied in a variety of practice settings such as inpatient palliative care/pain management consult services, community-based hospice, inpatient hospice units, and/or outpatient palliative care/pain management clinics. In these areas, residents gain experience managing patients with diseases and conditions such as acute pain, chronic malignant and nonmalignant pain, pain related to chronic diseases (i.e., rheumatologic and neurologic conditions), constipation, and nausea and vomiting. Identification and management of medication adverse effects, understanding psychosocial influences, identifying nutritional deficiencies, and understanding the patient's spiritual considerations are addressed during pain management and palliative care pharmacy residencies.[7]

Career opportunities continue to increase for individuals formally trained in pain management and palliative care. Healthcare providers are identifying the vital role pharmacists play as members of interdisciplinary treatment teams. Graduates may find pain management/palliative care clinical pharmacy specialist positions based in inpatient settings as part of a consult service or inpatient hospice unit or in outpatient settings serving community-based hospice groups or palliative care/pain management clinics. Some positions may have an opportunity to conduct pain management and palliative care in inpatient and outpatient settings. Opportunities also exist in academia and research. Providing palliative care and end-of-life care to patients in the last few years or months of their lives is a challenging yet rewarding experience.

Chapter Takeaways

▶ PGY-2 residency programs in special populations are designed to teach the generalist who completed the PGY-1 pharmacy residency to become a specialist in a specific population.

▶ A PGY-2 residency program provides learning experiences in both inpatient and outpatient settings and many provide opportunities to develop teaching skills.

▶ Pediatric and geriatric pharmacy are specialized areas that encompass a variety of disease states, disorders, and syndromes. Knowledge and skills learned in a PGY-2 pediatric or geriatric pharmacy residency program will provide you with numerous career opportunities in a variety of settings.

▶ PGY-2 solid organ transplant residencies prepare pharmacists to care for patients throughout all phases of their transplant: as they are selected for and prepare to receive a transplant, during the acute inpatient peri-transplant hospitalization, and after transplant in the ambulatory care setting.

▶ PGY-2 pain management and palliative care pharmacy residencies train a pharmacy resident to function as an authoritative medication resource on palliative care and pain management teams.

ROLE FOR THE MENTOR

Discuss specific characteristics of patient populations you would like to work with in the practice environment (such as children, elderly, transplant patients, cancer patients, critically ill, and those who can communicate with you [thus not infants or intubated patients]).

Emphasize unique pharmacist's activities of different patient populations (such as weight-based dosing in pediatrics, monitoring of transplant medications, renal or hepatic adjustments in the elderly).

Provide an overview of issues surrounding social and humanistic aspects of patient care in the population (such as abuse in pediatrics, organ rejection in transplant patients, death in geriatrics, and hospice patients).

FREQUENTLY ASKED QUESTIONS

Q: Can I focus on one area of the pediatric population during my PGY-2 pediatric residency?

A: The PGY-2 pediatric residency is designed to provide the pharmacy resident with exposure to a variety of pediatric patients and pediatric disease states. This includes seeing preterm neonates, neonates, infants, children, and adolescents in the inpatient and outpatient settings. Most programs will allow pharmacy residents to spend additional elective rotations in a specific area of interest after core rotations are completed.

Q: What type of transplants would a PGY-2 pharmacy resident see in a PGY-2 solid organ transplant residency?

A: Pharmacy residents may provide services for recipients of both abdominal (kidney, liver, pancreas/islet cell, intestinal) and thoracic (heart, lung) transplants. Other rotation opportunities may include bone marrow/ stem cell transplant, advanced critical care, transplant infectious diseases, and pediatric transplant.

Q: Do I need to complete a PGY-2 geriatric pharmacy residency to find a job as a consultant pharmacist?

A: Many consultant pharmacist positions don't require the completion of a PGY-2 geriatric pharmacy residency as a requirement for employment. However, the completion of the residency should make you more competitive in the job market and prepare you for future changes or directions in your career path.

Q: What opportunities are available for teaching in PGY-2 pharmacy residency programs?

A: Teaching opportunities are individualized for each PGY-2 pharmacy residency program. Some programs may offer opportunities for delivering didactic lectures, leading case/topic discussions, presenting to multidisciplinary groups of healthcare professionals and trainees, or precepting pharmacy students. Teaching certification programs may also be incorporated into some residency programs. If you have an interest in teaching, be sure to inquire about the opportunities available in a particular PGY-2 pharmacy residency program.

References

1. American Society of Health-System Pharmacists. ASHP Accreditation Standard for Postgraduate Year Two (PGY2) Pharmacy Residency Programs. http://www.ashp.org/DocLibrary/Accreditation/ASD-PGY2-Standard.aspx. Accessed January 16, 2012.

2. American Society of Health-System Pharmacists. Educational Outcomes, Goals, and Objectives for Postgraduate Year Two (PGY2) Pharmacy Residencies in Pediatrics. http://www.ashp.org/menu/Accreditation/ResidencyAccreditation.aspx. Accessed January 16, 2012.

3. American Society of Health-System Pharmacists. Educational Outcomes, Goals, and Objectives for Postgraduate Year Two (PGY2) Pharmacy Residencies in Solid Organ Transplant. http://www.ashp.org/menu/Accreditation/ResidencyAccreditation.aspx. Accessed February 27, 2012.

4. Alloway RR, et al. Evolution of the role of the transplant pharmacist on the multidisciplinary transplant team. Am J Transplant. 2011;11(8):1576–1583.

5. American Society of Health-System Pharmacists; prepared in collaboration with the American Society of Consultant Pharmacists. Educational Outcomes, Goals, and Objectives for Postgraduate Year Two (PGY2) Pharmacy Residencies in Geriatrics. http://www.ashp.org/menu/Accreditation/ResidencyAccreditation.aspx. Accessed February 17, 2012.

6. American Society of Consultant Pharmacists. Geriatric Pharmacy Curriculum Guide. http://www.wgec.org/resources/art/pharmacy.PDF. Accessed February 26, 2012.

7. American Society of Health-System Pharmacists. Required and Elective Educational Outcomes, Goals, Objectives, and Instructional Objectives for Postgraduate Year Two (PGY2) Pharmacy Residencies in Pain Management and Palliative Care. http://www.ashp.org/menu/Accreditation/ResidencyAccreditation.aspx. Accessed February 17, 2012.

PGY-2 Programs in Health-System Administration, Drug Information, Medication-Use Safety, Informatics, and Outcomes and Policy

22

Brad S. Fujisaki

"There are two types of pharmacists: those that directly care for patients and those that support those that directly care for patients."

Cae Ryan   PharmD

The majority of Postgraduate Year Two (PGY-2) residency programs aim at producing pharmacists with specialized knowledge, skills, and abilities, with the intent of caring for a targeted group of patients such as those critically ill, having an infectious disease, or with age-based needs (pediatric and geriatric populations). Then there are PGY-2 residency programs that could be categorized by some as being focused on "non-patient care" or follow a "management track" within the specialties of health-system administration, drug information, medication-use safety, and informatics. For you, this grouping of specialized residencies may conjure up feelings of aversion as your explicit goal for becoming a pharmacist was likely to *one day be able to help and care for patients* (note: you may have actually written this in your application for pharmacy school or responded as such during interviews). If this is the case, for the next few minutes, please suspend any apprehension you may have with regard to pursuing these types of PGY-2 programs and reflect on the following scenario:

Imagine that you are currently on an Internal Medicine rotation in your last year of pharmacy school. You just completed the second week of your rotation at Boxer Medical Center, and you are currently following three patients assigned by your preceptor. Your team has had many interesting patients, but by far, the majority of your time has been either working up patients with pneumonia, heart failure, or "mental status changes"— all three of which have provided you numerous opportunities to recommend interventions surrounding medication therapy. Your preceptor has noted that you have been managing your workload well and has challenged you to take on additional responsibilities. She suggests increasing your workload by having you choose one of the following items:

1. double your patient load to six patients total;
2. develop a drug monograph for a new antibiotic;
3. draft a protocol or an order set for community acquired pneumonia;
4. conduct a chart review of patients with "mental status changes" to evaluate for possible drug-related causes; or
5. assist the Heart Failure Nurse Practitioner in developing patient education materials (including information about medications) to provide at discharge.

Which one would you choose and why?

If you chose (a), to increase your patient load, it is likely that you genuinely find the most reward in making individual patient interventions since you probably enjoy working closely with patients and other care providers to optimize the health of individuals. If you chose any of the other options, your reasoning could be that your efforts today would likely impact many patients over time, even though you may never actually interact one-on-one with the patients that would benefit from your work. So rather than helping patients individually, you help support the system that cares for your patients.

The PGY-2 residency programs in health-system administration, drug information, medication-use safety, and informatics have in common a larger emphasis on *systems-based practice* with foundational roots in organizational thinking and population-based decision making. As a resident in these types of programs, you will specialize in "the system" or a component of the system rather than caring for a specialized group of patients. This chapter is intended to provide you with additional detail regarding these postgraduate training programs, likely career paths for those completing these types of PGY-2 programs, and practical advice for navigating your roadmap in this realm of pharmacy practice. Fellowships focused on outcomes/pharmacoeconomics/drug policy also have overlapping themes with PGY-2 programs in systems-based practice and will be briefly discussed.

Aren't these already areas that I will be exposed to as a PGY-1 resident?

The purpose of a Postgraduate Year One (PGY-1) residency is to provide a broad and diverse experience with required elements in acute and ambulatory patient care, drug information, and practice management. In some ways, these PGY-1 experiences are "small plate" portions, whereas a PGY-2 experience is an expanded "full course meal" in a very focused and/or subspecialty area. In this analogy, the required practice management and drug information experiences in a PGY-1 program would give you an initial "taste" of what would be expanded upon in more depth in a PGY-2 system-based practice program. That being said, the patient care components in a PGY-1 are extremely important in providing a well-grounded understanding of the medication-use process as well as solidifying a practice philosophy that always puts the patient at the forefront of everything you do.

What do these PGY-2 programs have in common?

In addition to the systems-based aspect of these practices, there are also other overlapping commonalities among these PGY-2 programs. In actuality, all PGY-2 programs have some degree of advanced practice management components that involve further development in areas such as self-regulated learning, project management, quality assurance, and fiscal justification for clinical service. As a PGY-2 resident focused on systems-based practice, more time will be spent in organizational and operations meetings compared with your counterparts completing PGY-2 residencies focused on the care of specialized patient populations. Your skills will be honed in developing policies and procedures that will be communicated system-wide. A larger component of your training will focus on regulatory and accreditation aspects of the institution. Continuous quality improvement will become part of everything you do, and you will almost automatically begin with the end in mind. Close working relationships with other system-based members of the healthcare team including service-line managers, department directors, and "C-suite" administrators will be a normal part of your day. Many opportunities to evaluate the financial impact and return on investment of various system-based interventions including human capital, technology, and educational programming will be in abundance. Improvements in the system are synonymous with implementation of new processes; thus, you will lead others through various types of organizational change. All PGY-2 residencies have elective opportunities that relate to the development of skills necessary to function in an academic setting with an emphasis on teaching, both in the didactic (classroom) and experiential (precepting) environments.

What are unique opportunities or key differences between these PGY-2 programs?

PGY-2 IN HEALTH-SYSTEM PHARMACY ADMINISTRATION

As a health-system pharmacy administration (admin) resident, you will develop into a leader with knowledge, skills, and attitude to effectively oversee the medication-use system in the health-system setting. Many PGY-2 admin residencies are designed as 2-year programs, having the outcomes of a PGY-1 general residency also achieved at the end of the 2 years. Depending on the program, you may also be enrolled to complete a master's degree concurrently with your residency. In order to maximize positive patient outcomes, you will spend time learning to manage day-to-day departmental operations utilizing principles of continuous quality improvement to gain experience in leveraging available resources (human and technology). Your expertise will expand in legal, regulatory, and accreditation requirements pertaining to medication provision and use within the institution. Along these lines, you can also expect to utilize your expertise to shape the profession by taking on early leadership roles in pharmacy organizations at the state and national levels (e.g., ASHP). As an admin resident, financial management skills around budgets, contracts/supply chain, revenue cycles, and productivity metrics will be honed. Compared with other PGY-2 residents, you will become more involved with human resources and personnel management that pertain to recruitment and hiring, performance evaluation, and progressive discipline of departmental employees.

PGY-2 IN DRUG INFORMATION

As a drug information resident, you will excel in the location, retrieval, and provision of information that is accurate, valid, and timely. Most PGY-2 drug information programs provide staffing opportunities within a Drug Information Center as well as learning how to manage the operations of the center. Depending on the design of the program, you may have the opportunity to spend additional time in the medical information department of a pharmaceutical (or biotechnology) company. You will also learn to manage the institutional drug formulary and Pharmacy and Therapeutics (P&T) Committee-related activities such as preparing drug monographs, conducting drug-use evaluations (DUE), and developing appropriate criteria for drug use. Opportunities to train and staff in an Investigational Drug Service may also be available to you. Drug information residents tend to have more emphasis on medical writing compared with other PGY-2 residents; so, you can expect more formalized feedback regarding your skill and style in written communication. Some PGY-2 programs in drug information are designed to have the resident spend some of their time at a publisher of a drug/medical information company (i.e., Facts & Comparisons, Lexi-Comp, and FirstDataBank). Many drug information centers are also affiliated with a Poison Control Center, in which elective opportunities for a rotation in toxicology may be available.

PGY-2 IN MEDICATION-USE SAFETY

As a medication-use safety resident, you will become a leader in the safe use of medications. Focused training and experiences will allow you to become proficient in the principles underlying human factors engineering and its contribution to medication errors. Experiences will prepare you to organize a response team to evaluate medication-related events utilizing methods such as failure mode, effects, criticality analysis (FMECA), and root cause analysis (RCA). These advanced methods will provide you with tools for detection of latent system errors and at-risk behaviors that go beyond the basic "5 rights" of medication administration. For institutional decisions involving evaluation of technology and automation affecting the medication-use system, you will be the advocate for safeguarding patients from potential and unintended consequences of such implementation. An integral component of your experience will be learning to manage the medication error-reporting program for your institution by evaluating key metrics or triggers to identify error-prone areas as well as track institutional improvements made to the medication-use system.

PGY-2 IN INFORMATICS

As an informatics resident, you will become a leader in managing projects involving automation and technology that results in a safe medication-use system. Expertise will develop in the information architecture supporting the medication-use system—understanding exactly how medication information flows in and out of the system. The focus of your training will allow you to be intimately involved in all phases of a project's life cycle from initiation to close. You will develop skills to effectively assess systems and processes for technology needs and readiness. As liaison between the information technology (IT) department and the pharmacy department, your communication skills will be honed in translating between "tech speak" and "pharm speak." You can expect to be an active participant in the interdisciplinary development of evidence-based decision support tools that maximize the quality and efficiency of care provided to patients. Skills in risk management and contingency planning will be further developed, particularly as it relates to implementing technology within a healthcare system.

OUTCOMES AND POLICY FELLOWSHIPS

In addition to specialized postgraduate residency training, fellowships are another option for those interested in system-based practice with an emphasis on outcomes research, pharmacoeconomics, and healthcare policy. Compared with PGY-2 residencies, fellowships have a larger emphasis on systematic research, and often require teaching responsibilities within an affiliated college of pharmacy. Many fellowships will require either a PhD degree or completion of a residency as a program prerequisite. For highly competitive programs, completion of a PGY-2 residency may actually be the norm for the pool of fellowship applicants. There are also policy-based fellowship programs administered through pharmaceutical industry or government agencies (e.g., FDA) and these usually have a larger focus on regulatory aspects of drug product.

What opportunities should I look for in a PGY-2 program focused on systems-based practice?

Patient care. Although this may sound counterintuitive, the further you move away from being in the frontline, the less informed you likely become about the processes and systems that you are helping to make decisions about. In other words, continuing to have some clinical and distribution responsibilities during your PGY-2 program will further complement your development in systems-based practice; you can more effectively contribute at the systems level when you clearly can describe what happens at the individual patient level. This is not to say that you should let your $n = 1$ frontline experiences overpower systematically collected evidence, but having the ability to fully appreciate the impact your decisions have on others will be invaluable as a leader. This is mentioned here as practice management outcomes are clearly defined for "patient-focused" PGY-2 residency programs, but individual patient care outcomes are not defined for "management-focused" PGY-2 programs; therefore, it has the potential to be forgotten.

When should I start thinking about applying to a PGY-2 program in systems-based practice?

If possible, you should be ready to talk about your specific plans for completing a PGY-2 residency during your interview for your PGY-1 program. All accredited programs go through the match and because of the possibility for "early commitment" by a current PGY-1 resident, it is imperative that you evaluate whether specialized residency training is right for you. Moreover, some programs such as a PGY-2 in admin may be 1-year in design while others are more extensive and require a 2-year commitment.

CAREER PATHS FOLLOWING SYSTEMS-BASED PRACTICE PGY-2 PROGRAM–A SHORT STORY

There once was a pharmacist named Braden who just completed his PGY-1 program and was beginning a PGY-2 program in drug information at a nearby Academic Health Center. Shawna was the outgoing PGY-2 Drug Information Resident and Katie was the Residency Program Director. Danny, a PGY-1 coresident with Braden, was also starting a 2-year fellowship in pharmacoeconomics and outcomes at that local school of pharmacy. Upon completion of his PGY-2 program in drug information, Braden was hired on at the Academic Health Center as an Informatics Pharmacist. Kimiko was the incoming drug information resident and Katie remained the program director. Braden, Katie, and Kimiko all reported to Mitchell, the Assistant Director of Pharmacy, who recently completed a 2-year combined masters' PGY-2 health-system pharmacy administration residency. A few years later, Braden became the Residency Program Director for a new PGY-2 in pharmacy informatics with his first resident being Jonah. So, let us fast forward a few years and see where the characters of the story ended up and what they are doing now:

- Shawna (PGY-2 in Drug Information)—Clinical Pharmacy Manager at Managed Care Organization
- Kimiko (PGY-2 in Drug Information)—Investigational Drug Pharmacist at a Cancer Research Center
- Katie (PGY-2 in Drug Information)—Medication Safety Coordinator at a different Health System
- Danny (Fellowship in Outcomes)—Faculty Member at School of Pharmacy; Medicaid Drug Utilization Review Board
- Jonah (PGY-2 in Informatics)—Informatics Pharmacist at the Academic Health Center

- Mitchell (PGY-2 in Health-System Admin)—Director of Pharmacy at Academic Health Center
- Braden (PGY-2 in Drug Information)—Assistant Dean and Faculty at School of Pharmacy; Director of the Drug Information Service

Though this short story lacked a true plot, the intent was to provide you with actual examples of career paths for graduates of PGY-2 programs in systems-based practices. Clinical coordinator positions often require the knowledge and skill set provided through these PGY-2 programs, thus a common "first job out of residency" stepping-stone in becoming an institutional leader. In addition, some graduates from PGY-2 programs take positions in industry (pharmaceutical, publishing, technology/automation) and/or also become independent consultants.

Chapter Takeaways

▶ PGY-2 residency programs in health-system administration, drug information, medication-use safety, and informatics prepare pharmacists for specialized systems-based practice.

▶ There is considerable overlap between the PGY-2 programs in system-based practice, however, there are areas of emphasis and unique opportunities for each type of program, which sets them apart from the other types of programs.

▶ There are many different career paths and job options available to graduates from PGY-2 programs in systems-based practice.

ROLE FOR THE MENTOR

Discuss with mentor whether you will thrive more in directly caring for patients or supporting those who directly care for patients. Those who express interest in wanting to help to develop solutions to problems (vs. "someone needs to fix this") should consider whether systems-based practice is in their future.

Talk with a mentor about why you would like to pursue that specific area rather than another systems-based area as there is much overlap between the PGY-2 programs in systems-based practice. For example, why pursue a PGY-2 in informatics rather than drug information or medication-use safety?

Seek out a mentor who should try to connect you with a current resident or recent graduate from a systems-based practice type of program to allow you to gather as much information as possible.

PGY-2–Other Specialty Residency Programs– Pharmacotherapy, Nuclear, Veterinary, Association/ Executive, and Combination Residencies

23

Ola Oyelayo

PHARMACOTHERAPY

Are you interested in a residency that provides the training of a generalist while also offering the opportunity of a specialist training? Do you want to receive a residency training that allows for incorporation of individual career goals and plans (e.g., practice site and subspecialty)? Then a pharmacotherapy residency might be the perfect program for you.

The overarching objective of a pharmacotherapy residency is to develop a specialist that is able to navigate across different practice sites with confidence due to the extensive breadth of experience gained during residency training. The scope of the residency is perhaps best illustrated by the American Society of Health-System Pharmacists (ASHP) definition of a pharmacotherapy residency as being "...designed to produce a specialized practitioner with an advanced degree of proficiency and expertise in working with interdisciplinary teams to deliver pharmaceutical care to diverse inpatient and outpatient populations presenting with varied and complex health problems."[1] As such a pharmacotherapy specialist should be comfortable managing both acute and chronic medical problems in various practice sites such as clinics, critical care settings, academia, and acute care settings. During a pharmacotherapy residency, you should expect to be exposed to a variety of internal medicine topics such as cardiology, critical care, oncology, infectious

> "I always thought residency training was just all about perfecting clinical skills, but I have learned it is also a great time to form networks, friendships, and memories that will last a lifetime."
>
> *Maria T. – Pharmacy Resident, Georgia*

diseases, and endocrinology etc., at sufficient depth to become a clinical specialist.

If you still find yourself asking why choose this program over other programs with a more narrow focus, there is a simple answer—flexibility. While there is a core set of rotations and experiences expected, it also allows for additional training and experience in a specialized area of practice depending on individual career goals. Nothing illustrates this better than a recent editorial describing career choices of graduates from ASHP-accredited pharmacotherapy residencies.[2] The editorial found that the graduates practiced in a variety of settings ranging from academia to acute care hospitals to ambulatory care clinics to the pharmaceutical industry. Practice areas of past graduates included critical care, cardiology, infectious diseases, internal medicine, and pain and palliative care. Interestingly, the graduates were from only eight programs yet practiced in such a variety of settings demonstrating the breadth and depth of the training offered by a pharmacotherapy residency.

Most pharmacotherapy residency programs are designed as either a 12-month or 24-month program, often with the flexibility to accommodate specialization in an area of practice. The 12-month programs are designated as PGY-2 programs, whereas the 24-month programs are designated as combined PGY-1 and PGY-2 program. Upon completion of a pharmacotherapy residency, a graduate should be qualified to take the board examination required to become a Board Certified Pharmacotherapy Specialist (BCPS). Therefore, if you possess a broad-based knowledge and want a program designed to harness such skills with practice experience, you should consider a pharmacotherapy residency as the ideal program.

NUCLEAR PHARMACY

Quiz time, what was the first pharmacy specialty recognized by the board of pharmacy specialties? Don't look at the chapter subheading for the answer, but if you said nuclear then you guessed right. Your reward is a follow-up question. In what year was nuclear pharmacy recognized as a specialty? The answer is buried in the text, so read along. Although it was the first specialty to be officially recognized in the pharmacy profession, nuclear pharmacy is seldom covered in-depth at most pharmacy schools. If you are like me, you probably had a lecture or two from a speaker who discussed the benefits and uniqueness of a career in nuclear pharmacy. Indeed you can consider yourself part of the lucky few, if you had any concrete exposure to nuclear pharmacy practice and extremely lucky if you had faculty members specialized in nuclear pharmacy. The lack of attention to nuclear pharmacy is not due to lack of importance, but a testament to the specialized skills required to become a nuclear pharmacist.

Radiopharmaceuticals, also known as radioactive medications, are widely used in hospitals for various testing, imaging, and treatment modalities such as cardiac stress tests, positron emission tomography (PET) scans, and thyroid ablation. Examples of radiopharmaceuticals include but are not limited to radioactive iodine, technetium-99m, and thallium. A nuclear pharmacist ensures the safe and effective use of radiopharmaceuticals.

Let's imagine you are the nuclear pharmacist at a local hospital and you receive an order for a radiopharmaceutical for a patient undergoing thyroid ablation. You will fulfill such an order by interpreting the prescription, compounding, or preparing from bulk the agent requested and having it delivered to the requesting unit. The process is quite comparable to a prescription for a nonradiopharmaceutical. Therefore, a nuclear pharmacist acts similarly to any other pharmacist with the difference being the type of medication dispensed.

No special license is required to become a nuclear pharmacist; however, the Nuclear Regulatory Commission (NRC) has licensing requirements to become an "authorized nuclear pharmacist." This designation is required to independently manufacture, produce, acquire, receive, possess, prepare, use, or transfer radiopharmaceuticals without supervision from an authorized user or nuclear pharmacist.[3]

The majority of nuclear pharmacists are trained by their employer through in-house training, or through certificate programs offered by certain pharmacy schools. Another option is through a nuclear pharmacy residency. At a minimum, residency programs in nuclear pharmacy should provide the 700 hours of training required by the NRC to become an "authorized nuclear pharmacists." They should also provide operations training such as checking and testing of instrumentation, safe preparation of radiopharmaceuticals, waste disposal, decontamination of the preparation area, storage, and ensuring appropriate shielding during administration.[4] Residency training hours can also be applied toward becoming a Board Certified Nuclear Pharmacist (BCNP). As with other specialty residency programs, a nuclear pharmacy residency provides much more in terms of clinical, research, and educational training required to become an expert in radiopharmaceuticals.

Upon completion of the residency, you should be qualified to obtain employment at an independent or chain nuclear pharmacy; you may even decide to open your own nuclear pharmacy. Additionally, some large healthcare institutions directly employ nuclear pharmacists to prepare and dispense radiopharmaceuticals for use at the facility. Another potential career option is academia, teaching at one of the few pharmacy schools with an active nuclear pharmacy program or potentially establishing a new program. Now back to the earlier question about the year nuclear pharmacy was recognized as a specialty of pharmacy practice. That would be 1978.

VETERINARY PHARMACY

Do you love providing individualized care, compounding medications, and animals? Then a career as a veterinary pharmacist is a great opportunity to combine all of the above. Veterinary pharmacists do a lot of mixing, concocting, and formulating because there are few standardized veterinary medications available on the market. However, the role of a veterinary pharmacist is not limited to compounding alone; they are also an integral part of the medication selection process. In a recent role delineation study, the role of a veterinary pharmacist specialist (a pharmacist who practices exclusively in a veterinary setting) was considered to be much broader by incorporating clinical practice, research, and education than expected of a veterinary pharmacist (any pharmacist supporting the need of a veterinarian).[5] A residency or fellowship training was considered in the study, to be crucial for acquiring the broad training needed to be a veterinary pharmacy specialist.[5]

The concept of a veterinary residency is relatively new as most veterinary pharmacists acquired their knowledge through work experience and on-the-job training. The scope and nature of training activities and topics required in a veterinary pharmacy residency are not well defined or standardized, as no national standards are available yet. A resident can, however, expect exposure to the administrative component of pharmacy operations such as purchasing and formulary management as well as the clinical component such as rounding experiences with small or large animals, pharmacokinetic consulting, and others.[6] The training is typically provided as either a 12-month or 24-month experience. A 24-month program allows for further subspecialization. The few programs available have a direct affiliation with a veterinary school to provide sites for clinical practice and research. Such affiliations provide an opportunity for collaborative practice and research with veterinarians.

Upon completion, a veterinary pharmacy residency certificate can be used as a qualification criterion for certification as a Diplomate in the International College of Veterinary Pharmacy. A Diplomate in International College Veterinary Pharmacy denotes a specialist in veterinary pharmacy who has passed through a credentialing and examination process. Job opportunities following the residency include working in academia at pharmacy or veterinary medicine schools, animal hospitals, animal research, industry, and regulatory agencies.[7]

COMBINATION OR "SLASH" PROGRAMS

The phrase to "kill two birds with one stone" could apply to pharmacy residency training. In general, specialty programs are designed to offer training and exposure to a particular area of pharmacy or medicine however; there is often room for secondary or additional areas of focus. In theory, the combinations that can be offered are limitless. In reality, the need for considerable areas of overlap in the subject matter limits the possible combinations. This is particularly important given the time restraints of completing a residency program in 1 or 2 years.

Certain areas of pharmacy practice such as critical care, administration, or academia lend themselves to additional specialty/subspecialty training. Combinations of critical care medicine with infectious diseases, emergency medicine, or nutrition are common as they involve a similar patient case mix. For example, it is not uncommon for an infection to be the cause for admission to a critical care unit or for a critically ill patient to require enteral or parenteral nutrition. By utilizing the related patient population, training can be provided in multiple areas that prepares the resident for independent practice in the different specialties. Another common example is combination programs involving academia. Such programs can be offered as a teaching certificate program or adjunct faculty position with mentoring from senior faculty and is often available as an option with most specialty programs.

A major drawback to combination programs is the lack of standards or training expectations as ASHP currently does not have set standards for these programs. Clearly, the more combinations that are added to a program, the greater the chance of an unwieldy program failing to meet its program objectives. Therefore, if you are considering a combination program, it is important that you carefully evaluate the curriculum and learning objectives to ensure that adequate time and resources are dedicated to achieving the desired level of competence in all of the specialties offered. Remember it is important that residency programs maintain a clear focus with accomplishable objectives.

A major advantage of a combination program is the career flexibility it offers upon completion. Depending on the type of combination program you complete, you may have the opportunity to pursue a career in multiple specialty areas. An example could be obtaining a faculty position specializing in oncology with clinical responsibilities upon graduation from a combination program involving academia and oncology. The additional training could also benefit you by providing unique skill sets that differentiate you in an increasingly competitive job market.

ASSOCIATION LEADERSHIP/EXECUTIVE

Residencies are also offered by pharmacy associations and advocacy organizations. You are/were probably a member of one or more pharmacy organizations as a student. You may have even participated in selecting the leadership team of the association or organization either as a candidate or as a voting member. It should come as no surprise that organizations at the pharmacy school level also exist on a state, regional, and national basis. Organizations such as American Pharmaceutical Association (APhA), American College of Clinical Pharmacy (ACCP), National Community Pharmacy Association (NCPA), and ASHP, and others have national offices that coordinate activities for their chapters and chapter members. A residency with a pharmacy association offers the resident an opportunity to participate in the day-to-day operations of the association at a national level.

An association leadership or executive residency provides the opportunity for a first-hand experience at expanding the mission and goals of the selected organization. It is an ideal program for someone with strong communication, leadership, and organizational skills. A resident should expect to lead or develop initiatives to be implemented nationwide as part of the mission and goals of the organization.[7] It also offers the opportunity to travel across the nation to introduce such initiatives or to gather ideas from local chapters. The resident also serves as an ambassador for the organization. As a student, I remember visits from residents from the NCPA, who explained the benefits of independent pharmacies and how to become engaged with the organization.

Pharmacy associations are at the forefront of advocacy for the profession and health care in general. As a resident, you will have countless opportunities to advocate for the profession at legislative bodies, governmental agencies, inter-professional meetings, and other venues. This active role enhances the communication skills of the resident while also providing an excellent opportunity to network with key thought leaders in the profession. Upon completion, the resident will be well prepared for a career in pharmacy organizations, academia, advocacy, government relations, or other administrative-type positions.

Chapter Takeaways

▶ There are a limited amount of programs available nationwide for veterinary, nuclear, and association leadership/executive residencies.

▶ The overarching goal of a pharmacotherapy residency is to develop a specialist that is able to navigate across different practice sites with confidence due to the extensive breadth and depth of experience gained during training.

▶ A nuclear pharmacy residency provides the training hours required to become an "authorized nuclear pharmacist" while also enhancing research and teaching skills to develop a well-rounded nuclear clinical pharmacist.

▶ Combination programs are designed to provide training in more than one area/specialty by utilizing complementary patient cases or experiences.

ROLE OF THE MENTOR

Review career opportunities with a mentor after successful completion of a residency.

Discuss expectations during the residency year and the typical profile of daily activities with a mentor.

Speak with a mentor about eligibility for board certification or recognition by specialty organization.

Discuss travel requirements particularly with association or organizational residencies.

FREQUENTLY ASKED QUESTIONS

Q: What is the difference between an internal medicine residency and a pharmacotherapy residency?

A: If you review the diseases and conditions for which graduates of both programs are required to have experience in managing, there is indeed a great deal of overlap. The major differences between both programs are related to duration and flexibility of the programs. A pharmacotherapy residency is available as a combined PGY-1 and 2 24-month experience and also allows for individualization of program objectives.

Q: **What areas of pharmacy can I practice in with my pharmacotherapy residency training?**

A: The options for career choices are varied with a pharmacotherapy residency. As a pharmacotherapy specialist, your training should allow you to confidently practice in a wide variety of areas. As discussed earlier, a review of graduates of 24-month ASHP-accredited pharmacotherapy residency programs revealed that graduates upon graduation accepted positions in diverse areas of pharmacy including critical care, academia, ambulatory care, and cardiology.

Q: **Is a nuclear pharmacy residency required to practice as a nuclear pharmacist?**

A: No, however a nuclear residency does allow for a more in-depth understanding of the role of a nuclear pharmacist including operations, research, and clinical practice.

Q: **Do I need to complete a residency to work in a veterinary hospital or practice?**

A: No, veterinary pharmacy residency is a relatively new area of postgraduate training. In the past, veterinary pharmacists received the bulk of their training from on-the-job training and mentorship. The advent of residency training however allows for a formalized learning experience.

References

1. American Society of Health-System Pharmacists. Required Educational Outcomes, Goals and Objectives for Postgraduate Year Two Pharmacy Residencies in Pharmacotherapy. http://www. ashp.org/menu/Accreditation/ResidencyAccreditation.aspx. Accessed February 14, 2012.

2. Nappi J, Haase K, Kessels A, Fink J. What is a pharmacotherapy residency? Benefits of a 24 month program [editorial]. Pharmacotherapy. 2008;28(7):819–820.

3. United States Nuclear Regulatory Commission. NRC Regulations (10CFR) §35.11. http://www.nrc. gov/reading-rm/doc-collections/cfr/part035/part035–0011.html. Accessed February 14, 2012.

4. American Society of Health-System Pharmacists. Required Educational Outcomes, Goals and Objectives for Postgraduate Year Two Pharmacy Residencies in Nuclear Pharmacy. http://www. ashp.org/menu/Accreditation/ResidencyAccreditation.aspx. Accessed February 14, 2012.

5. Ceresia ML, et al. The role and education of the veterinary pharmacist. Am J Pharm Educ. 2009;73(1):16.

6. Residency Program in Veterinary Clinical Pharmacy. School of Veterinary Medicine, University of California, Davis, Web site. Available at http://www.vetmed.ucdavis.edu/vmth/pharmacy/residency_program.cfm. Accessed February 16, 2012.

7. National Community Pharmacists Association. Executive residency brochure. http://www. ncpanet.org/index.php/internship-opportunities. Accessed February 16, 2012.

Pursuing Pharmacy Fellowships 24

Melissa D. Johnson

American Society of Health-System Pharmacy (ASHP) defines a fellowship as:

"a directed, highly individualized, postgraduate program designed to prepare the participant to become an independent researcher."[1]

The first thing many students say when hearing about fellowship programs is "oh no ... not more years of training! I'm too poor, and have spent numerous years in school already." Yet, the time commitment spent in a fellowship program can pay off exponentially during your career. Ultimately, pharmacists with postgraduate training are more productive in publishing papers and are more satisfied with their careers than their peers.[2,3] With an increasingly competitive job market and emphasis on more specialized training, fellowship opportunities have expanded. There are more than 100 fellowship opportunities across the United States, in a variety of specialties.

While fellowships have often traditionally had a research focus, more practice-based fellowship experiences are now available. As a fellow, you work closely with an established research mentor throughout the program to develop expertise in a focused area. Ultimately, this experience is aimed at developing you as an independent researcher and/or collaborator at the end of the fellowship program.

Fellowship programs may be offered with accreditation from a professional organization, such as American College of Clinical Pharmacy (ACCP), or on a nonaccredited basis. At this time, ACCP is the only professional pharmacy organization that conducts peer-review of fellowship programs, although others have published guidelines of suggested program requirements. In general, the duration of fellowships varies from 1 to 2 years. Requirements for prior clinical experience and/or residency (i.e., Postgraduate Year One [PGY-1] and/or Postgraduate Year Two [PGY-2]) training vary among the programs as well.

STANDARDS AND OUTCOMES OF FELLOWSHIP PROGRAMS

Fellowship programs can be broadly divided into two main categories: (1) traditional fellowships that are focused on a particular area of expertise and

TABLE 24-1 • Program Focus

Ambulatory Care	Nephrology
Cardiology	Oncology
Community	Outcomes Research
Critical Care	Pediatrics
Drug Development	Pharmacoeconomics
Drug Information	Pharmacogenomics
Family Medicine	Pharmacokinetics
Geriatrics	Toxicology
Infectious Diseases	Transplant
Medication Safety	

Areas of Focus for Traditional Fellowship Programs.[5]

prepare the trainee to become an independent researcher in an academic setting and (2) industry fellowships that often provide a broad-based experience in areas relevant for a career in pharmaceutical industry.

Traditional fellowship programs are those intended to prepare you to become a future faculty member and conduct independent research. Most faculty positions require postgraduate training including a PGY-1 residency and preferably a PGY-2 specialty residency and/or a fellowship. While this may seem like a lot of additional training, this experience is often necessary to teach you how to transition from a student learner to someone who can lead a research team, gain funding necessary to support that research team, and teach others about that specialty area.[4]

Fellowships programs may differ in terms of the therapeutic focus, as depicted in Table 24-1.[5] These programs may also vary in terms of clinical involvement and laboratory components of the training experience, as well as in time requirements, teaching opportunities, and resources available to support your research. While some programs may offer mostly laboratory-based research, others may have more clinical (patient-oriented) or translational (bringing laboratory advances to the bedside) research. Many programs share one or more of the components recommended by ACCP in its formal guidelines for peer-reviewed clinical research fellowship programs. However, only seven programs have undergone and met the ACCP peer-reviewed criteria.[6]

ACCP recommends programs last at least 2 years in duration and includes at least 3000 hours of time spent on research-related activities.[7] In addition to the time requirement, the site must have certain resources available to support the program, including adequate research facilities, administrative support, and easy access to computer resources and scientific literature. The program needs to provide personnel qualified to teach the fellow research skills. ACCP states that fellowship preceptors should be clinical scientists who have a demonstrated track record of accomplishments in their respective area of research, including fellowship and/or graduate degree, experience as principal investigator on research projects and/or grants, and primary or senior authorship on peer-reviewed published scientific papers. Furthermore, the preceptor is expected to have ongoing research collaborations with others in the field. In addition to personnel, the program should facilitate training opportunities in research methods via graduate-level coursework or other experiences in areas such as biostatistics, ethics, and pharmacokinetics/pharmacodynamics.[7]

ACCP also states you should expect to complete at least one original research project during a fellowship, but this is not necessarily required. You should gain research experience through one or multiple projects by generating and testing a scientific hypothesis, writing and submitting protocols/grants, designing research studies, collecting/analyzing/interpreting data, preparing abstracts and posters for presentation at scientific meetings, writing/submitting manuscripts for publication, and participating in educational opportunities such as journal clubs, workshops, and seminars regarding research methods as well as ethics.[7] Research experiences can vary widely between fellowship programs, so careful research during the application process will help determine the best research experience for you.

Industry fellowships are another category of postgraduate fellowship training, with less emphasis on developing an individual as a principal investigator. Rather, these programs aim to develop a skill set that will prepare the fellow for a career in pharmaceutical industry. These programs are typically 1 or 2 years in duration. Experience may be gained in a variety of areas including clinical research, regulatory affairs, pharmacovigilance, drug safety, marketing, and health outcomes. Drug information fellowships may also be included in this category. Many of these industry-sponsored programs are affiliated with academia, but some are offered solely by the pharmaceutical company.

Larochelle et al. reviewed 131 fellowship programs offered in 2007, of which 58 (44.3%) met their definition of postgraduate industry fellowships.[8] Given the lack of accreditation of such programs, inconsistency between these industry fellowship experiences, and their different focus from traditional pharmacy research fellowship programs, Larochelle et al. recommended a set of standards for such programs. These included cosponsorship by an academic institution, with appropriate administrative and financial support; a dedicated and qualified fellowship preceptor with a position in the pharmaceutical industry and training in the fellowship's focus; access to adequate workspace, computer technology, and scientific literature; program duration of 1 to 2 years; at least 75% of fellow's time spent on program's area of focus; completion of at least two scholarly activities (poster presentation at a national meeting, textbook or journal article publication) by the fellow; fellow attendance at ≥ one national meeting in area of focus; fellow training on drug development; and fellow experience in the educational setting including didactic and/or experiential teaching of pharmacy students.[8]

Although at this time, none of the professional pharmacy organizations have adopted these criteria for assessing industry-based fellowship programs, you should carefully assess these important areas when considering an industry-based fellowship.

Pharmacoeconomics and outcomes research fellowships are another specialized category of fellowships. There are more than 50 of these programs. They are typically 2 years in duration, have pharmaceutical industry sponsorship, include training on research design and analysis, and have available resources such as scientific literature, computer technology, and software applications. These programs vary most in qualifications of program preceptors and time spent on experiential activities and didactic coursework. In 2008, ACCP and the International Society of Pharmacoeconomics and Outcomes Research (ISPOR) Fellowship task force recommended the following training program requirements[9]:

- Fellows spend at least 3000 hours engaged in pharmacoeconomics and outcomes research (PEOR) over a minimum of 2 years.

- Training programs have prespecified goals and objectives with adequate personnel/data resources to support the fellow's research.

- The program provides formal instruction in PEOR topics that may include didactic coursework through an advanced degree or certificate program completed during the fellowship.

- The program has structured evaluations of fellows as well as preceptors.

- The program provides a primary advisor for the fellow as well as a team of qualified preceptors with an established track record of experience, education, and collaboration in PEOR.

The task force recommends that fellows have clinical experience prior to initiation of the PEOR fellowship, via residency or work experience. Given the goal of becoming an independent investigator, fellows should complete at least one but ideally numerous research projects during their training. The fellow should be the lead investigator on at least one of these projects, although that may not be universally possible (particularly in the industry setting). Additional proficiencies for the fellow are outlined in the task force recommendations, and include participation in all aspects of study design/implementation/analysis, understanding measurements of economic, clinical, and patient-reported outcomes; comprehension of aspects of healthcare delivery system, communication skills, literature evaluation; and participation in research seminars and workshops.[9]

Fellowships may also be sponsored by governmental agencies (such as the FDA) or professional societies.[10,11] Some of these are cosponsored by academic institutions, and focus on specialty areas such as drug information or regulatory aspects of pharmaceutical industry. These programs aim to prepare the fellow for a career in academia and/or government. There are no standards of formal guidelines specific to these types of training programs, and therefore requirements and outcomes may vary for each program.

CAREER OPTIONS AND OPPORTUNITIES AVAILABLE FOR FELLOWSHIP-TRAINED PHARMACISTS

When considering postgraduate training, ask yourself, "Where do I see myself in 5 years?" What about 10 years from now? Without additional training, you may be relegating yourself to a very narrow area of practice. With fellowship training, there are numerable career opportunities available. Traditionally, most fellows would pursue academic faculty positions at colleges of pharmacy. They would conduct research and perhaps also teach. The faculty member would also likely write grants and pursue promotion on the basis of their scholarly activity, teaching, and service to the college. Clinical practice may also be a component of some of these positions.

With the increase in industry and other fellowship programs, fellows may pursue a career path that is less focused on independent research, and more focused on collaborative work or work conducted in a clinical setting. Outcomes research is particularly hot at the moment and offers positions in managed care organizations, academia, or industry settings.[12] Within industry, a myriad of positions are available in drug development, regulatory affairs, pharmacovigilance, medical information, pharmacology, pharmacokinetics/pharmacodynamics, toxicology, clinical operations, promotion, market research, business analytics, and medical affairs. In a recent survey, 90% of industry fellowship graduates remained in industry positions 1 to 5 years after completion of their fellowship program.[12]

PROCESS OF APPLYING AND OBTAINING A FELLOWSHIP POSITION

So, where do you start researching and applying to fellowship programs? Unlike PGY-1 residencies, the application process requires applicants to contact each program individually because there is no centralized directory of all fellowship programs and no match process. However, Rutgers Institute for Pharmaceutical Industry Fellowships coordinates fellowships with more than 12 biotechnology and pharmaceutical corporations.[13] There is one centralized application process for these programs through Rutgers. Additional industry fellowships are offered directly by biotechnology and pharmaceutical corporations. Applicants should contact those companies directly for materials. In addition, professional organizations such as ASHP, ACCP, and ISPOR maintain a directory of fellowship programs.

The timing of when to apply for fellowship depends on the types of program you are considering. It is never too early to start collecting information and researching various programs. You can meet program directors and current fellows at professional meetings such as the ASHP Midyear Clinical Meeting (MCM) and the ACCP Annual Meeting. In addition, Rutgers offers an on-campus Fellowship Information Day annually in November.

Given the extra time necessary to complete fellowship training, students often ask if it is possible to shorten the training time line and enter a fellowship program directly after obtaining their Doctor of Pharmacy degree. If you are considering a career in academia, you should strongly consider gaining clinical experience first through a PGY-1 and/or PGY-2 residency program. Since these programs are more clinically oriented, you will gain valuable experience that helps provide a basis for research and teaching later in your career. Likewise, even if your end goal is a career in pharmaceutical industry, having clinical expertise in your therapeutic area will help you in the long run. Long-term vision is incredibly important in planning your moves at this stage in your career.

The application process for fellowship is quite competitive, and there are several things you can do to make yourself more attractive as a candidate for these programs:

a. Maximize your GPA in pharmacy school courses and rotations by maintaining focus and dedication throughout your curriculum.

b. Select your clinical rotations carefully. Try to take an elective or extra rotation in your therapeutic area of interest. If you can do a rotation at the site where you later plan to apply for fellowship, this can be helpful if you perform well since then you would be a "known" entity.

c. Develop strong relationships with preceptors in your area of interest, who can mentor you and guide you through the process. You can ask these preceptors to review your portfolio and CV to identify areas of potential weakness that you can address prior to applying for postgraduate training.

d. Pursue a leadership position in at least one organization that is meaningful to you, rather than joining all the student organizations you can and having no leadership positions.

e. Obtain as many unique professional experiences as you can that will set you apart from the field of other candidates. These will be your talking points in your personal statement and future interviews! Seek industry internships, research clerkships, drug information experience, medical writing opportunities, etc.

f. Complete research projects as a student and get these published as posters at national society meetings and articles in peer-reviewed journals. This demonstrates your ingenuity and dedication to following a project through to completion, as well as develops your basic research skills.

g. Consider pursuing a joint degree while in pharmacy school or a postgraduate degree program such as a master's degree in clinical research, public health, global health, health sciences, pharmacy administration, statistics, pharmacoeconomics, health policy, or health outcomes research. If your ultimate career goals include conducting research, the practical research skills learned in these programs and collaborations you make with program faculty will vault your career even further.

h. Give careful thought to whom will provide future letters of recommendation for your application once you are ready to apply. It is never too early to start thinking about this, and too few students recognize the importance of selecting the best people to write the letters. You may be surprised to know: not all preceptors/faculty are good writers! Generally it is best to get letters from those who can assess your recent performance in a research setting, as well as your performance on relevant clinical rotations. It is substantially *less* helpful to have a letter from a professor who taught you 3 years previously in a large classroom setting. If you have several mentors to choose from, prioritize those who know you best, who can *critically* evaluate your performance (i.e., have worked with you on research or on rotations), and have extensive experience precepting fellows and residents. These individuals typically know what type of information selection committees are looking for in the letters. Likewise, if the recommenders have a track record of research in your field of interest, that is quite helpful.

PREPARING YOUR APPLICATION

Once you have decided to apply for fellowships, contact each of your potential references (you don't have to wait until you have the application in hand to ask them generally if they would write you a letter of recommendation!).

> "Keep in touch with your references and keep them posted on your status. It's a great way to thank them for their help regardless of the outcome."
>
> *Ngoc-Diep P. – P4 Forest Grove, Oregon*

Since some faculty members have so many students asking for letters, it is a good idea to ask references early in the process and then send them relevant materials as it gets closer to the application period. You should make your request in person, or at least with a phone call rather than a generic email. Make sure you speak to each recommender candidly about your interests in each program that you are considering, and ask them if they will be able to recommend you. Further details regarding letters of recommendation are available in Chapter 9. As with residency applications, you should provide your references with a comprehensive sheet outlining the program details and contact information (see Chapter 9, Table 9-2).

Many programs require additional site-specific forms that the student signs and then gives to the preceptor for evaluation. Make sure to sign your forms in advance in the appropriate area of the form to avoid unnecessary delays. If a program application is in electronic format, you typically need to gather email addresses from your references to input into the electronic system. The system will then generate an email to each recommender requesting the letter. Some email programs automatically place such emails into a spam folder as soon as they are received, so it is a good idea to alert your references that you have submitted their email address to the system and they should anticipate receiving a request for a letter of recommendation from that particular site. As the program deadline approaches, it is alright to follow up with each of your references to make sure they have submitted your letters. It is also a good idea to check with each site to ensure that your application is complete.

THE ON-SITE INTERVIEW

Programs will typically wait a few weeks after the application deadline to start inviting candidates for on-site interviews. The on-site interview is a great opportunity to get more information about the resources available to the fellow and speak to preceptors who would mentor the fellow throughout the program. It is very important for you to be well prepared before the interview. Using published resources to research typical interview questions is a good idea, but you don't want to seem too practiced or robotic in your answers. You should also talk with preceptors, residents, and other students about their interviewing experience. If a faculty member is willing to perform a mock interview with you, this is generally a good idea. Mock interviews can give you valuable experience answering questions under pressure, as well as feedback on areas where you might need improvement.

The key feature of the interview is taking the opportunity to let programs know what makes you stand out from the field of applicants. If you have completed a research project or published something in the past, expect to be asked about it during the interview. If you are not asked, then you can refer to this accomplishment during your interview as an example of your ability to follow something successfully through to completion. Chapter 10 offers excellent tips on a successful interview.

In addition to the traditional types of interview questions, you should take this opportunity to ask the program about the types of experiences and resources available to you as a fellow. If pursuing a traditional fellowship program, it is a good idea to do a literature search for the work of the program director, preceptors, and past fellows. This will give you an idea of the scope of their work, as well as some of their successes. You can then ask about opportunities within this line of work, or if there are other kinds of opportunities available for you at that site. You may also want to ask about the grants that the program personnel have obtained, as an indicator of the type of projects they generally perform (i.e., industry vs. government supported work) and their success in the funding arena. As you transition to an independent researcher, gaining funding from granting agencies is increasingly important.

It's also a good idea to ask what kinds of positions former trainees have obtained after completing the fellowship program at that site. This can provide insight on your potential future opportunities by completing that particular program. It is fair to ask about what challenges past fellows faced, and how they were able to overcome these challenges. This will give you valuable insight on some stumbling blocks that you may face, or allow the program to show you how they can respond and make changes to help you be successful.

SUMMARY

While it might seem daunting to enter into additional years of training after the education you have already received, investing your time in a fellowship program will pay dividends for the rest of your career. There are many different fellowship opportunities that offer experience in a wide variety of areas.

Although applying to fellowships is a competitive process, careful planning and attention throughout your time in pharmacy school will help prepare you to be the best possible candidate. Take the time to research programs and career options to find the best fit for you. Starting the process early will enable you ample time to gain experiences that set you apart from other applicants, seek valuable advice from career mentors that will guide you through the process, and secure interviews at your chosen sites. This chapter has given you an idea of what to look for in each program. Use this information to compare and contrast the programs as you decide which path to pursue. You are about to embark on the most exciting phase of your career!

Chapter Takeaways

▶ It's never too early to start thinking about and researching fellowship programs.

▶ Requirements and activities vary between fellowship programs so research each program carefully.

▶ Maximize your ability to be an attractive fellowship candidate by performing well in the classroom and seeking unique leadership and experiential activities that help you stand out.

▶ Work with a mentor throughout the process; prepare your applications carefully, and make sure you get the best possible letters of recommendation.

▶ Use the interview process to fully investigate the unique research and career aspects of each program.

ROLE FOR THE MENTOR

Ask your mentor to review your CV and portfolio to identify gaps in your experience, considering the types of fellowship programs that you are interested in. Try to gain additional experiences in these focus areas *before* you apply for fellowship programs.

Ask your mentor about their experiences with particular fellowship programs and past students that applied for fellowships. Ask them if there's anything the students wished they had known when they started the process that they had maybe overlooked.

Ask your mentor for feedback on your personal statement, as well as feedback on who you will ask for your letters of recommendation.

FREQUENTLY ASKED QUESTIONS

Q: Do fellowship programs last one or 2 years?
A: The duration of each fellowship program varies according to the type of program and preferences at each site.

Q: Do fellowship programs require a PGY-1 or PGY-2 residency to be completed prior to entering the fellowship program?

A: Requirements for previous clinical experience and training vary according to each fellowship program, although it is helpful to have some clinical and research experience prior to entering a fellowship program.

Q: How are fellowship programs different than residencies?

A: Although some fellowship programs are practice-oriented, fellowships generally have more of a research component than residencies, which are more clinically oriented.

References

1. Definitions of pharmacy residencies and fellowships. Am J Hosp Pharm. 1987;44(5):1142–1144.

2. Padiyara RS, Komperda KE. Effect of postgraduate training on job and career satisfaction among health-system pharmacists. Am J Health Syst Pharm. 2010;67(13):1093–1100.

3. Pleasants DZ, et al. Academic-drug industry fellowships. Drug Intell Clin Pharm. 1987;21(1): 112–114.

4. Murphy JE, Hawkey L. Education, postgraduate training, board certification, and experience requirements in advertisements for clinical faculty positions. Am J Pharm Educ. 2010;74(4):73.

5. American College of Clinical Pharmacy. Directory of Residencies, Fellowships & Graduate Programs; 2012. http://www.accp.com/resandfel/search.aspx. Accessed January 17, 2012.

6. American College of Clinical Pharmacy. Peer Review of Fellowships; 2012. http://www.accp.com/resandfel/peerReview.aspx. Accessed January 17, 2012.

7. American College of Clinical Pharmacy. ACCP Guidelines for Clinical Research Fellowship Training Programs; 2004. http://www.accp.com/resandfel/guidelines.aspx. Accessed January 17, 2012.

8. Larochelle PA, et al. Post-PharmD industry fellowship opportunities and proposed guidelines for uniformity. Am J Pharm Educ. 2009;73(1):20.

9. Kane-Gill S, Reddy P, Gupta SR, Bakst AW. Guidelines for pharmacoeconomic and outcomes research fellowship training programs: Joint guidelines from the American College of Clinical Pharmacy and the International Society of Pharmacoeconomics and Outcomes Research. Pharmacotherapy. 2008;28(12):1552.

10. Cunningham JE, Sheehan AH. Proposed guidelines for uniformity of postgraduate industry-affiliated fellowships. Am J Pharm Educ. 2009;73(5):93.

11. US Food and Drug Administration. Commissioner's Fellowship Program; 2012. http://www.fda.gov/AboutFDA/WorkingatFDA/FellowshipInternshipGraduateFacultyPrograms/CommissionersFellowshipProgram/default.htm. Accessed February 1, 2012.

12. Melillo S, et al. Postdoctoral pharmacy industry fellowships: A descriptive analysis of programs and postgraduate positions. Am J Health Syst Pharm. 2012;69(1):63–68.

13. Rutgers Institute of Pharmaceutical Industry Fewllowships. Rutgers Pharmaceutical Industry Fellowship Program; 2012. http://pharmafellows.rutgers.edu/home/index.php. Accessed January 17, 2012.

Advanced Degree Programs 25

Morton P. Goldman

You have been working diligently with your mentor to discuss career options. For your classmates who aren't going retail, everyone is talking about residency training. You think that might be the direction you want to go, but you are wondering if there are other post-PharmD options for you.[1]

> "It's exciting to consider all of the different areas of science and healthcare I can access after I graduate pharmacy school."
>
> *Cyle W. – Pharmacy Student, Tennessee*

This chapter will give you some introductory insight into advanced degrees that provide expanded career opportunities for individuals with a PharmD. Many of the programs described are intimately related to the pharmacy world.[2] Some may take you outside of the profession completely. We will focus here on those degrees that are most related to pharmacy or may take you to one or two degrees of separation. Table 25-1 lists the various areas of study that will be discussed and potential career opportunities.

A great way to begin is by visiting the American Association of Colleges of Pharmacy (AACP) Web site where they have a listing of all colleges of pharmacy that offer advanced degrees.[3] According to the site of the 126 accredited colleges of pharmacy, there are at least 69 colleges that offer a wide variety of graduate degrees. There are also a number of degree opportunities that are not associated with colleges of pharmacy. For some career goals, it would be wise to look at programs with a relationship to a college of pharmacy, but this is not necessary in all cases.

PHARMACY ADMINISTRATION, HEALTHCARE ADMINISTRATION, AND BUSINESS MANAGEMENT

We can start with a few common options. These include Masters of Science (MS) in pharmacy administration, Masters of Business Administration (MBA), and Masters of Healthcare Administration (MHA). These degrees will relate most to your pharmacy degree if your future interests are in management and leadership in pharmacy or health care.

The MS in pharmacy administration is not a uniform degree as some programs are geared toward the business and leadership of pharmacy, while

TABLE 25-1 • Advanced Degree Programs and Career Opportunities

Degree	Career Opportunity
Management-related degrees including MS pharmacy administration, MBA, MHA	Pharmacy administration, business (including managed care or retail pharmacy) healthcare administration, pharmaceutical industry, academia, government healthcare agencies
MS (science focus)	Research (basic science or clinical) in industry or academia
Public health or health policy (MPH or PhD)	Governmental agencies (e.g., Centers for Disease Control and Prevention), state and local health departments, nonprofit organizations, pharmaceutical industry, insurance companies, academia.
Regulatory affairs, industrial pharmacy, drug development (MS or PhD)	Pharmaceutical industry, governmental agencies, academia
Clinical research, clinical, and translational research	Academia, pharmaceutical industry, health-systems

MS, Masters of Science; MBA, Masters of Business Administration; MHA, Masters of Healthcare Administration; MPH, Masters of Public Health; PhD, Doctor of Philosophy.

others are science, statistics, and research based. Some programs focus on the understanding of pharmacoeconomics and outcomes research, while others are more social science based. You will need to take a significant amount of time researching the specifics of the programs. The easiest way may be to look online at the area that is most interesting to you. If it is pharmacoeconomics you are looking for, use that in your search terminology.

The MS in pharmacy administration that is *management* based will provide a specific curriculum dealing with the management and leadership required in pharmacy, with typical coursework including pharmacy operations, pharmacy finance, and research methods used in pharmacy practice. The accounting, budgeting, and leadership courses often have a pharmacy flavor to them. Many of these programs collaborate with the universities' business college, college of public health, or other appropriate programs.

There are specific MS programs in health-system pharmacy administration available as well. These programs have a significant focus on hospital practice, medication use systems, management, and leadership. There are also a growing number of MS health-system pharmacy administration programs that have teamed up with affiliated medical centers to provide a combined MS plus a 2-year residency in health-system pharmacy administration. These have become extremely competitive, as there are only 30 to 40 residency positions available nation-wide for these programs. Pharmacy-specific MS programs are best suited to prepare graduates for careers in pharmacy management and administration. There are also a number of graduates of these programs that have successful careers as vice presidents, presidents, chief operating officers or chief

"Consider your faculty and preceptors as valuable resources for learning about postgraduate training opportunities. For example, if you are interested in pursuing an MBA, make an appointment to speak with someone in your university's college of business. They will appreciate your interest."

Cyle W. – Pharmacy Student, Tennessee

executive officers of hospitals or health systems, and leaders in other career venues. There are a handful of programs that are available online. These offerings continue to grow in number.

The MBA provides students with exposure to most areas of business including accounting, finance, marketing, operations, and human resources. These are essential elements for careers in any type of management or administration. In pharmacy, these skills are key components in pharmacy management and leadership. Most MBA programs allow a concentration in a specific discipline, such as accounting, marketing, health care, and information systems. Many programs offer dual degrees that combine an MBA with a variety of other degrees. Several programs combine the MBA with an MHA. These combined programs typically have all of the components of an MHA program with added coursework in finance, marketing, and legal issues.

The MHA provides students with the tools and fundamentals for careers in healthcare administration. Typical coursework includes health finance and economics, health policy, healthcare management, operations and leadership, health information technology, and more. Most programs will either require or allow a focus in one of these areas. The MHA provides a more focused course of study in the arena of health systems and health as compared with the typical MBA, but a broader healthcare focus than a degree in pharmacy administration. The combined MBA/MHA programs typically provide both depth and breadth in health care and business.

Participation in an MBA or MHA program outside of pharmacy may have the benefit of meeting classmates with different business or healthcare perspectives. Interacting with physicians, nurses, health administrators, and other business people may help to define your view of the role of pharmacy. Completion of any of these administrative degrees will allow you to pursue management and leadership positions ahead of those individuals who have a PharmD degree only. If you also have a PGY-1 residency, you may even be more marketable. Those degrees with combined health-system pharmacy administration residencies open the doors even faster, but are clearly specific for health-system pharmacy.

OTHER MASTERS AND DOCTOR OF PHILOSOPHY DEGREES

There are a wide variety of paths you can take if you are interested in the basic sciences and research. As described above, the nomenclature in this area is confusing where the basic science, pharmacoeconomics, statistics, and health policy degrees may be listed under pharmacy administration or pharmaceutical sciences. The MS degrees most related to pharmacy include the pharmaceutical sciences (pharmaceutics, pharmaceutical chemistry, pharmacognosy, toxicology, etc.), pharmacoeconomics/outcomes research, public health, clinical research, or industrial/regulatory pharmacy.

The Doctor of Philosophy (PhD) is the highest academic degree that anyone can pursue. It requires the true mastery of a subject and trains you in research and research methods. Most of the programs that offer basic science, pharmacoeconomics/outcomes research, and industrial pharmacy MS degrees, also offer the ability to obtain the PhD in that discipline. PhD degrees are also available in pharmacy administration programs. They meet all of the criteria for a PhD as a research-based discipline. There are also master's degrees and PhDs available for all basic science disciplines (chemistry, biology, etc.). Suffice to say that the PhD degree is geared toward those individuals aspiring to have careers in research, academics, or industry and could possibly take you far from the practice of pharmacy.

PHARMACOECONOMICS AND OUTCOMES RESEARCH

An MS or PhD in pharmacoeconomics and outcomes research is a growing area of interest in industry and academia. Determining the cost and related outcomes in healthcare is extremely complex and takes a specific knowledge of pharmacoeconomics methods, biostatistics, and clinical knowledge. The coursework involved in these programs may include coursework in biostatistics, pharmacoeconomics, modeling and design, research methods, epidemiology, public health, and a project or thesis. Some of the MS programs may also include coursework in marketing and management. The PhD curriculum is a deeper and broader dive into these areas of study with the completion of a major thesis. For some employers in industry or academics, the PharmD in combination with an MS in this area may be better than the PhD without the PharmD degree. The clinical knowledge plus the MS degree is a very marketable combination.

PUBLIC HEALTH AND HEALTH POLICY

Master's degrees in public health (MPH) or health policy are also excellent choices for individuals with a PharmD. Degrees in public health and health policy are focused on what is done collectively to assure that there are conditions and services in place to improve and protect the health of a community. Public health practice spans from small communities, to larger populations, to solving public health dilemmas on a global basis. The curricula may include coursework or practical experience in community health, economics and finance, epidemiology, biostatistics, infectious diseases, global health, and environmental health. Many programs have the ability to choose an area of concentration. The MPH or PhD in public health or health policy can either have a practice or academic direction. Careers can include governmental organizations, nongovernmental organizations, and universities. Any organization or business that looks at populations has the need for individuals with these degrees. The combination of the pharmacy background puts you in a unique position.

CLINICAL RESEARCH

The MS in clinical research provides education and training to doctoral level health professionals interested in developing skills in clinical research. Typically, a 2-year program includes practical (research) and didactic components and may include a final research project, presentation at a national meeting, or a completed grant proposal. Most of these programs are not usually housed within colleges of pharmacy (there are a few), but may be in the university's college of graduate studies, medical college, college of public health, and others. Some universities offer dual degree programs aligned with a PharmD or MD degree. In addition, there are programs that offer MS and PhDs in clinical and translational research. Translational research has the goal of taking basic science research and making it applicable to clinical situations (from bench to bedside). These degrees set you up nicely to be able to perform clinical research either as a clinician in a hospital setting or as a faculty member or in industry.

REGULATORY SCIENCE, INDUSTRIAL PHARMACY, AND DRUG DEVELOPMENT

MS and PhD degrees are available that send you directly to the pharmaceutical industry. Although the degrees do vary slightly, curricula typically will include drug development, research, biostatistics, regulatory, finance, and manufacturing. They provide students with all aspects of pharmaceutical industry processes from chemical entity development to clinical trials to marketing of new products. Careers can also include working for governmental agencies or academia.

PHARMD COMBINED PROGRAMS

All of the advanced degrees discussed in this chapter are available in combined programs with a PharmD degree. If you have started the thought process of post-PharmD opportunities early enough, you may need to look no further than your present college of pharmacy. The AACP Web site has a complete 2012 to 2013 listing of combined programs that are offered within the colleges of pharmacy and in cooperation with other programs. Some of these programs do not take additional time to complete, but many of them do have add-on components that require additional time. Typically, the combined degrees take less time than doing the PharmD followed by the next degree. These are great options for those of you who already have specific career direction.

REQUIREMENTS FOR GRADUATE PROGRAM ADMISSION

The basic requirement for admission to graduate programs can be found in Table 25-2. Although each program may have its own prerequisites, you will likely be required to take one of two standardized tests: the Graduate Management Admission Test (GMAT) or the Graduate Record Exam (GRE).

The GMAT is owned and administered by the Graduate Management Admission Council (GMAC) that is a nonprofit organization for graduate business schools around the globe.[4] The test is used to determine whether prospective students have the ability and skills to succeed in a typical business school curriculum. It is made up of three sections: verbal (reading comprehension, critical reasoning, sentence correction), quantitative (problem solving and data sufficiency), and analytical writing assessment. Most students score between 400 and 600 (on a scale of 200 to 800) with the higher-ranking MBA programs requiring scores in the 600 to 750 range.

The Educational Testing Service (ETS) is a nonprofit organization that develops, administers, and scores the GRE now called the GRE revised general test.[5] This exam is also made up of verbal, quantitative, and analytical writing

TABLE 25-2 • Advanced Degree Program Requirements and Availability

Degree	Testing Requirements[a]	Previous Degree Requirements	Available Totally Distance Learning	Combined Programs Available with PharmD
MBA	GMAT (or GRE)	Bachelors	Yes	Yes
MS (administration)	GMAT or GRE[b]	Bachelors	Yes	Yes
MS (basic science, other)	GRE[b]	Bachelors	Yes	Yes
MHA	Variable[a]	Bachelors	Yes[d]	Yes
MPH	GMAT/GRE/ LSAT/MCAT[c]	Bachelors	Yes	Yes
MSCR	Variable[a]	Most often professional doctorate degree	Yes	Yes
PhD	Variable[a]	Bachelors	Yes[d]	Yes

[a]Check with the individual program for testing requirements; programs combined with PharmD degrees may accept PCAT.
[b]GRE/GMAT may or may not be required for some programs—some programs may allow PCAT or MCAT in lieu of GRE or GMAT.
[c]A program may accept any of these.
[d]Not all MS or PhD degree types will be available as online or distance learning.

MS, Masters of Science; MBA, Masters of Business Administration; MHA, Masters of Health Care Administration; MPH, Masters of Public Health; MSCR, Masters of Science, Clinical Research or Clinical and Translational Research; PhD, Doctor of Philosophy.

assessments, with some additional emphasis on word relationships and basic mathematics (including algebra and geometry). The new scoring system (as of August, 2011) separates out the verbal and quantitative, each on a scale of 130 to 170. The writing section is scored on a scale of 1 to 6. Many MBA programs will accept either the GMAT or the GRE. Many colleges offering MS degrees in basic sciences require the GRE.

These tests are generally administered at local testing centers. The GRE is available only in October, November, and February. The GMAT is available on a rolling basis with time stipulations for retesting. More information can be found on the ETS and GMAC Web sites.

ADVANTAGES AND DISADVANTAGES OF ADVANCED DEGREE PROGRAMS

As you have a specific career goal in mind, advanced degree programs may be the right directions for you to take. In addition, some employers may have tuition incentive programs that are part of your benefit package to encourage you to advance your training, especially if they are interested in grooming you for management or leadership roles. If you keep your pharmacy license current, there is no downside to advanced training. If you find that you are not happy with the program or career path you chose, you can easily return to a typical pharmacy career.

Students with PharmD and MBA typically can expect to earn approximately 10% more in compensation than individuals without an MBA.[6] In general, faculty members at universities tend to make less money than practicing pharmacists, but this gap is narrowing. The gap is even wider for individuals with PhDs in academia.[7] But it is not all about the money. The advanced degree programs discussed in this chapter will either broaden your career options, or narrow them to a focused and fulfilling career choice. There is never a downside to more education.

The PharmD curriculum, which includes significant basic sciences, communication, literature evaluation, therapeutics, and business knowledge, has prepared you quite well for careers both inside and outside of pharmacy practice. Pursing an advanced degree program is among the many excellent choices you can make to enhance your skills in a variety of areas.

Chapter Takeaways

▶ There are tremendous opportunities to expand the value of your PharmD degree by participating in additional advanced degree programs.

▶ Many advanced degree programs are available as combined programs with the PharmD degree.

▶ Some advanced degrees will take you away from the typical careers in pharmacy practice, administration, academics, etc.

▶ Many advanced degrees are offered online, and employers may have tuition reimbursement plans for relevant degrees.

ROLE FOR THE MENTOR

The mentor should be able to advise students regarding postgraduate training other than residency training.

The mentor should be aware of dual degree programs and other graduate program available at his/her own university.

Encourage students with various career aspirations to pursue their goals.

FREQUENTLY ASKED QUESTIONS

Q: **What postgraduate degrees are available online or distance learning?**

A: Most of the master's degrees discussed are available as online or distance learning programs. There are large numbers of the management-related MS degrees available online. There are few MS or PhD degrees in the basic sciences available as online learning.

Q: **How do I know if my future employer will pay for an advanced degree?**

A: Tuition reimbursement programs will be part of your benefits package. You will need to check with the human resources department to determine availability.

Q: **Do advanced degree programs take the place of postgraduate residency training?**

A: Although this may be considered a debatable issue, there is never a downside to residency training. For specific career goals in research-based academics or industry, most MS and PhD programs will be sufficient. The experience of having completed residency training may give you an edge over other candidates who have not. This is particularly true in the management track.

References

1. Hagemeier NE, Murawski MM. Economic analysis of earning a PhD degree after completion of a PharmD degree. Am J Pharm Educ. 2011;75(1) article 15:1–10.

2. Chumney ECG, Ragucci KR, Jones KJ. Impact of a dual PharmD/MBA on graduates' academic performance, career opportunities, and earning potential. Am J Pharm Educ. 2008;72(2) article 26:1–6.

3. Schommer JC, Brown LM, Sogol EM. Work profiles identified from the 2007 pharmacist and pharmaceutical scientist career pathway profile survey. Am J Pharm Educ. 2008;72(1) article 2:1–7.

4. American Academy of Colleges of Pharmacy: Is Pharmacy for You? http://www.aacp.org/resources/student/pharmacyforyou/Pages/default.aspx. Accessed March 12, 2012.

5. American Society of Health-System Pharmacists. Job Market Perceptions Report. December 2011. http://www.ashp.org/jobmarketperceptions. Accessed March 12, 2012.

6. Graduate Management Admission Council. http://www.gmac.com. Accessed March 12, 2012.

7. Educational Teaching Services. http://www.ets.org. Accessed March 12, 2012.

SECTION IV

Road Under Construction: The Future of Postgraduate Pharmacy Residency Training

• Kelly M. Smith

INTRODUCTION

If you've reached your destination of postgraduate training, what can be left? As you read about in Chapter 1, today's residency training model is much different from that of years past. We can only expect that the future will continue to hold changes in how we view postgraduate training, especially residencies, where we will find them, and how they will be delivered. Section IV gives you an early glimpse of those future changes to your career development map. Read on to learn how the world approaches pharmacy residency training, and if obtaining a passport or visa (no, not the credit card) in the name of your own career training should be on your to-do list. If training outside your home country is not on your bucket list, this section still holds important lessons for you. Chapter 27 provides a gaze into the future of residency training, including thoughts on your role as an attending pharmacist, the support your college of pharmacy may provide in coordinating your residency program conducted 300 miles away, and how a practicing pharmacist can also join the ranks of resident trainees. It's important for you to update your car's GPS to account for changes in the highway system, and the same can be said for the need to continually update your career GPS. So, buckle up and let's complete the journey.

Beyond Borders: Postgraduate Pharmacy Training from an International Perspective

26

Charles E. Daniels

Did you know there is an American Society of Health-System Pharmacists (ASHP)-accredited residency program in Saudi Arabia? And, did you know that program is accredited under a different residency standard? Although international pharmacy residency training is not a common consideration for US pharmacists, knowing how the rest of the world approaches residency training, and how you may fit into that international perspective, may be helpful. Consider this chapter to be a journey down the residency road less traveled.

PROFESSIONAL DEGREE PATHS

Before you examine international residency training, you first must understand global approaches to professional pharmacy education. There is no internationally uniform professional degree or curriculum for the profession of pharmacy. As an early proponent of the clinical pharmacy practice model, the United States has long-established training programs to support that goal. Since the 1970s, that goal has attracted international students and practicing pharmacists to the United States to pursue PharmD degrees. As clinical pharmacy has taken hold in many other global regions, many countries have developed corollary formal educational programs. The master's degree in clinical pharmacy is offered in some countries, while others now offer a PharmD degree. Those with emerging clinical degree offerings may send their pharmacy faculty to the United States to grow their clinical skills and learn how pharmacy students are educated and trained, so that they may return to their home country to implement these newly learned skills and educational approaches. You may be on one of these educational paths, or you may have classmates who bring these professional motivations to your pharmacy classroom.

Because there is no uniform international model for pharmacy education, there is no global accreditation process for specific degree programs. However, non-US-based programs can ascribe to the American accreditation model, as evidenced by Lebanese American University, the first and currently only non-US pharmacy school with ACPE accreditation. This could open the door for additional ACPE-accredited PharmD programs across the globe.

RESIDENCY TRAINING BEYOND US BORDERS

Formal pharmacy residency training programs are conducted in many countries around the globe. Most pharmacy residency training programs in the international setting are designed to prepare pharmacists for a career in that specific country. As in the United States, these programs are also individually linked with unique license or examination requirements for entering residents.

As with pharmacy degree training, there is no singular international vision for the nature, operations, or accreditation of pharmacy residency programs. However, in 2009, ASHP's COC approved its first international pharmacy residency accreditation standard (see Chapters 1 and 3).[1] That accreditation standard is much the same as the Postgraduate Year One (PGY-1) standard used in US institutions, with modifications to entering resident qualifications and specific elements of the recruitment process. A hospital residency program in Saudi Arabia is the first and only to have been accredited under the ASHP International Standard, with the emergence of others likely in the future.

In order to best understand specific residency opportunities in any individual country, you should contact pharmacy societies, pharmacy schools, or major hospitals in the country of your interest. Your current pharmacy faculty may even have international colleagues who can assist you in identifying residency-training opportunities.

> "Ask your mentors and preceptors if they have any experience with pharmacy outside of the United States. Pharmacy can be a small world, and you may be surprised by who they know!"
>
> *Morgan H. – Pharmacy Student, Tennessee*

Another source of information about both international pharmacy practice and residency training is the International Pharmaceutical Federation (FIP), a global membership organization that brings together pharmacy practitioners through its Community Pharmacy and Hospital Pharmacy Sections.[2] The networking provided by FIP's Young Pharmacists Group may also help you set up contacts for international training. Don't overlook US gatherings of international pharmacists at meetings of the American College of Clinical Pharmacy, American Pharmacists Association, and American Society of Health-System Pharmacists, as these too provide excellent networking venues.

Now it's time to grab your passport for this quick tour of pharmacy residency programs that span the globe. While this is not a comprehensive tour, you can easily conduct a quick Internet search for a listing of both PharmD and pharmacy residencies across the world.

CANADA

Residency training in Canada is a broad-based and integral component of professional training, and is most commonly sponsored by the country's hospitals or hospital regions. Information about Canadian programs can be found on the Internet, particularly through the Canadian Society of Hospital Pharmacists' catalog of residency programs accreditation by the Canadian Hospital Pharmacy Residency Board (CHPRB).[3] A national matching program is offered and can also be accessed through the CHPRB site. These elements resemble those of the American approach to accreditation conducted by ASHP. However, one striking difference from the US process is that pharmacists who successfully complete programs accredited by the CHPRB are entitled to include "ACPR" (Accredited Canadian Pharmacy Residency) as part of their official pharmacy title.

EUROPE

Postgraduate training is closely linked to the pharmacy degree process in many European countries. In some settings, practice regulations and customs require specialized training of an additional 2 to 6 years beyond the entry-level pharmacy degree. For instance, hospital specialization in the Netherlands requires completion of a 4-year post-PharmD residency. In addition to clinical specialization, other areas for specialty training include pharmaceutical industry, regulatory, and medicinal biology. Each country is unique in its requirements for practice credentials and models of training.

MIDDLE EAST

Structured residency training programs are offered at several hospitals in the Kingdom of Saudi Arabia.[4] Saudi programs are accredited by the Saudi Commission on Health Specialties. These 2-year programs that provide hospital-based pharmacy training allow a new pharmacy graduate to learn about operations and clinical aspects of pharmacy service. King Faisal Specialist Hospital (Riyadh, KSA) is the first, and currently only, internationally conducted, ASHP-accredited residency program.

ASIA

Formalized residency training is in its early stages but developing rapidly in Singapore. Clinical residency programs are currently offered in pharmacy infectious disease at Singapore General Hospital,[5] and hematology/oncology at the National University of Singapore Hospital.[6] Both programs are 1 year in length and are suited to pharmacists entering with experience in hospital pharmacy. Completion of a PGY-1 program prior to application to these specialized programs may provide you with the needed pharmacy background. There is a well-described process for graduates of non-Singapore pharmacy schools to become licensed in order to meet that prerequisite for the residency. Residency programs are also offered at several university teaching hospitals in

Japan and in other Asian countries. You can learn more about each program by directly contacting its sponsoring organization (e.g., hospital).

OTHER REGIONS

Pharmacy training throughout Africa is less formalized. Some programs are conducted by individual hospitals, while other post-PharmD clinical training programs are linked to international partners. For example, Rutgers University supports HIV/AIDS clinical training programs in South Africa.[7] While there are no clinical pharmacy residency training programs currently in Mexico or Latin America, some may emerge by the time you begin your residency search.

FINDING YOUR PATH

Now that your global tour is complete, are you ready to forgo the Montana winters for a few years of training in Spain? Or, do you dream of traveling to the United States for your residency training? Before you pack your bags, consider what may be the most important message of this chapter: the knowledge you gain and the credentials you obtain from a residency in one country are not likely suitable for the credentials for your dream job in another country. A training path in Spain cannot be interchanged for a training path in the United States. Thus, you should carefully consider all elements of your own situation when evaluating international training opportunities.

US RESIDENCY PATH FOR GRADUATES OF NON-US PROGRAMS

Residency training in the United States is an attractive proposition for many pharmacists from across the globe, but the path can be rocky.[8] The journey to pharmacist licensure for you as a graduate of a non-US college of pharmacy includes successful completion of standardized examinations in language skills and pharmacy knowledge before becoming eligible for a pharmacist intern permit in a US state. Following that, you must meet the internship experience requirements (e.g., 1500 hours) of the state in which you will pursue licensure. Once you have the requisite experience, you are then eligible to undertake the National Pharmacy Board (NAPLEX) examination and relevant law examinations in your pursuit of licensure as a pharmacist. This journey toward US licensure can be a long one, often exceeding 1 year. Most US programs are unwilling to consider your application if you are not immediately eligible for US licensure, as you would have to wait until your licensure is imminent before you could begin the residency program. This element alone often stops a foreign pharmacy graduate's dreams of pursuing a US residency.

Beyond licensure, perhaps a bigger challenge is your ability to legally pursue training in the United States. If you are a foreign national, you must now overcome the visa hurdle.[8] There are multiple visa types (e.g., H1B), and they can be applied for different steps in your path toward pharmacy practice.

Obtaining a visa to enroll in a PharmD degree program (e.g., F1 visa) is generally easier to obtain than approval for nondegree programs, like most residencies and many fellowships. Additionally, the visa requirements may be different for the type of training you seek. A single additional year of training (e.g., PGY-1 residency) following graduation from an ACPE-accredited US college of pharmacy is readily attainable through the optional practical training provision of an F1 visa. However, if you are a foreign national on a F1 visa seeking additional training (e.g., Postgraduate Year Two [PGY-2] residency), or you are a graduate of a non-US college of pharmacy seeking entry into the country solely for PGY-1 residency training, you will likely be required to seek an H1B visa that requires official sponsorship by your employer (your residency program), a process that entails financial investment and a lengthy paperwork process. Because many residency programs lack experience with this process, you may wish to consider those sites with strong connections to graduate medical education or international student education, as they likely will have local resources or expertise in the visa process. Programs with these resources often are conducted at large academic medical centers or universities. Training programs that are tied to graduate degrees lack this additional visa hurdle.

Any way you look at it, the journey to a US residency for a foreign national is a long one. Yet, for many, the benefits far outweigh the challenges. If your career goal is to practice in a progressive US setting, your US training will increase your competitiveness for employment. If your career dream is to be your country's first board-certified clinical specialist in oncology, you can certainly garner the necessary credentials by pursuing a PGY-2 oncology residency in the United States. And, don't forget the growing role for US residency trained pharmacists who wish to develop clinical pharmacy practices or clinical training programs outside of the United States.

INTERNATIONAL TRAINING PATH FOR US PHARMACY GRADUATES–*CAVEAT EMPTOR*

The world has become "smaller" in many ways, and pharmacists are following this shift as they participate in global health initiatives. Additionally, international APPE rotation offerings may be paralleling your university's growing number of international students. You have much to gain from training experiences beyond the American border. Such a value has been recognized by AACP, which is currently working to standardize best practices, orientation, and evaluation of international training rotations for US pharmacy students. Yet, your yearning for international training may far surpass an APPE rotation, and instead extend to your determination to pursue a residency outside of the United States. Understand that there is no clear track record for a pharmacy career that includes a PharmD degree from a US pharmacy school, followed by residency training abroad. The Latin phrase *Caveat emptor* (buyer beware) certainly applies, as you will be blazing your own trail with few examples of how a future career will unfold. If you desire a *career abroad*, then you may be well served by international residency training, as the training may serve as an entry into practice into your country of destination. Alternatively, if you are considering residency training abroad to expand your global perspectives as you pursue an eventual *US pharmacy career*, you should carefully examine more traditional and established paths. Consider alternatives such as obtaining a graduate degree (e.g., masters degree in public health), participating in medical missions or brigades, or employment with international agencies (e.g., World Health Organization).

If you remain undeterred from seeking international residency training, closely examine the nature of the credential you will obtain and the type of additional training or practice for which you will be qualified. As a pharmacist with residency training from abroad, you will not likely be qualified for ASHP-accredited PGY-2 training programs. Residency programs not accredited by ASHP, which to date includes nearly all international residencies, often do not provide sufficient credentials for many US practice settings. If you are fully committed to international residency training, completing an ASHP-accredited PGY-1 pharmacy residency prior to undertaking international training may be advisable. Regardless of your motives for international training, you should review your plan with your mentor or a trusted advisor, as you will indeed be venturing into foreign territory.

BON VOYAGE

There is great value in understanding pharmacy from an international perspective, and much to be learned and applied through life-changing international experiences. US-educated pharmacy students considering international residency training should approach the issue thoughtfully, and be certain that the programs pursued will provide strong value in their career and personal goals. It is not certain how much the training itself will enhance your skills as a pharmacist, though you will undoubtedly expand your view of the world that will impact you forever. International pharmacy students or pharmacists who are thinking about pharmacy residency training in the United States need to expect an uphill course. You should review the rules for participation in residency or other programs prior to application to minimize frustration with the obstacles you will encounter. Don't consider taking the road less traveled unless you are confident that it is the best option for your personal and professional plans.

Chapter Takeaways ....

▶ International pharmacy education and training models vary, and the credentials are generally not interchangeable.

▶ There is no comprehensive directory of international pharmacy residency training opportunities. Individual communications and networking with pharmacists and pharmacy organizations in the country of interest may provide the most complete picture.

▶ Not all residency programs have been subject to quality review through an accreditation process. Accreditation may be provided by local or national review boards, though there is an ASHP international accreditation standard and process for non-US programs to become accredited.

▶ US residency training for foreign nationals or non-US trained pharmacists is a long and winding road with many obstacles to the applicant.

▶ US trained pharmacists should carefully review the objectives and content of international programs to ensure they align with their own career plans.

ROLE FOR THE MENTOR

Assist the student in aligning the scope, nature, and setting of advanced training options with his/her career plan.

Discuss the potential merits of international training for the student, and how he/she may fit into global health practices.

FREQUENTLY ASKED QUESTIONS

Q: Can I apply to an accredited PGY-2 residency program in the United States after completing a residency program outside the United States?

A: ASHP-accredited PGY-2 programs require that the resident complete an accredited PGY-1 residency prior to beginning the specialized program. There is a process for a nontraditionally trained applicant to submit credentials of equivalent experience for review by the ASHP Accreditation Services Division, which may clear the applicant to participate in the matching program and be qualified for a PGY-2 program. However, there is no guarantee that such an exception will be granted.

Q: Will I receive "credit" for my international residency training if I go on to practice pharmacy in a different country?

A: That is entirely dependent on the employing organization that you wish to work in. A transfer of credentials between countries is highly unlikely at this point, given the variability in pharmacy education and training models.

References

1. ASHP International Accreditation Standard for Postgraduate Year One (PGY-1) Pharmacy Residency Programs. http://www.ashp.org/DocLibrary/Accreditation/ASDInternationalStd010410. Accessed March 3, 2012.

2. International Pharmaceutical Federation. http://www.fip.org. Accessed March 1, 2012.

3. Canadian Society of Hospital Pharmacists. Canadian Hospital Pharmacy Residency Board and Canadian residency matching service. http://www.cshp.ca/programs/residencyTraining/index_e.asp. Accessed February 20, 2012.

4. Saudi Commission for Health Specialties. Accredited Directors/Centers in Programs. http://english.scfhs.org.sa/index.php?option=com_content&view=article&id=699&Itemid=5510. Accessed February 20, 2012.

5. Singapore General Hospital. Infectious Disease Pharmacy Residency. http://www.sgh.com.sg/subsites/pgahi/Programmes/Postgraduate/Pages/infectious-disease-pharmacy-residency.aspx. Accessed February 13, 2012.

6. National University of Singapore. Clinical Pharmacy Residency. http://www.pharmacy.nus.edu.sg/programmes/ClinPharmResid/. Accessed February 13, 2012.

7. Collins KD. Facing the reality of AIDS in Africa. Rutgers Focus; July 2010. http://news.rutgers.edu/focus/issue.2010-07-01.2257001546/article.2010-07-07.2930951369. Accessed February 13, 2012.

8. Traynor K. Non-U.S. pharmacists face residency hurdles. Am J Health Syst Pharm. 2012;69:450–452.

On the Horizon: The Future of Pharmacy Residency Training 27

Kelly M. Smith

While Benjamin Franklin's assertion that, "In this world nothing can be said to be certain, except death and taxes," is generally viewed as a commentary on the role of government in our lives, it too reflects the inevitability of change. Such change extends to postgraduate pharmacy training; what you see today may be just that—what residency training is today. Predicting the specific seminal events and changes in residency training that will occur over the rest of your professional career is impossible, yet you can be prepared for changes that are feasible over the next 5 to 10 years. These changes, as summarized in Table 27-1, may be transparent to you as a student or eager residency candidate, while others will touch you directly. Regardless of those most affected, these changes can be illustrated by some age-old idioms, so brace yourself for what lies ahead.

THERE'S MORE THAN ONE WAY TO SKIN A CAT

While that sentiment evokes a frightening (and fortunately, unimaginable) scene, it does illustrate the concept that differing approaches to a number of life's quandaries exist, and the same holds true for pharmacy residency training. Today's stand-alone Postgraduate Year One (PGY-1) and Postgraduate Year Two (PGY-2) programs may become tomorrow's multiyear programs. In your desire to become a transplant pharmacist, you may commit to 2 years of training during your initial match process, rather than the current 1 + 1 model. That approach is seen with some areas of specialization currently, including residencies in pharmacotherapy and administration. The integration of graduate degree programs (e.g., Master of Science and Master of Business Administration) into residency training, a current feature of many health-system pharmacy administration residency programs, may also grow in numbers. And, as pharmacy grows in its intricacy and complexity, who knows if 1 year or 2 of training will be sufficient? The rate of discovery and innovation in pathophysiology, diagnosis, and therapeutic regimens is expected to escalate, or at the least not diminish during the 40+ years of your pharmacy career (gulp). Our medical colleagues have learned over the years that more time is needed

TABLE 27-1 • Pharmacy Residency Changes on the Horizon

- Multiyear (e.g., 2-year) residency programs
- Graduate degree pursuit integrated with residency training
- Working professional (nontraditional) residency programs
- Staggered residency start dates
- New residency training environments
- Expanded residency "class" size
- Regional program administration
- Team-based experiential education and training—the attending pharmacist model
- Simulation in training
- Centralized residency application process (PhORCAS) - effective Fall 2012

to train a highly skilled physician, and the likelihood that the same is true for pharmacy is quite high. Do I hear Postgraduate Year Three (PGY-3), anyone? While such a concept has not been fully vetted by the profession, do not be surprised if you hear about it soon.

Speaking of new training models, who says you have to be a resident for 12 consecutive months? Residents bring tremendous value to a practice site, one measure of which is the pipeline of well-trained pharmacists who can be retained as full-time employees upon residency graduation. Unfortunately, not every practice site has a complement of pharmacists who completed residency training. Maybe they had differing career goals upon graduation or were unable to find a residency that fit their needs. For those who go on to desire advanced skills or have new practice interests that require residency training, this has usually meant the need for the pharmacist to resign from his job to seek a residency, only then to return to the market in search of a new job. This leaves the employer without the services of a pharmacist who was an excellent contributor to the pharmacy team. Now, both the practice site and pharmacist can benefit from developing a nontraditional residency program.[1] In such a structure, pharmacists assume the role of a resident during defined time periods, rather than 12 consecutive months. This take on interval training, which still likely increases the heart rate but not from aerobic activity, allows a pharmacist to serve as a resident during short periods of time (e.g., month-long rotations alternating between pharmacist and resident roles), while retaining their employment as a pharmacist. In addition to gaining advanced patient care skills, the pharmacist can focus on cultivating his practice leadership, administrative, and project management skills, which are other components of residency training that are not easily integrated into staff development programs offered by employers. In this scenario, the pharmacist and the practice site do not have to sever ties, as the practitioner gains additional skills and the employer retains a pharmacist who soon is able to contribute to the site at a much higher level, yielding a win-win situation.

Sequencing program activities so that each member of the residency class begins and completes the program at the same time each year may make their oversight and management easier for program administrators, but is it optimal for everyone?[2] We are starting to see a handful of residencies with training dates well apart from the traditional July through June calendar. Directors are realizing that some new graduates need a bit of time following graduation to take care of life's issues. (Do I hear wedding bells, anyone? How about backpacking across Europe?) Practitioners who wish to return to residency training, whether they bypassed a residency immediately upon graduation or failed to match to a program, may also be great candidates to begin a residency program in January, rather than July. Some hospital employees note that July is the worst time of the year to be admitted to a teaching hospital, a nod to the large turnover in resident physicians at that time. As those who are well trained and familiar with the institution's practices depart, a new crop of naïve physicians arrives, increasing the likelihood of medical errors and cases gone awry. That is yet another justification for staggered start and stop times for residency training. And, a large turnover in well-trained pharmacists, especially in the summer when many veteran pharmacists may be taking personal leave, may not be in the best interests of the department or patient care.

LOCATION, LOCATION, LOCATION

Do you ever wonder who envisioned the day when you could stroll into a grocery store to grab freshly carved turkey breast from the deli counter, a gallon of milk, replacement contact lenses, cash a check at the local bank branch, file your income tax return, have your car's oil changed, and pick up your prescription refills? Such a confluence of daily conveniences is commonplace in today's big-box superstores. How does this relate to pharmacy residencies? Well, much of our profession and where we are today has been the result of visionaries who saw the need for us to do more, and the opportunities for us to indeed demonstrate the unique things we as pharmacists can do. That means that the pharmacy specialties of today may be different from those of the future. For instance, once a stalwart of clinical pharmacy specialization, nutrition support pharmacy has somewhat diminished in its role as a specialty, with more advanced practitioners (e.g., critical care pharmacists) incorporating nutrition support into their daily practices. While there is still a role for specialists in that arena, the extent of the need has changed. Exactly where future pharmacy specialty areas will be remains to be seen, but you can surmise many of them will follow growth areas in the practice of medicine. Pain and palliative care (see Chapter 21) is an example of an emerging pharmacy specialty, and its development has followed in the footsteps of emergency medicine pharmacy training.

Along with new pharmacy specialties may come the presence of pharmacy residencies in locations today unimaginable, or at least uncommon. Residencies in local health departments? Check (see Chapter 23). Hospice centers? Check. Ambulatory surgery centers? Why not? Wherever there is a need for someone with a pharmacist's training and skill set, there is an opportunity to train a generation of others to serve in those roles. So, be open to not only the specialties of today but also the unique opportunities of tomorrow.

BIGGER IS BETTER

While the concept of bigger being better does not always hold true, there is something to be said for economies of scale and the likelihood that having more than one resident in a program means that residents are integral for the practice site's functioning. At this point, the United States still has too many residency programs that have the potential to grow, but do not yet train at their full capacity. Leaders in our profession are encouraging each residency program director (RPD) to assess their program's structure, recognizing that many institutions could easily increase the number of residents trained by at least one.[3] In 2011, if 50% of the residency programs grew by one position, an additional 500 residency graduates would result each year.[4] This rather simplistic growth model could certainly go a long way to ease our current capacity challenges.

WHO'S IN CHARGE?

Take a moment to think about what it takes to create, implement, and maintain a residency program. Since that is probably not something you have given much thought to, here is some help. A quick review of the residency accreditation standard shows you that a residency program requires the combination of skills in professional education (e.g., pedagogy, learning styles, and assessment), human resources (e.g., personal leave policies, licensure requirements, and salary structure), staff development and employee advancement, facilities maintenance, leadership and visioning for the future as well as today, adherence to practice standards, quality assurance, and a commitment to excellence. The likelihood that every pharmacy practice site has the requisite resources to pull off all of that in an efficient and highly commendable manner is almost laughable. Pharmacists are pharmacists, not experts in all it takes to conduct a residency. So, why does our profession expect a pharmacist who is well prepared to motivate, inspire, and ensure a great experience for residency training to be an expert in Bloom's taxonomy, employee separation policies, and sterile compounding facility maintenance? Why not leave certain elements to the experts?

Let's trot out the medical model again. In medicine, academic (e.g., colleges of medicine) or training units (e.g., graduate education departments in academic medical centers) dedicated to education and professional training conduct medical residency training. Employees in those settings have the expertise and resources to conduct the "business" of residency training, including ensuring paperwork is completed for revenue streams, assuring learning experiences are of a sufficient quality, ensuring preceptors are well trained, and providing valuable feedback to residents, measuring resident learning and making adjustments when the resident does not seem to "get it." They are in the business of residency training, and they are good at it. Should we as pharmacists at least consider the benefits of such an approach? There is now a move afoot to see how we do just that, recognizing that colleges of pharmacy, for instance, are well positioned to provide the infrastructure to conduct residency training.[5] In 2011, 50% of US colleges of pharmacy conducted pharmacy residencies, yet only a handful assisted in the conduct of residency training outside of their own facilities. Why reinvent the wheel when you can simply reach out to a neighborhood partner who can take care of what is admittedly for most program directors tedious and time consuming work of running a residency? This model does not obviate the need for the actual practice site to maintain its commitment to quality by partnering to offer a fertile training environment. Rather, it allows an independent community pharmacy owner to provide the training ground and preceptors for the resident to learn from while letting the college of pharmacy handle some of the minutiae.

PHARMACY IS A TEAM SPORT

You hear it everywhere you turn—teamwork is important. Yet, why are you learning about patient care only with fellow pharmacy students, when in your final year of pharmacy school you will be thrust into a world in which you must play well with others? Our pharmacy educational model is slowly evolving to embrace the notion that those already in practice have known for some time; taking care of patients requires a team. Pharmacy schools are using interprofessional approaches to your education not only to enhance your abilities, but those of others (e.g., nurses, physicians, dentists, and social workers) who will one day be part of your team. So, if we expect you to practice with other professions within a team, and we are teaching you how to do that during pharmacy school, why do we often isolate you from working with other emerging pharmacists? The combination of a second-year student, fourth-year student, PGY-1 resident, PGY-2 resident, and practicing pharmacist sounds like too many cooks in the kitchen. There may be more to this team thing than you realize, however. Consider that much of how we as pharmacists have been taught, trained, and practiced has relied upon traditional roles and values of our profession; in short, "we've always done it that way." We have now begun asking ourselves if there is another way to do things, in this case residency training.

Practice sites often lament the demands placed upon them to offer more experiential education slots for IPPE and APPE, on top of existing residency programs they support or rotations they offer. This reaction is often in response to the paradigm that only one fully-fledged pharmacist may precept one student or resident at a time. After all, that sentiment is found in each state's pharmacy regulations, correct? Well, not exactly. Pharmacy licensure is necessary for care, but there are elements of direct and indirect supervision, as well as the fact that pharmacy residents are licensed practitioners. Imagine the passion and enthusiasm you as a PGY-2 critical care resident can bring to an APPE student's first acute care patient experience. After all, that APPE student is not expected to be a critical care expert at the conclusion of her rotation, and there is clearly much she can learn from you. In turn, you will benefit greatly from mentoring a young, eager student, from refining your own teaching skills to learning how to prioritize activities, manage others, and deal with different personalities, all expectations of any established and seasoned practitioner. And yes, our medical colleagues have recognized this tenet for decades.[5] Attending physicians sit atop the hierarchy of students and trainees, with each person on the ladder providing guidance and mentorship to the person on the rung below, all the way down to the third-year medical student.[6] This hierarchical, attending pharmacist, or team-based model to training was embraced by the 2011 Pharmacy Residency Capacity Stakeholders' Conference, and some practice sites have begun their own approaches to implementing it.[5,7]

PRACTICE MAKES PERFECT

You can never devalue the importance of repetition in enhancing your ability to do something. As a pharmacist you may never have the opportunity to care for a patient with Fabry's disease or have monitored the effects of gold salts in a patient with refractory rheumatoid arthritis, yet that does not diminish your ability to possess the specific knowledge and needed skills to complete those challenges. Colleges of pharmacy realize this, and they use simulation to provide students the opportunities to practice and demonstrate they have what it takes to care for patients. Simulation models include activities like conducting mock medication history interviews, with a classmate serving as your patient, and the use of mannequins to demonstrate your ability to select the proper antiarrhythmic agent and dose for a 68-year-old anephric patient with ventricular fibrillation. This concept could easily extend to the residency environment.[8] Some PGY-2 RPDs struggle with assuring their residents have the opportunity to care for patients with every major disease state within the corresponding specialty; think about how a simulation activity could be of value to both you as the resident (confidence in your abilities to do this, should you one day encounter such a patient) and the preceptor (ability to provide specific guidance to you on how you could approach such a patient). Bringing disease states and patient factors to life, but still in an artificial manner, far surpasses a dry, boring disease state discussion or case presentation. This use of simulation is embraced by pharmacy schools, the national pharmacy licensure body in Canada, and many other health professions. And, it is not only limited to rare situations. Simulation can have tremendous utility in ensuring to both the "examinee" (you as a resident or student) and "examiner" (preceptor), that you can provide consistent care to situations that are especially common, fraught with a high degree of difficulty or complexity, or are highly prone to error.

THE POWER OF ONE

RPDs, faculty members, employers, and residency candidates have more in common than you may know, especially when it comes to the challenges of the residency application process (see Chapter 9). In years past, as a candidate you seemingly needed a smartphone application or personal assistant to keep track of the various submission approaches (e.g., mail, electronic file upload, submit all materials together, email the application and follow with a hard copy, and deadline for receipt versus postmark deadlines), recommendation letter requirements (e.g., a customized candidate evaluation form and your signature acknowledging your permission for an individual to write a letter of recommendation on your behalf), and elements that compose the residency application process. Your personal references too needed a scorecard to keep track of which applications require a letter, comparison table, structured evaluation or form letter, and the corresponding deadlines and submission processes. If only there were a better way ... like a common application process. Much like the centralized application service you likely used to apply to pharmacy school, entering the pharmacy residency application world has recently harnessed technology long used in other professions and markets. ASHP created Pharmacy Online Residency Centralized Application System (PhORCAS), a Web-based, electronic submission portal with common program features and options for a residency program to customize what you as a potential resident must upload.[9] If you are familiar with Pharmacy College Application Service (PharmCAS), the process will seem somewhat similar as the company, Liaison International, will also manage this service. While there may still be small differences between application requirements of individual programs, think about how nice it will be for you to have a single, secure Web site to submit and maintain a record of your application components. To get started, you create a PhORCAS account, and then you are transferred to the National Matching Service site to insure that you register for the match. Much like applying to pharmacy school, you will incur nominal fees to use PhORCAS, based upon the number of applications you submit. As an applicant, you can begin assembling the primary components of your application in mid-Fall. In late Fall, the entire site is open to allow you to view each residency program's application requirements, respond to any extra application features of each program, and trigger your full application to each program you have selected. You can even craft cover letters specific to each residency program you are pursuing.[10] Your personal references will have access to the portal too, allowing them to upload their letter of recommendations in the same system you use to apply. This system, which launched in late 2012, will also come in handy for programs or applicants who do not match and are engaged in the residency scramble, because it links each applicant to their match code. Both programs and applicants who participate in the scramble will be able to see updated lists of availabilities, and you still can use your original application components to apply to different programs during the scramble.

THE MIRAGE AHEAD

Hopefully, you as an astute reader have realized that these residency changes share a common impetus—we need to increase pharmacy residency training capacity without sacrificing the quality of the experience for the trainee, the site, and the patient. While this chapter highlights several major changes that are likely to occur in the residency world, even the most expert of pharmacy preceptors or the most accomplished fortune teller cannot accurately predict the future of the residency world. There may be dozens of other advances in our process (e.g., structured approach to what many affectionately call the residency scramble[8] [see Chapter 12] and changes in residency program funding streams from the federal government[3]). Conversely, the changes listed in the figure may be overshooting the eventual reality. Whatever the nature of the changes to come, know that we as pharmacists are committed to continually improving and reinventing ourselves, always holding to the importance of doing what is best for our patients.

Chapter Takeaways

▶ Changes to the pharmacy residency training model are inevitable, yet difficult to accurately predict.

▶ A common impetus for impending changes is to increase pharmacy residency capacity to meet the needs of the workforce, the healthcare system, and the patient.

ROLE OF THE MENTOR

Discuss the future vision you have of pharmacy practice and residency training.

Based on your vision of the future, how would you approach residency training if you were a student today?

Share the advice you have for a practicing pharmacist who is considering the pursuit of residency training.

References

1. Winegardner ML, Davis SL, Szandzik EG, Kalus JS. Nontraditional pharmacy residency at a large teaching hospital. Am J Health Syst Pharm. 2010;67:366–370.

2. Fuller PD, et al. Value of pharmacy residency training: A survey of the academic medical center perspective. Am J Health Syst Pharm. 2012;69:158–165.

3. Johnson TJ, Teeters JL. Pharmacy residency and the medical training model: Is pharmacy at a tipping point? Am J Health Syst Pharm. 2011;68:1542–1549.

4. Kent SS. Closing the residency training gap. Am J Health Syst Pharm. 2011;68:1293–1294.

5. Zellmer WA. Expanding the number of positions for pharmacy residents: Highlights from the Pharmacy Residency Capacity Stakeholders' Conference. Am J Health Syst Pharm. 2011;68: 1843–1849.

6. Allen DD, Smith KM. A hand and glove approach to pharmacy experiential education and residency training. Am J Pharm Educ. 2010;74(4): Article 65.

7. Ashby DM. Permission granted. Am J Health Syst Pharm. 2011;68:1497–1504.

8. May JR, et al. Coping with the residency scramble: Need for national guidelines. Am J Health Syst Pharm. 2012;69:253–255.

9. Pharmacy Online Residency Centralized Application Service Information. http://www.ashp.org/phorcas. Accessed November 13, 2012.

10. Pharmacy Online Residency Centralized Application Service Applicant Log-in. https://portal.phorcas.org/. Accessed November 13, 2012.

APPENDIXES

APPENDIX 1 • Comparison of Residency Program Characteristics[a]

Characteristic	Where Can I Find It?	How Important Is This Characteristic to Me? (1 [low] to 5 [high])	Programs/Notes
Institution			
Type (e.g., academic, community, VA)	Web site	_____	_____
Institution size (# beds, average census, # annual patient visits, daily prescription volume, etc.)	Directory Web site	_____	_____
Location (e.g., urban, rural, local)	Directory		
Complexity and diversity of patient population	Web site, showcase	_____	_____
Scope of services	Web site		
Automated dispensing devices	Showcase	_____	_____
Chart documentation	Showcase	_____	_____
Code response	Showcase	_____	_____
Collaborative practice/ prescriptive authority	Showcase	_____	_____
Electronic medical record/computerized prescriber order entry	Showcase	_____	_____
Pharmacokinetics/ anticoagulation consult services	Showcase	_____	_____
Other		_____	_____

(continued)

APPENDIX 1 • Comparison of Residency Program Characteristics[a] (continued)

Characteristic	Where Can I Find It?	How Important Is This Characteristic to Me? (1 [low] to 5 [high])	Programs/Notes
Program			
Accredited	Directory	_____	_____
Affiliations	Web site	_____	_____
College of pharmacy			
Program size	Directory	_____	_____
# PGY-1 residents	Directory	_____	_____
# PGY-1 + PGY-2 residents	Directory, Web site	_____	_____
Preceptor: Resident ratio	Showcase	_____	_____
PGY-2 program in area of interest	Web site	_____	_____
Rotations and programs	Web site	_____	_____
Rotations in areas of interest	Web site, showcase	_____	_____
On-call program	Web site, showcase	_____	_____
Advanced cardiac life support certification	Web site, showcase	_____	_____
Teaching certificate program	Web site	_____	_____
Graduate certificate	Web site	_____	_____
Off-site elective rotations	Web site	_____	_____
Staffing	Web site, showcase	_____	_____
Teaching opportunities	Web site	_____	_____
Experiential (precepting)	Web site, showcase	_____	_____
Facilitation/laboratory instruction	Web site, showcase	_____	_____
Didactic	Web site, showcase	_____	_____
In-services/other	Showcase	_____	_____

APPENDIX 1 • Comparison of Residency Program Characteristics[a] (continued)

Characteristic	Where Can I Find It?	How Important Is This Characteristic to Me? (1 [low] to 5 [high])	Programs/Notes
Scholarship opportunities		____	____
Poster presentation	Showcase		
Grand rounds/CE presentation	Web site, showcase	____	____
Publications	Showcase, Pubmed	____	____
Other		____	____
Professional organization involvement	Web site, showcase	____	____
Meeting attendance	Showcase	____	____
Other opportunities		____	____
Training environment			
RPD		____	____
RPD board certified	Web site	____	____
Local/regional/ national offices and appointments	Web site, Internet	____	____
Track record of presentations at meeting and publications in literature	Pubmed, Web site	____	____
Faculty appointment	Web site	____	____
Frequency of RPD meetings	Showcase	____	____
Preceptors		____	____
% board certified	Web site	____	____
Local/regional/ national offices and appointments	Web site, Internet	____	____
Track record of presentations at meeting and publications in literature	Pubmed, Web site	____	____

(continued)

APPENDIX 1 • Comparison of Residency Program Characteristics[a] (continued)

Characteristic	Where Can I Find It?	How Important Is This Characteristic to Me? (1 [low] to 5 [high])	Programs/Notes
% faculty appointment	Web site	_____	_____
Precepting style	Showcase	_____	_____
Positions taken by former residents	Web site, showcase	_____	_____

[a]For a completed example of this table, see Chapter 5.

How to Use This Table
Column 1—Characteristic: Specific characteristics have been listed and categorized as discussed in the chapter. There is also space at the bottom of each category to write in characteristics that are important to you.

Column 2—Location of information: This column tells you where to look to find the characteristic for each program. In some cases, more than one place is recommended. In many cases, preliminary information can be found in a residency directory or on their Web site. However, detailed information can be determined only after talking to representatives of the program, such as the RPD/preceptors/residents at the residency showcase.

Column 3—Importance of characteristic: This column provides a place to rank the importance of each characteristic to you. For example, if the institution type, complexity of patient population, and teaching certificate are important to you, these characteristics should be ranked as a four or five out of five.

Columns 4 and 5—Specific program information: The next several columns provide places for you to list specific programs for comparison. Two examples have been provided for you in the table.

APPENDIX 2 • Resident Candidate Self-Assessment Tool[a]

Factor	Aspect	Self-Evaluation
Experiential training	Number of clinical experiences	
	Acute care or ambulatory care experience	
	Specialty populations, diverse experiences	
	Experiences in the candidates stated area of interest	
	Level of responsibility during experience	
Professional organization Involvement	Membership in pharmacy organizations	
	Attendance at state or national pharmacy conferences	
	Leadership positions	
	Accomplishments	
Leadership activities	Informal leadership roles in organizations	
	Formal leadership roles in organizations	
Community service and extracurricular activities	Volunteer activities	
	Community service	
	Neighborhood activity	
	Shadowing experiences	
Academic performance	Transcripts	
	GPA and class rank	
	Trends in grades	
	GPA in therapeutics/pharmacology courses	
	Previous degrees	
	NAPLEX pass rate of your college	
	Prestige of college of pharmacy	
Scholarly activities	Participation in research or projects	
	Presentation of a poster at a regional, state, or national meeting	
	Publications	
Honors and awards	Membership in honorary societies	
	Local, state, or national awards and honors	
	Merit-based scholarships	
Professional work experience	Pharmacy: community, health system	
	Internship experience	
	Length of employment	
	Duties	
	Accomplishments	
Other employment experience	Nonpharmacy employment	
	Length of employment	
	Duties	
	Accomplishments	

(continued)

APPENDIX 2 • Resident Candidate Self-Assessment Tool[a] (continued)

Factor	Aspect		Self-Evaluation
Communication	Written—Letter of intent	Knowledge of specific program	
		Interest and enthusiasm in residency	
		Grammar, punctuation	
	Written—Essay of goals	Motivation for residency	
		Organized, style, logical flow of thoughts	
		Mature and open-minded goals	
	Verbal—Presentation	Professional, communicative	
	Verbal—Interview	Poised, thoughtful, insightful	
	Verbal—Informal	Conversational, warm, friendly, thankful	
	Written—Follow-up	Thank you note timely and sincere	

[a]This table includes typical screening questions used by the interview selection committee when reviewing resident candidate application packets. For more information, see Chapter 6.

INDEX

Note: Page number followed by f and t indicates figure and table respectively.